Review for Intensive Care Medicine

Review for Intensive Care Medicine

Mark W. Sebastian, M.D.
Assistant Professor of Surgery
Department of Surgery
Duke University Medical Center
Durham, North Carolina

William J. Fulkerson, M.D.
Professor of Medicine
Director, Medical Intensive Care
Department of Medicine
Duke University Medical Center
Durham, North Carolina

R. Lawrence Reed II, M.D.
Associate Professor of Surgery
Director, Surgical Intensive Care
Department of Surgery
Duke University Medical Center
Durham, North Carolina

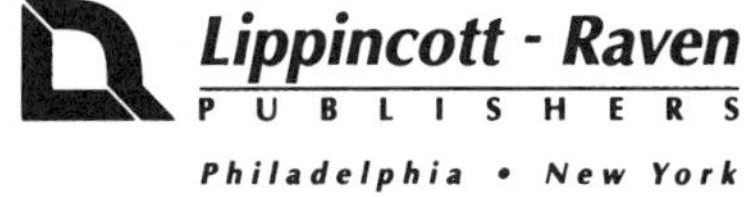
Lippincott - Raven
PUBLISHERS
Philadelphia • New York

Manufacturing Manager: Dennis Teston
Production Editor: Rita Madrigal
Compositor: Eastern Composition
Printer: Maple Press

Printed in the United States of America

9 8 7 6 5 4 3 2 1

ISBN: 0-316-73633-3

Contents

Foreword

The *Review for Intensive Care Medicine* by Drs. Sebastian, Fulkerson, and Reed is a welcomed and much needed addition to the literature in critical and intensive care. The three authors, all of whom are highly skilled and well-regarded clinician-scientists, have done a masterful job of distilling key information from the third edition of *Intensive Care Medicine* and linking this knowledge to over 700 multiple choice and true/false questions based on the parent book. While this book will be extremely valuable to all practitioners of intensive care, it will be particularly useful for individuals who are preparing for the critical care boards. The book will also be invaluable to those individuals whose learning style favors responding to questions, rather than simply reading text material.

The practice of intensive care is becoming increasingly multi-disciplinary in nature—a fact recognized and reflected in the critical care boards. The diverse backgrounds of the authors of this book mirror this multi-disciplinary approach and add to the great strength of this book.

In the ten years since the first edition of *Intensive Care Medicine* appeared, both the field of intensive care medicine and the literature and knowledge used by practitioners of intensive care have undergone great change. New techniques and therapies are constantly emerging. The challenge in editing books in this area has always been to provide readers with state-of-the-art, user-friendly, and clinically relevant information.

Now, with the addition of this book, the basic body of information contained in the third edition of *Intensive Care Medicine* can be viewed from a slightly different perspective through answering board review–type questions. The accuracy and timeliness of this book are assured not only by the experience and knowledge of the authors of this fine new book, but also by the participation of all the contributors to the parent book. *Review for Intensive Care Medicine* thus joins *Intensive Care Medicine* as a useful, authoritative resource to guide the practice of modern intensive and critical care.

James M. Rippe, M.D.
Boston, MA

Review for
Intensive Care Medicine

I. Procedures and Techniques

1. Airway Management and Endotracheal Intubation

1. True or False. The hard palate defines the beginning of the oropharynx, which extends inferiorly to the epiglottis.

2. True or False. The thyroid, cricoid, epiglottic, cuneiform, and corniculate cartilages comprise the laryngeal skeleton.

3. True or False. The cricoid cartilage defines the narrowest portion of the airway in an adult.

4. Select the best answer. Regarding alternative airway management:

A. Proper positioning of the head and neck rarely aids in airway management in oropharyngeal or nasopharyngeal airways.
B. Nasotracheal intubation should always be utilized after attempts at endotracheal intubation.
C. The laryngeal mask airway can be positioned without direct visualization of the vocal cords.
D. Nasotracheal intubation should be performed in the obtunded and apneic patient.

5. True or False. The indications for endotracheal intubation can be divided into four basic categories: acute airway obstruction, excessive pulmonary secretions or inadequate ability to clear secretions, loss of protective reflexes, and respiratory failure.

6. True or False. Acute airway obstruction is most often due to foreign body in the mouth with aspiration.

7. Select the best answer. Regarding endotracheal tubes:

A. Endotracheal tubes are measured utilizing both millimeters and French units to measure the external diameter of the endotracheal tube.
B. In the United States, the French units are most commonly used.
C. Tracheal ischemia can occur when the cuff pressure is less than the capillary arterial pressure, which is usually approximately 32 mm Hg.

D. Modern endotracheal tubes are equipped with high-volume, low-pressure cuffs to minimize the danger of tracheal ischemia.

8. Select the answer that is **false**. Regarding techniques of endotracheal intubation:

A. When the laryngeal scope blade is in place, the operator should lift at the handle, keeping the left wrist stiff.
B. The endotracheal tube is held in the right hand and is inserted at the right corner of the mouth in a plane that intersects with the laryngeal scope blade at the level of the glottis.
C. If the vocal cords cannot be visualized, no attempt at intubation can be made.
D. A stylet can be utilized with a light to aid in intubation.

9. True or False. The nasotracheal tube operator must continually monitor for the presence of air movement through the nasotracheal tube by listening for breath sounds with the ear near the open end of the tube.

10. Select the best answer. Regarding intubation in a patient with suspected cervical spine injury:

A. Cervical spine injury must be confirmed radiologically before manipulation, and airway management should be performed.
B. Nasal intubation is uniformly preferred in the patient with suspected cervical spine injury.
C. If oral intubation is required in the patient with suspected cervical spine injury, an assistant is required to maintain the neck in the neutral position.
D. Cervical collars should be discontinued prior to oral or nasotracheal intubation in the patient with suspected cervical spine injury.

11. Select the best answer. Regarding complications of endotracheal intubation:

A. The most serious complication of extubation is laryngeal spasm.
B. The decision to extubate a patient is based on multiple laboratory parameters.
C. Females are more likely than males to experience vocal cord paralysis after intubation.
D. Laryngeal edema rarely accompanies smooth endotracheal intubations.

2. Central Venous Catheters

1. Select the answer that is **false**. Regarding the basic principles of central venous catheterization:

A. Volume resuscitation alone is not an indication for central venous catheterization.
B. Peripheral vein cannulation may be impossible in the hypovolemic patient.
C. The femoral vein may be a reasonable alternative for resuscitation in the hypovolemic patient.
D. Central venous access may be required for infusion of irritant medications such as potassium chloride or for infusion of vasoactive agents.

E. The external jugular vein is a simple conduit for positioning a catheter in the central venous circulation.

2. Select the best answer. Regarding emergency transvenous pacemaker insertion:

A. Emergency transvenous pacemakers are best inserted through the right subclavian vein.
B. In patients with coagulopathy, the external jugular vein, although accessible, should not be utilized.
C. Catheters inserted from the right subclavian vein follow a more natural curve than the left subclavian vein, traversing the right ventricle into the right pulmonary artery.
D. Emergency transvenous pacemakers are best inserted through the right internal jugular vein because of the direct path to the right ventricle.

3. True or False. The ideal location for the catheter tip for central venous catheterization is in the distal innominate or proximal superior vena cava, 3 to 5 cm proximal to the caval atrial junction.

4. True or False. Once properly placed, migration of the catheter tip is uncommon.

5. True or False. After utilizing ECG leads to ensure accurate catheter tip location, a chest x-ray is not necessary.

6. True or False. An important complication resulting from antecubital central venous catheterization includes pericardial tamponade.

7. Select the **false** answer. Regarding the structures neighboring the internal jugular vein:

A. The internal carotid artery runs medial to the internal jugular vein, in general.
B. The stellate ganglion and the cervical sympathetic trunk lie within the carotid sheath posterior to the internal carotid artery.
C. The dome of the pleura, which is higher on the left, lies caudal to the junction of the internal jugular vein and subclavian vein.
D. The cholinergic and vagus nerves course posteriorly at the route of the neck.
E. The thoracic duct lies behind the left internal jugular vein and enters the superior margin of the subclavian vein near the jugulosubclavian junction.

8. Select the best answer. Regarding catheter-related bacteremia and septicemia:

A. Every catheter should be removed in a febrile patient.
B. Catheter sites should be covered and only examined in the septic patient.
C. Catheter exchange over a guidewire may be a feasible alternative in the febrile patient.
D. Antibiotic therapy is usually continued for 3 days when catheter-related bacteremia does develop.

3. Arterial Line Placement and Care

1. True or False. When Allen's test is utilized, it reliably predicts that the blood supply to the hand will not be compromised by percutaneous radial placement of an arterial line.

2. True or False. Brachial artery catheterization is commonly performed in major medical centers.

4. Pulmonary Artery Catheters

1. True or False. Pulmonary artery catheters, as invented by Swan and associates in 1970, are able to predict occult blood loss in trauma victims.

2. True or False. Hemodynamic monitoring has three central objectives: to assess left and/or right ventricular function, to monitor changes in hemodynamic status, and to guide treatment with pharmacologic and nonpharmacologic agents.

3. True or False. The inflation of the distal balloon in the pulmonary artery catheter can be with air or liquid.

4. Select the correct answer. Regarding catheter placement for pulmonary artery catheters:

A. With the balloon inflated in the superior vena cava, catheter advancement is continued until a right ventricular pressure tracing is seen on the monitor.
B. The initial access of the pulmonary artery catheter to the central venous circulation proximal to the right atrium is the most risky time for generation of arrhythmias.
C. If arrhythmias are encountered in passage of the right ventricle, transient deflation of the balloon will minimize right ventricular irritation.
D. With the catheter in the right pulmonary artery position, chest x-ray should be ordered to confirm catheter position and, whatever the placement of the catheter, it should be documented and confirmed with daily chest x-rays.

5. True or False. Anticoagulation or deranged coagulation parameters are a contraindication for hemodynamic monitoring.

6. Select the best answer. Regarding right atrial pressures:

A. Normal resting right atrial pressure is 10 to 14 mm Hg.
B. Two major positive atrial pressure waves, the A wave and B wave, can usually be recorded.
C. Once a multilumen pulmonary artery catheter is in position, it is possible to sample right atrial blood and monitor right atrial pressure using the proximal lumen.
D. The V wave represents the pressure generated by venous filling of the right atrium with the tricuspid valve open.

7. Select the best answer. Regarding the right ventricle and right ventricular pressure:

    A. The normal resting right ventricular pressure is 30 to 35 mm Hg over 6 to 10 mm Hg recorded when the pulmonary artery catheter crosses the tricuspid valve.
    B. The right ventricular systolic pressure should always equal the pulmonary artery systolic pressure.
    C. Right ventricular monitoring is being increasingly utilized in the surgical critical care setting.
    D. The right ventricular pressure exceeds the mean right atrial pressure during diastole when the tricuspid valve is open.

8. Select the best answer. Regarding the pulmonary artery during pulmonary artery catheter utilization:

    A. Normal resting pulmonary artery pressure is 15 to 30 mm Hg over 5 to 13 mm Hg with the normal mean pressure of 10 to 18 mm Hg.
    B. The pulmonary artery waveform is characterized by systolic peak and diastolic trough with a smooth decline from the peak to the trough.
    C. The peak pulmonary artery systolic pressure occurs within the QRS complex of a simultaneously recorded ECG.
    D. Pulmonary artery diastolic pressure is closely related to mean pulmonary artery wedge pressure and can be reliably utilized as an index of left ventricular filling pressure.

9. Select the best answer. Regarding pulmonary artery wedge pressure:

    A. Pulmonary artery wedge pressure correlates poorly with left ventricular filling pressure.
    B. A valid pulmonary artery wedge pressure is obtained if the catheter tip lies in zone one of the lung.
    C. Pulmonary artery wedge pressure is an acceptable measurement for estimating capillary hydrostatic filtration pressure and is an absolute indication for the formation of pulmonary edema.
    D. Pulmonary artery wedge pressure should be measured at end expiration for a reliable reference point for interpretation.

10. True or False. Regarding interpretation of pulmonary artery wedge pressure with a patient on ventilatory support and utilization of positive end-expiratory pressure (PEEP): Since it is difficult to precisely estimate the true transmitted vascular pressure when a patient is on PEEP, disconnecting the PEEP to measure the wedge pressure is recommended.

11. True or False. Within the setting of acute mitral regurgitation, a V wave is generated, which will impact on the pulmonary artery waveform, creating a bifid pulmonary artery waveform that persists with catheter wedging.

12. Select the answer that is **false**. Regarding right ventricular infarction:

    A. Right ventricular infarction typically occurs in the setting of anterior myocardial infarction.
    B. In the event that hemodynamics of right ventricular infarction are present, they may be confused with cardiac tamponade or constrictive pericarditis.
    C. Right ventricular end-diastolic pressure and volume are increased, and right ventricular stroke volume is decreased.

D. The hemodynamics of right ventricular infarction result in a narrowed pulmonary artery pulse pressure.

13. True or False. A mean pulmonary arterial pressure of greater than 40 mm Hg defines pulmonary hypertension.

5. Temporary Cardiac Pacing

1. Select the best answer. Regarding utilization of temporary cardiac pacing in acute myocardial infarctions:

A. Bradyarrhythmias unresponsive to medical treatment, resulting in hemodynamic compromise, are an indication for temporary pacing.
B. Patients with anterior infarction and bifascicular block, or second degree atrioventricular block, do not require a temporary pacemaker.
C. Ventricular pacing may be essential for preservation and maintenance of effective stroke volume in certain patients and should be the mode of choice.
D. Prophylactic transvenous cardiac pacing is indicated in patients who are to undergo thrombolytic therapy.

6. Cardioversion and Defibrillation

1. True or False. The term *cardioversion* is utilized to describe electrical countershock to terminate ventricular fibrillation.

2. True or False. Defibrillation is the process of electrically depolarizing the myocardium in an effort to terminate ventricular fibrillation.

3. True or False. Cardioversion of paroxysmal supraventricular tachycardia or atrial fibrillation is contraindicated in pregnancy.

7. Echocardiography in the Intensive Care Unit

1. True or False. The use of transthoracic echocardiography in the intensive care unit (ICU) is not indicated due to considerations of mechanical ventilation, chronic obstructive pulmonary disease, and the presence of bandages on the thorax.

2. True or False. Ejection fraction estimated by visual inspection of the two-dimensional echocardiographic images has been found to be inferior to computation of left ventricular end-diastolic and end-systolic volumes.

3. Select the best answer. Regarding echocardiography of the left ventricle:

A. Left ventricular chamber dimensions and volumes may be estimated visually or by quantitative analysis.

B. Echocardiography cannot be utilized to diagnose hypovolemia.
C. Echocardiography in patients who are hypotensive and have undergone valve replacement for aortic stenosis can aid in changes in management.
D. Echocardiographic findings rarely lead to dramatic changes in management of the hypotensive patient.

4. Select the answer that is **false**. Regarding use of echocardiography in the evaluation of congestive heart failure:

A. Studies on patients with congestive heart failure referred for echocardiogram show findings that are worse than clinically suspected in some patient populations.
B. Echocardiography leads to changes in clinical management in approximately one-third of patients.
C. In clinical heart failure in patients suffering from acute myocardial infarction, there is a restricted mitral inflow pattern indicative of abnormally elevated left ventricular diastolic pressure.
D. In clinical congestive heart failure, diastolic filling variables become unrelated to systolic function.

5. Select the answer that is **false**. Regarding echocardiography for the assessment of cardiac valves:

A. Continuous wave Doppler may be utilized to measure peak velocity and estimate pressure gradients.
B. Doppler-derived gradients correlate closely with invasive determinants.
C. Transesophogeal echocardiography is more sensitive than transthoracic echocardiography for sensitivity and specificity in bacterial endocarditis.
D. Transesophogeal echocardiography has replaced transthoracic echocardiography as a diagnostic technique in endocarditis.

8. Pericardiocentesis

1. Select the best answer. Regarding the anatomy of the pericardium:

A. The multiple attachments of the parietal pericardium are attached directly to the epicardium at the borders of the entrance at the inferior and superior venae cavae and pulmonary veins.
B. The anchoring of the parietal pericardium results in a distensible large space between the visceral and parietal areas.
C. The pericardial space, or sac, usually contains no fluid.
D. The effusions that collect slowly over days to weeks may cause hemodynamic compromise with volumes under 200 ml.

2. True or False. Regarding pericardiocentesis: Patient position has relatively little influence on successful aspiration of pericardial fluid.

3. Select the best answer. Following successful pericardiocentesis:

A. Recurrent tamponade is an infrequent event after successful pericardiocentesis.
B. A small effusion is associated with a decreased incidence of complications following pericardiocentesis.

C. A localized pericardial effusion is associated with an increased risk of complications.
D. A chest x-ray performed immediately after the procedure is the only monitoring necessary after pericardiocentesis.

4. Select the *surgical* indication that is **false** regarding long-term management after pericardiocentesis:

A. Pericardial disease with constrictive physiology.
B. Known loculated or posteriorly located effusions not amenable to pericardiocentesis.
C. Suspected purulent pericarditis.
D. Effusions not successfully drained by pericardiocentesis.
E. Metastatic disease of the pericardium.

9. The Intraaortic Balloon and Counterpulsation

1. True or False. The intraaortic balloon pump requires no minimum cardiac output to function effectively.

2. True or False. Intraaortic balloon counterpulsation is effective in stabilizing patients with mechanical intracardiac defects complicating myocardial infarction.

3. True or False. Other indications for intraaortic balloon counterpulsation include management of unstable angina, weaning from cardiopulmonary bypass, preoperative use as a bridge to transplantation, and during percutaneous coronary angioplasty.

4. Select the answer that is **false**. Regarding contraindications to balloon pump utilization:

A. The use of intraaortic balloon counterpulsation to control ventricular arrhythmia is decreasing in frequency.
B. Aortic valvular insufficiency is not a contraindication to intraaortic balloon pump counterpulsation.
C. Aortic dissection is an absolute contraindication to counterpulsation.
D. Severe aortoiliac disease is a contraindication to counterpulsation.

5. Select the best answer regarding weaning from counterpulsation:

A. Weaning from counterpulsation requires three steps: weaning, inotropic support, and removal of the device.
B. The only method of weaning involves counterpulsation ratios of 1:1, 1:2, and 1:3, based on the cardiac cycle.
C. Heparin infusion should be continued through removal of the intraaortic balloon pump to avoid reocclusion of the coronary arteries.

D. Once the patient has been weaned to a ratio of 1:3 and has been stable for a few hours, the intraaortic balloon pump may be removed.

10. *Temporary Mechanical Assistance of the Failing Left Ventricle*

1. True or False. Indications for use of a left ventricular assist device include criteria such as cardiac index of less than 1.8 liters/m^2/min, mean arterial pressure of less than 60 mm Hg, left atrial pressure or right atrial pressure of greater than 20 mm Hg, urine output of less than 20 ml per hour, and systemic vascular resistance greater than 2100 dyne/sec/cm^{-5}.

2. Select the answer that is **false**. Contraindications to a ventricular assist device include the following:

A. The presence of massive myocardial infarction.
B. Sepsis.
C. Coagulopathy.
D. The presence of a chronic debilitating disease.

3. Regarding left ventricular assist device weaning, signs of potential success include the following, **except**:

A. Less than 75 hours of left ventricular assist device pump support.
B. No evidence of postoperative myocardial infarction.
C. Some evidence of left ventricular recovery.
D. No evidence of bleeding diathesis.
E. Right ventricular failure.

11. *Chest Tube Insertion and Care*

1. True or False. The lung fills all but approximately 10 ml of the hemithorax in the normal physiologic state.

2. True or False. Up to 100 ml of fluid is present in the pleural space under normal conditions.

3. Select the best answer. Regarding timing of operation for traumatic hemothorax:

A. Pulmonary parenchymal hemorrhage is often life threatening due to the high volume of blood flow through the pulmonary vasculature.
B. Systemic arterial sources of bleeding, such as the intercostal, internal mammary, or subclavian arteries or the heart, rarely cause hemothorax.
C. Tube thoracostomy is not indicated in the initial management of hemothorax due to trauma.
D. Indications for open thoracotomy after thoracostomy include blood loss of over 1 liter, greater than 500 ml of blood loss over the first hour, greater

than 200 ml of blood loss per hour after 2 to 4 hours, or greater than 100 ml per hour after 6 to 8 hours, or in an unstable patient not responding to volume resuscitation.

4. Select the answer that is **false**. Regarding chylothorax:

A. The primary causes of chylothorax are trauma, malignancy, congenital abnormalities, and miscellaneous, such as infection.
B. The surgical procedures most often implicated in iatrogenic injuries include those involving mobilization of the aortic arch and esophageal resection.
C. The appearance of chyle in the pleural space is immediate after injury.
D. Treatment consists of tube drainage and aggressive maintenance of nutritional status.

5. True or False. The most important facet of chest tube insertion is insertion of the finger into the pleural space prior to placement of the chest tube to explore the anatomy.

13. Methods of Obtaining Lower Respiratory Tract Secretions in Pneumonia

1. True or False. Patients with bacterial pneumonia in the intensive care unit setting should be treated with broad-spectrum antibiotics at all times.

2. Select the best answer. Regarding expectorated sputum samples for diagnosis of pneumonia:

A. Routinely processed expectorated sputum samples are both sensitive and specific for diagnosis of pneumonia.
B. Homogenized expectorated sputum specimens are as sensitive and specific as transthoracic aspiration for diagnosis of pneumonia.
C. Expectorated sputum cultures may grow large concentrations of *Staphylococcus aureus* and various facultative gram-negative organisms while the patient is on antibiotic therapy.
D. Expectorated sputum cultures are unreliable, especially with the diagnosis of pneumococcal pneumonia.

3. True or False. To define an optimal expectorated sputum sample, both number of white cells and presence of epithelial cells are required.

4. True or False. Transtracheal aspiration is commonly performed in the intensive care unit for the isolation of anaerobic and aerobic pulmonary pathogens.

5. True or False. Bronchoalveolar lavage samples a smaller, but more representative amount of the lower respiratory tract than protected brush specimen does.

14. Thoracentesis

1. Select the correct answer. Regarding a cell count and differential for thoracentesis in a grossly bloody effusion:

A. A red blood count of 50,000 cells per cubic millimeter must be present for fluid to appear pink.
B. Effusions containing greater than 100,000 red blood cells per cubic millimeter are consistent with trauma alone.
C. To distinguish a traumatic thoracentesis from a preexisting hemothorax, blood from a preexisting hemothorax will form a clot on standing.
D. A traumatic thoracentesis is suggested when pleural fluid and blood hematocrit values are identical.

2. Select the answer that is **false**. Regarding malignant pleural effusions:

A. Malignancies can produce pleural effusions by two basic mechanisms: implantation of malignant cells on the pleural space or impairment of lymphatic drainage secondary to tumor obstruction.
B. The most common tumors that cause pleural effusions are lung cancer, breast cancer, and lymphoma.
C. Pleural fluid cytology should be performed for a translated effusion of unknown etiology.
D. Heparin should be added to a container where a suspected malignant effusion is present to prevent clotting of the fluid.

16. Tracheotomy

1. True or False. Tracheotomy performed in the intensive care unit is an uncommon procedure.

2. True or False. The placement of a tracheotomy minimizes the chance of tracheal stenosis from pressure necrosis, which can be a consequence of endotracheal intubation.

3. Select the best answer. Regarding delayed hemorrhage after tracheotomy:

A. Late hemorrhage after tracheotomy is usually caused by erosion into adjacent venous collaterals.
B. In some early series, it was reported that tracheotomy bleeding more than 48 hours after the procedure was due to rupture of the innominate artery.
C. Exsanguination has been virtually eliminated with the advent of low-pressure, high-volume cuffs.
D. Tracheal–innominate artery fistulas are still described in the literature and carry a mortality rate of 50 percent.

4. True or False. The cricothyroid space is larger in its vertical dimension than the diameter of most tracheotomy tubes.

5. Select the best answer. Regarding percutaneous dilatational elective tracheotomy in the intensive care unit setting:

A. A sterile operative field is necessary.

B. It is somewhat slower than standard conventional tracheotomy.
C. The kit is less expensive than operating room expense and personnel.
D. There is increased dissection when compared to operative tracheotomy.
E. Upper airway endoscopy is contraindicated during the procedure.

17. Extracorporeal Membrane Oxygenation and Carbon Dioxide Elimination

1. Select the best answer. Regarding extracorporeal life support:

A. Extracorporeal life support has made little progress in recent years.
B. Extracorporeal life support is more successful when utilized as an early intervention prior to appearance of irreversible organ damage.
C. Early clinical trials with extracorporeal membrane oxygenation (ECMO) compared conventional mechanical ventilation to ECMO as therapy for the adult respiratory distress syndrome and showed a survival advantage with ECMO.
D. To date, approximately 900 patients have been treated with extracorporeal life support in the United States at 90 centers.

18. Peritoneal Dialysis, Hemodialysis, and Hemofiltration Techniques in the Intensive Care Unit

1. Select the indication that is **false** as an absolute indication for dialysis, regarding hemodialysis:

A. Volume overload refractory to diuretic therapy.
B. Hyperkalemia.
C. Acidosis.
D. Specific drug overdose.

2. True or False. Dialysis may delay recovery of renal function.

3. Select the correct answer. Regarding movement of solute from blood to dialysate:

A. The movement of solute from blood to dialysate is accomplished by either diffusive or convective transport.
B. Diffusive clearance is achieved by ultrafiltration or flow-dependent phenomena.
C. Convective transport is achieved by the concentration-dependent movement of solute across the semipermeable membrane.
D. Smaller-molecular-weight solutes, such as urea and potassium, have low diffusive clearances, whereas larger molecules such as vitamin B_{12} and $beta_2$-macroglobulin depend on ultrafiltration for clearance.

19. Gastrointestinal Endoscopy

1. Select the answer that is **true**. Regarding lower gastrointestinal endoscopy:

   A. Lower gastrointestinal endoscopy is indicated as the primary diagnostic test in lower gastrointestinal bleeding.
   B. Colonic decompression is indicated as primary therapy in intensive care unit patients with cecal dilatation.
   C. Endoscopic colonic decompression has been advised for right colonic diameter dilatations exceeding 15 cm.
   D. Relapse is uncommon after colonic decompression.

21. Management of Acute Esophageal Variceal Hemorrhage with Gastroesophageal Balloon Tamponade

1. Select the best answer. Regarding complications of gastric balloon tamponade of variceal bleeding:

   A. The most common complication is acute laryngeal obstruction.
   B. The most severe complication is aspiration pneumonia.
   C. Migration of the tube may lead to esophageal perforation.
   D. Mucosal ulceration of the gastroesophageal junction is rare but related to prolonged traction time.

22. Endoscopic Placement of Feeding Tubes

1. True or False. Maneuvers used for clearance of clogged feeding tubes include irrigation with warm saline, with carbonated liquid, with cranberry juice, or with an enzyme solution.

23. Therapeutic Hemapheresis

1. True or False. Hemapheresis involves separation of the patient's whole blood into components, removal of a specific component, and reinfusion of the remaining blood.

2. Select the disease entity that is not indicated for treatment with therapeutic plasma exchange.

   A. Guillain-Barré syndrome.
   B. Idiopathic thrombocytopenic purpura.

C. Myasthenia gravis.
D. Thrombotic thrombocytopenic purpura.

25. Neurologic and Intracranial Pressure Monitoring

1. Select the best answer. Regarding cerebral ischemia:

A. The brain constitutes approximately 10 percent of the total body weight.
B. The brain receives 30 percent of cardiac output.
C. The brain accounts for 15 to 20 percent of the total body oxygen consumption.
D. Certain regions of the brain appear to be selectively vulnerable to hypercapnic injury.

2. True or False. Regarding measurement of mixed cerebral venous blood oxygen levels: Retrograde cannulation of the jugular bulb is a high-risk, technically demanding procedure that yields consistently sensitive analysis of cerebral oxygen demand.

27. Aspiration of Joints

1. Select the best answer. Regarding arthrocentesis:

A. Generalized joint inflammation is an indication for arthrocentesis.
B. Bursitis and tendonitis may mimic true joint arthritis.
C. A patellar tap may be useful with small effusions as a diagnostic technique.
D. Arthrocentesis is a diagnostic technique only.

2. True or False. The viscosity of synovial fluid is a measure of the protein present in the fluid.

28. Anesthesia for Bedside Procedures

1. True or False. Return of consciousness can be seen within minutes following termination of an 8-hour propofol infusion, although the elimination half-life of propofol is 5 hours.

2. Select the correct answer. Regarding the use of naloxone in the intensive care unit:

A. The effect of administering small doses of naloxone (0.04 mg) to patients to reverse respiratory depression of narcotic overdose is commonly seen in the intensive care unit (ICU) setting.
B. The practice of administering small doses of naloxone is advisable in the ICU setting to improve respiratory function.

C. The administration of small doses of naloxone is relatively contraindicated in the ICU setting due to the significant number and severity of side effects.
D. Naloxone levels decline more slowly than morphine levels, leading to complications of analgesia and respiratory status in the ICU setting.

3. True or False. Recent data suggest that reversal of opiods with an opioid agonist-antagonist such as nalbuphine may be safer than administration of naloxone.

4. True or False. Etomidate has beneficial effects on cerebral oxygen kinetics, similar to those seen with barbiturates; however, it has significantly increased risk of cardiovascular side effects.

5. Select the best answer. Regarding midazolam:

A. Midazolam provides excellent anterograde amnesia.
B. Midazolam produces significant pain on injection.
C. Midazolam is approximately one-half protein-bound.
D. The elimination half-life of midazolam is approximately 12 hours.

6. True or False. The most important aspect of pain and anxiety control in the ICU setting is sedative administration.

29. Routine Monitoring of Critically Ill Patients

1. Select the best answer. Regarding gastric intramucosal pH monitoring:

A. Intramucosal pH monitoring is used for trends in tissue pH in response to systemic oxygen delivery and metabolism.
B. These trends have not yet been utilized in predicting intensive care unit outcome.
C. The technique measures PCO_2 and pH in a gas state in a balloon placed in the lumen of a viscus, usually the stomach, the sigmoid colon, and the bladder.
D. Gastric intramucosal pH monitoring is currently being studied as an early predictor of multiple organ failure.

31. Interventional Radiology Drainage Techniques

1. True or False. The presence of infection with fluid accumulation is effectively treated by antibiotics.

2. True or False. After catheter insertion into a fluid collection requiring drainage, the aftercare of the catheter consists of continuous wall suction.

3. True or False. Regarding cholecystostomy: Cholestasis is uncommon in the intensive care unit setting.

Answers

Chapter 1

1. **False.** The soft palate defines the beginning of the oropharynx, which extends inferiorly to the epiglottis. The oropharynx connects the posterior portion of the oral cavity to the hyopharynx. (*See* Anatomy.)

2. **False.** The thyroid, cricoid, epiglottic, cuneiform, corniculate, and arytenoid cartilages comprise the laryngeal skeleton. The thyroid and cricoid cartilages are readily palpated in the anterior neck. The cricoid cartilage articulates with the thyroid cartilage and is joined to it by the cricothyroid ligament. With extension of the head, the cricothyroid ligament may be pierced with a scalpel or a large-bore needle, providing an emergency airway. (*See* Anatomy.)

3. **False.** The glottis is the narrowest space in the adult upper airway, and in children the cricoid cartilage is the narrowest portion of the airway. (*See* Anatomy.).

4. **C.** Often, proper positioning of the patient's head, especially utilizing the head-tilt and jaw-thrust maneuvers, may allow the patient to resume spontaneous breathing. If proper positioning of the head and neck or clearance of foreign bodies fails to establish an adequate airway, adjuncts may be utilized. These include an oropharyngeal or nasopharyngeal airway, which may be utilized when proper head positioning alone is insufficient. The laryngeal mask airway, which has recently been evaluated, can be positioned without direct visualization of vocal cords and conforms to the shape of the laryngeal inlet. (*See* Airway Adjuncts.)

5. **True.** Indications for endotracheal intubation can be divided into four basic categories, which consist of acute airway obstruction, excessive pulmonary secretions or desire for pulmonary toilet, loss of protective reflexes and inability to protect the airway, and respiratory failure. (*See* Indications for Intubation.)

6. **False.** Acute airway obstruction is most often due to posterior displacement of the base of the tongue. Other contributing factors could include injury to the mandible, smoke inhalation or chemical ingestion or inhalation leading to laryngeal edema, and aspiration of foreign bodies. Other considerations include rapidly expanding hematomas, rapidly growing tumors, and rare congenital lesions, such as laryngeal webs or superglottic fusion, which could cause obstruction in infants. (*See* Indications for Intubation.)

7. **D.** Endotracheal tubes are measured utilizing both millimeters and French units to measure the internal diameter of the endotracheal tube. In the United States, the internal diameter in millimeters is commonly used. Tracheal ischemia occurs when the inflated cuff pressure exceeds the capillary arterial pressure. Modern endotracheal tubes are equipped with high-volume, low-pressure cuffs, which are felt to minimize the danger of tracheal ischemia. (*See* Equipment for Intubation.)

8. **C.** Although it is desirable to visualize the vocal cords during intubation, it is occasionally impossible to do so. When this is true, it is helpful to insert the soft metal stylet into the endotracheal tube and bend it into a "hockey-stick" configuration. Alternatively, a control-tip endotracheal tube may be utilized,

which has a nylon cord running the length of the tube, attached to a ring at the proximal end. This allows the tip of the tube to be directed in an anterior fashion. Also, a stylet with a light or light wand is available. When the room lights are dimmed, the endotracheal tube containing the lighted stylet is inserted into the oropharynx and advanced into the midline. When it is just superior to the larynx, a glow is seen over the anterior neck. The stylet is then advanced into the trachea, and the tube is threaded over it. The light intensity is diminished if the wand enters the esophagus. (*See* Equipment for Intubation.)

9. **True.** Blind nasal intubation is more difficult to perform than oral intubation; however, it is more comfortable for the patient and is generally preferable in the awake and conscious patient. The tube operator must continually monitor for the presence of air movement through the tube by listening for breath sounds with the ear near the open end of the tube. The tube must never be forced or pushed forward if breath sounds are lost because damage to the retropharyngeal mucosa can result. If resistance is met, the tube should be withdrawn 1 to 2 cm, and the patient's head should be repositioned. Once positioned in the oropharynx, the tube should be advanced to the glottis while the tube operator listens for breath sounds through the tube. If breath sounds cease, the tube should be withdrawn several centimeters until breath sounds resume and the plane of entry is adjusted slightly. Passage through the vocal cords should be timed to coincide with inspiration. This is often signaled by a paroxysm of coughing and the inability to speak. The cuff should be inflated as described for oral intubation, and proper position of the tube should be ascertained. (*See* Nasotracheal Intubation.)

10. **C.** If oral intubation is required in the patient with suspected cervical spine injury, an assistant should maintain the neck in the neutral position by ensuring axial stabilization of the head and neck as the patient is intubated. Any patient with multiple trauma requiring intubation should be treated as if cervical spine injury is present. In the absence of maxillofacial trauma or cerebrospinal fluid rhinorrhea, nasal intubation may be the preferable technique. However, orotracheal intubation is more commonly performed, even in the setting of a cervical spine injury. (*See* Intubation of Difficult Airways.)

11. **A.** The most serious complication of extubation is laryngeal spasm. This is much more likely to occur if the patient is not fully conscious. If laryngeal spasm occurs, the application of positive pressure can sometimes relieve the problem. Succinylcholine, IV or IM, can be administered, bearing in mind that severe hyperkalemia may occur in a variety of clinical settings. Mechanical ventilation is required until the patient has recovered from the succinylcholine. The decision to extubate a patient is based on favorable clinical response to a carefully planned regimen of weaning, recovery of consciousness following anesthesia, or sufficient resolution of the initial indications for intubation. (*See* Extubation.)

Chapter 2

1. **E.** The external jugular vein, although meeting the goal of causing fewer complications during venipuncture, may not allow catheter tip placement in the central venous circulation with ease. Technical advances and a better understanding of anatomy have made insertion of central venous catheters safer,

but there still is a risk-to-benefit ratio, and some locations are more logical for certain therapeutic and diagnostic indications. Volume resuscitation alone is not an indication for central venous catheterization. A 16-gauge catheter in a peripheral vein can infuse two times the amount of fluid as a longer 16-gauge central venous catheter. However, peripheral vein cannulation can be impossible in the hypovolemic individual. In this case, the subclavian vein may be more reliable because of its attachments to the clavicle, allowing for cannulation even in a hypovolemic state. The femoral vein is also a reasonable alternative. Central venous access is often required for the infusion of irritant medications or vasoactive medications, for diagnostic or therapeutic radiologic procedures, and in a patient in whom peripheral access is impossible. (*See* Indications and Site Selection.)

2. **D.** Emergency transvenous pacemakers are best inserted through the right internal jugular vein because of the direct path to the right ventricle. This route is associated with the fewest catheter tip malpositions and the fewest complications of catheter and sheath introduction. With an indication for transvenous pacemaker insertion in a coagulopathic patient, the external jugular vein, if readily apparent on the surface, may be a good alternative. When the subclavian vein is utilized for pulmonary artery catheterization, the left subclavian vein is appropriate because of the greater distance from the venipuncture site to the subclavian vein. In addition, a catheter inserted from the left subclavian vein follows a natural curve that traverses the right ventricle into the right pulmonary artery. (*See* Indications and Site Selection.)

3. **True.** Catheter tip location is a very important, often ignored consideration in central venous catheterization. The ideal location of the catheter tip is in the distal innominate or proximal superior vena cava 3 to 5 cm proximal to the caval atrial junction. Positioning of the catheter tip within the right atrium or right ventricle must be avoided. (*See* General Considerations and Complications.)

4. **False.** Migration of catheter tips can be impressive. Migration of 5 to 10 cm has been reported with antecubital catheters and 1 to 5 cm with internal jugular vein or subclavian vein catheters. (*See* General Considerations and Complications.)

5. **False.** Utilizing an adapter while inserting the catheter and utilizing lead II on the standard ECG to monitor advancement of the catheter tip into the right atrium can aid in proper catheter placement. Regardless of whether this technique is used, a chest radiograph should be obtained following every initial central line catheter insertion to ascertain catheter tip location and to detect complications. Withdrawal of the catheter tip 3 to 5 cm after utilizing ECG monitoring with verification of P waves usually ensures correct positioning. (*See* General Considerations and Complications.)

6. **True.** Although phlebitis is more common with antecubital central venous catheterization, thrombosis, infection, limb edema, and pericardial tamponade can occur. Phlebitis is more common with antecubital central venous catheters, probably due to impaired blood flow as well as the proximity of the venous puncture site to the skin. Risk of pericardial tamponade is noted and may be increased because of greater catheter tip migration that occurs during arm movements. (*See* Routes of Central Venous Cannulation.)

7. B. Knowledge of the structures neighboring the internal jugular vein is essential for avoidance of complications during central venous catheterization. The internal carotid artery runs medial to the internal jugular vein and rarely may lie directly posteriorly. Behind the internal carotid artery, just outside the carotid sheath, lie the stellate ganglion and the cervical sympathetic trunk. The dome of the pleura, which is high on the left, lies caudal to the junction of the internal jugular vein and the subclavian vein. Posteriorly through the neck, the cholinergic and vagus nerves course, and the thoracic duct lies behind the internal jugular vein and enters the superior margin of the subclavian vein near the jugulosubclavian junction. (*See* Routes of Central Venous Cannulation.)

8. C. Central venous catheters should always be considered a possible source of infection in the febrile or septic patient. If all catheter sites appear normal and a noncatheter site can be implicated as the source for infection, the catheter can be left in place. For patients with excessive risks for new catheter placement, a guidewire exchange of the catheter is justifiable after obtaining two peripheral blood cultures and a quantitative culture of the catheter segment. The catheter may then remain pending culture results. The most common situation that is faced in the intensive care unit is a stable febrile patient with a central venous catheter in place. If a catheter has been in place for less than 72 hours and the indication persists for central venous catheterization, observation is reasonable, as it is very unlikely that the catheter is already infected. For catheters in place more than 72 hours but less than 120 hours, guidewire exchanges may be rational. Catheters of this duration are still not likely to be a source of fever, but the risk also cannot be ignored. An appropriately conducted guidewire exchange allows comparison of catheter tip cultures to other clinical cultures without subjecting the patient to repeat venipuncture. If within the next 24 hours an alternative source of fever is identified or the initial catheter segment culture is negative, then the guidewire catheter can be left in place. (*See* Infectious Complications.)

Chapter 3

1. False. The technique of diagnosing occlusive arterial disease of the hand was described by Allen as an easily understood and performed test to document the intact nature of the collateral circulation of the hand. It consists of compression of both radial and ulnar arteries as the patient is asked to clench and unclench the fist repeatedly until pallor of the palm is produced. One artery is then released, and the amount of time until blushing of the palm is noted. Normal palmar blushing is completed before 7 seconds; 8 to 14 seconds is considered equivocal, and 15 seconds or more is considered abnormal. This test is not an ideal screening procedure, with a sensitivity of 87 percent and a negative predictive value of only 18 percent. In other words, only 18 percent of patients with no collateral flow by Allen's test have this confirmed by Doppler study. (*See* Technique of Arterial Cannulation.)

2. False. Brachial artery catheterization is infrequently performed in major medical centers because of the concern of a lack of effective collateral circulation at that location in the arm and the fear of median nerve palsy due to bleeding into fascial plains and compression of the median nerve. For this reason, coagulopathy is considered a contraindication to brachial artery cannulation. (*See* Technique of Arterial Cannulation.)

Chapter 4

1. **True.** Since its introduction in 1970 by Swan and associates, the pulmonary artery catheter has grown to be a common tool for physiologic monitoring in the intensive care unit. Pulmonary artery catheters allow the direct measurement of several major determinants and consequences of cardiac performance such as preload, afterload, and cardiac output. Scalia and Palase have described using the mixed venous or central venous oxygen saturation as an early accurate measurement of occult blood loss in trauma victims. Current pulmonary artery catheters with the ability to measure mixed venous oxygen saturation on a continuous basis have been utilized for resuscitation and for inotropic management.

2. **False.** In general, within the literature, hemodynamic monitoring has been cited as having four central objectives: to assess left and/or right ventricular function, to monitor changes in hemodynamic status, to guide treatment with pharmacologic and nonpharmacologic agents, and to provide prognostic information. The conditions in which pulmonary artery catheterization may be useful are characterized by clinically unclear or rapidly changing hemodynamic status. (*See* Indications.)

3. **False.** A standard pulmonary artery catheter is approximately 110 cm in length. A balloon is fastened 1 to 2 mm from the tip, and when inflated, it guides the catheter by virtue of fluid dynamic drag from the greater interthoracic veins through the right heart chambers into the pulmonary artery. The balloon, when fully inflated in vessels of sufficiently large caliber, is designed to protrude above the catheter tip, with the progression of the catheter stopping when the balloon encounters a pulmonary artery slightly smaller in diameter than the fully inflated balloon. From this position, the pulmonary artery wedge pressure is obtained. The usual balloon inflation medium is air, but filtered carbon dioxide should be used in any situation in which balloon rupture might result in access to the arterial system. Periodic deflation and reinflation may be necessary, since carbon dioxide diffuses through the latex balloon. Liquids should never be used as the inflation medium.

4. **A.** Regarding placement of pulmonary artery catheters with the balloon inflated, catheter advancement is continued until a right ventricular pressure tracing is seen on the monitor. Catheter passage into and through the right ventricle is the most risky time in terms of generation of arrhythmias during this procedure. Maintaining the balloon inflated will minimize ventricular irritation, although ECG monitoring is important throughout the entire procedure. Catheter advancement is continued until the diastolic pressure tracing rises above that seen in the right ventricle, indicating pulmonary artery placement. With the catheter in the correct pulmonary artery position, it is secured, and subsequently a chest x-ray should be ordered to confirm catheter position, which should show the catheter tip no more than 3 to 5 cm from the midline. (*See* Insertion Techniques.)

5. **False.** Generally, patients should have normal coagulation parameters prior to attempting central venous access. However, it is not possible in some patients to discontinue heparin for 3 hours to allow the partial thromboplastin time to normalize. Although techniques for normalization of the prothrombin time in patients on warfarin can be accomplished with infusion of fresh frozen

plasma, it may be imprudent or impossible to correct these coagulation profiles prior to pulmonary artery catheterization. In these patients, techniques can be utilized to minimize hemorrhagic risks, including cannulation of the basilic vein or the internal or external jugular veins as a secondary approach. The subclavian approach should generally be avoided in patients with coagulopathies, since this site is inaccessible to direct pressure. (*See* Insertion Techniques.)

6. C. With the tip of the pulmonary artery catheter in the right atrium, normal resting right atrial pressure should be 0 to 6 mm Hg. Two major positive atrial pressure waves, the A wave and the V wave, can usually be recorded. The A wave is due to atrial contraction, and the V wave represents the pressure generated by venous filling of the right atrium while the tricuspid valve is closed. It is possible to sample right atrial blood and monitor right atrial pressure utilizing the proximal lumen once the pulmonary artery catheter is placed. (*See* Physiologic Data.)

7. C. Right ventricular monitoring is being increasingly utilized in the surgical critical care setting. The normal resting right ventricular pressure is between 17 and 30 mm Hg over 0 to 6 mm Hg, recorded when the pulmonary artery catheter crosses the tricuspid valve. The right ventricular systolic pressure should equal the pulmonary artery systolic pressure, except in cases of pulmonic valve stenosis or right ventricular outflow tract obstruction. The right ventricular pressure should equal the mean right atrial pressure during diastole when the tricuspid valve is open. (*See* Physiologic Data.)

8. A. Normal resting pulmonary artery pressure is 15 to 30 mm Hg over 5 to 13 mm Hg with a normal mean pressure of 10 to 18 mm Hg. The pulmonary artery waveform is characterized by systolic peak and diastolic trough with a dicrotic notch due to closure of the pulmonic valve. The peak pulmonary artery systolic pressure occurs within the T wave of a simultaneously recorded ECG. The pulmonary vasculature is normally a low-resistance circuit, and the pulmonary diastolic pressure is closely related to mean pulmonary artery wedge pressure and can be used as an index of left ventricular filling pressure in patients in whom a wedge pressure is unobtainable. However, if pulmonary vascular resistance is increased, such as with pulmonary embolism, pulmonary fibrosis, or reactive pulmonary hypertension, pulmonary artery diastolic pressure may markedly exceed mean pulmonary artery wedge pressure and thus be rendered an unreliable index of left heart function. (*See* Physiologic Data.)

9. D. Pulmonary artery wedge pressure is an important application in pulmonary artery catheterization. This measurement is obtained when the inflated balloon impacts into a slightly smaller branch of the pulmonary artery. In this position, the balloon stops the forward flow, and the catheter tip senses pressure transmitted backward through the column of blood from the pulmonary venous circulatory bed. The lung is divided into three physiologic zones, depending on the relationship of the pulmonary arterial, pulmonary venous, and alveolar pressures. In zone three, the pulmonary arterial and pulmonary venous pressures exceed the alveolar pressure, ensuring an uninterrupted column of blood between the catheter tip and pulmonary veins. If on radiograph the catheter tip is below the level of the left atrium, in posterior position in the supine patient, it can be assumed to be in zone three. With a few exceptions, estimated capillary hydrostatic filtration pressure from pulmonary artery wedge pressure is acceptable. This measurement does not take into account capillary permeability, serum colloid osmotic pressure, interstitial pressure, or actual pulmonary capillary resistance. These factors all play a role in the formation of pulmonary edema and should be interpreted in context. End expiration provides the most consistent readily identifiable reference point for pulmonary artery wedge pressure interpretation because pleural pressure returns to baseline at the end of passive deflation, approximately equal to atmospheric pressure. (*See* Physiologic Data.)

10. **False.** Pleural pressure can exceed normal resting value in patients, even at end expiration, with active expiratory muscle contraction or with the use of PEEP. How much PEEP is transmitted to the pleural space cannot be estimated with simplicity; however, it is felt that when normal lungs deflate passively, end-expiratory pleural pressure increases by approximately one-half of the applied PEEP. In patients with reduced lung compliance, the transmitted fraction is felt to be less, on the order of one-quarter or less. Although it is difficult to precisely estimate the true transmitted vascular pressure in a patient on PEEP, temporarily disconnecting the PEEP to measure pulmonary artery wedge pressure is *not* recommended. The abrupt removal of PEEP causes hypoxia, which may not reverse quickly on reinstitution of PEEP. (*See* Physiologic Data.)

11. **False.** Acute mitral regurgitation should be considered when a systolic murmur develops in the setting of acute ischemia or severe left ventricular failure of any origin. Left ventricular blood floods a normal-size noncompliant left atrium during ventricular asystole, causing giant V waves in the wedge pressure tracing. The giant V wave may be transmitted to pulmonary artery tracing, yielding a bifid pulmonary artery waveform, composed of a pulmonary artery systolic wave and the V wave. As the catheter is wedged, the pulmonary artery systolic wave is lost, but the V wave remains. Prominent V waves may occur whenever the left atrium is distended and noncompliant due to left ventricular failure from any cause. (*See* Clinical Applications.)

12. **A.** Although the hemodynamic findings of right ventricular infarction are characteristic, they may be confused with cardiac tamponade or constricted pericarditis. Right ventricular infarction typically occurs in the setting of inferior myocardial infarction. The right atrial pressure is elevated and is often disproportionately increased relative to the pulmonary artery wedge pressure. The right atrial pressure does not decline with inspiration, and the abnormalities noted may become exaggerated as right atrial pressure increases during volume expansion therapy. Right ventricular end-diastolic pressure and volume are elevated, and right ventricular stroke volume is decreased, resulting in a narrowed pulmonary artery pulse pressure. Tricuspid regurgitation may complicate right ventricular infarction if right ventricular dilatation or pathway muscle dysfunction occurs. (*See* Clinical Applications.)

13. **False.** A mean pulmonary arterial pressure of greater than 20 mm Hg defines pulmonary hypertension. Pulmonary hypertension can be classified as passive (i.e., increases in left atrial or left ventricular end-diastolic pressure), active, or reactive. (*See* Clinical Applications.)

Chapter 5

1 A. Temporary pacing may be used therapeutically or prophylactically in acute myocardial infarction. Bradyarrhythmias unresponsive to medical treatment that result in hemodynamic compromise may be such arrhythmias. Further, patients with anterior infarction and bifascicular block, or type II second degree atrioventricular block, although hemodynamically stable, may require a temporary pacemaker, as they are at risk for development of complete heart block. Coordinated atrial contraction may be essential for preservation and maintenance of effective stroke volume, and therefore, atrioventricular sequential pacing may be the modality of choice in these patients. As an example, when there is right ventricular involvement complicating an inferior and posterior infarction, transvenous atrioventricular sequential pacing may be necessary to ensure adequate cardiac output. Prophylactic temporary cardiac pacing is an area of considerable controversy. The administration of thrombolytic therapy should take precedence over placement of prophylactic cardiac pacing. Transthoracic cardiac pacing is a safe and usually effective alternative in patients who are to undergo thrombolytic therapy.

Chapter 6

1. **False.** The term *cardioversion* is utilized to describe electrical countershock to terminate cardiac arrhythmias other than ventricular fibrillation.

2. **True.** Defibrillation is the process of electrically depolarizing a critical mass of myocardium to terminate ventricular fibrillation. Cardioversion differs from defibrillation in that in cardioversion the electrical shock is synchronized. This is a process whereby the electrical unit is able to recognize the R or S wave to avoid shock during the period of electrical activity in the myocardium when it is vulnerable to generation of malignant tachyarrhythmias.

3. **False.** Synchronized direct-current cardioversion has been performed successfully in all trimesters of pregnancy without apparent adverse fetal effects. Cardioversion of paroxysmal supraventricular tachycardia with 100 joules and of atrial fibrillation with 300 joules has been reported with effective results and without substantial risk to either fetus or mother. Multiple studies have shown that electrical countershock does not induce premature labor, although in one instance a cesarean section was performed for fetal distress. Fetal rhythms should be monitored during cardioversion to ensure safety. Clearly, defibrillation of unstable tachyarrhythmias in a pregnant woman poses no ethical dilemma, as this is lifesaving to both mother and fetus. Current recommendations are that if the maternal arrhythmia is serious and refractory to other nonteratogenic treatments, synchronized direct-current cardioversion should be performed with fetal monitoring.

Chapter 7

1. **False.** Although transthoracic echocardiography, or TTE, has limitations in the ICU setting, it is still the initial screening procedure of choice for consideration of pericardial tamponade and to assess ventricular function in the ICU.

The widespread use of transesophogeal echocardiography has extended the capabilities of echocardiography in the ICU setting by permitting high-quality diagnostic images for consideration of valvular vegetation in the febrile patient and for other considerations where a high-quality diagnostic image is desired.

2. **False.** Recent studies suggest that simple visual estimate of ejection by an experienced physician compares favorably with results of more labor-intensive off-line computer computation of ejection fraction from the same images.

3. **B.** Left ventricular analysis by echocardiography is commonly utilized in the ICU setting, since left ventricular chamber dimensions and volumes may be estimated visually or by quantitative analysis. Echocardiography can be utilized to diagnose hypovolemia. In this setting, the echocardiogram will demonstrate small end-diastolic and end-systolic left ventricular volumes and a normal or elevated ejection fraction. Echocardiography is an essential part of the evaluation and postoperative management of patients with aortic valve replacement for stenosis or outflow obstruction. Generally, echocardiography in these patients who become hypotensive in the ICU suggests the presence of marked ventricular hypertrophy, small chamber volumes, and an elevated ejection fraction. These findings can have a dramatic impact on management decisions.

4. **D.** In clinical congestive heart failure, it has been demonstrated that Doppler transmitral flow profile correlates with the presence of clinical heart failure in patients suffering from acute myocardial infarction. These findings are due to the fact that the restrictive inflow pattern is indicative of abnormally elevated left ventricular diastolic pressures. Therefore, in clinical congestive heart failure, diastolic filling variables complement systolic function, permitting a comprehensive assessment of ventricular function. In studies by Echeverria, 50 consecutive patients were referred for echocardiography for congestive heart failure. In patients with ejection fraction below 50 percent, echocardiography revealed findings that were worse than clinically expected in 40 percent of patients. Echocardiography led to changes in the clinical management of these patients. The clinical impact of echocardiography was greater in the 40 percent of patients with congestive heart failure and normal ejection fraction. In these patients, there was generally the presence of hypertensive heart disease, and unexpectedly a normal ejection fraction was found in 90 percent of these patients. In these individuals, echocardiographic findings led to changes in the clinical management of 90 percent of the patients.

5. **D.** Transthoracic echocardiography and transesophogeal echocardiography are complementary diagnostic techniques in infective endocarditis. A negative high-quality transthoracic echocardiography examination provides strong evidence against the diagnosis of bacterial endocarditis, particularly when valvular regurgitation is minimal. Transesophogeal echocardiography offers an important increase in diagnostic sensitivity and specificity when the transthoracic echocardiography is of poor quality or when the transthoracic echocardiography examination is negative or equivocal in the setting of high clinical suspicion. Transthoracic echocardiography also appears to identify endocarditis patients who are at an increased risk of complications. Patients with maximal vegetation diameters exceeding 10 mm were at a higher risk for development of emboli, congestive heart failure, the need for surgical intervention, and death than those with smaller vegetations. Besides improving the diagnostic

sensitivity of cardiac ultrasound in infective endocarditis, transesophogeal echocardiography may demonstrate clinically unsuspected intracardiac disease such as intracardiac abscess or infective endocarditis of both native and prosthetic valves.

Chapter 8

1. **A.** An understanding of the anatomy and anatomic relationships of the pericardium begins with the visceral pericardium, which is closely, but loosely adherent to the epicardial surface. The parietal pericardium is a fibrous structure defining the outer membrane. Anatomic, physiologic, and pathophysiologic definition of a pericardial pathophysiology is derived from the multiple attachments of the parietal pericardium within the thorax. At the posterior margin of the parietal pericardium above the esophagus and pleural sacs where the visceral pericardium is absent, the parietal pericardium attaches directly to the epicardium at the borders of the entrance of the inferior and superior venae cavae and pulmonary veins. These multiple attachments limit the inherent elasticity and distensibility of the pericardium. This complex anatomic arrangement provides an anchor for the contracting myocardium and results in a small space between the visceral and parietal layers. This space usually contains a small volume of clear serous fluid, chemically similar to a plasma ultrafiltrate. Pericardial effusions that collect rapidly, over minutes to hours, may cause hemodynamic compromise with volumes of less than 250 ml. In contrast, effusions developing slowly, over days to weeks, allow for both hypertrophy and distention of the fibrous parietal membrane. Volumes of 2 liters may accumulate without significant hemodynamic compromise.

2. **False.** The patient should be in a supine position with the head of the bed elevated to approximately 45 degrees from the horizontal plane. Elevation of the thorax will allow free-flowing effusions to collect inferiorly and anteriorly, which are the sites that are easiest and safest to access using a subxiphoid approach.

3. **C.** Factors associated with an increased risk of complications after pericardiocentesis include a small effusion of less than 250 ml, a posteriorly located effusion, a localized effusion, and a maximum clear space by echocardiography of less than 10 mm in an unguided approach. All patients undergoing pericardiocentesis should have a portable chest x-ray performed immediately after the procedure to exclude pneumothorax. In addition, a repeat transthoracic, two-dimensional echocardiogram should be obtained within several hours to evaluate the adequacy of pericardial drainage and to confirm catheter placement. Close monitoring is required on a constant basis following pericardiocentesis to detect evidence of recurrent tamponade and to detect procedure-related complications.

4. **E.** Long-term management of patients with significant pericardial fluid collection is dictated by ease of drainage and underlying pathophysiology. The indications for surgical intervention are established and include pericardial disease with constrictive physiology, known loculated or posteriorly located effusions not amenable to pericardiocentesis, suspected purulent pericarditis, and effusions not successfully drained by pericardiocentesis. Nonsurgical management of chronically debilitated patients with metastatic disease of the pericardium may be indicated. Even in busy tertiary care and intensive care

units, unguided pericardiocentesis is rarely indicated, and surgical drainage may be the preferred approach to pericardial drainage in patient populations after initial pericardial decompression.

Chapter 9

1. **False.** Intraaortic balloon counterpulsation improves left ventricular performance with an increase in coronary perfusion and a decrease in myocardial oxygen consumption. In contrast to other types of circulatory assist devices, the intraaortic balloon pump requires a minimum cardiac index of 1.2 to 1.4 liters/min/m^2 to be effective. Thus, the intraaortic balloon pump cannot assist in the patient who is asystolic or in ventricular fibrillation.

2. **True.** Intraaortic balloon counterpulsation is very effective in the initial stabilization of patients with mechanical intracardiac defects complicating myocardial infarction such as acute mitral regurgitation, ventricular septal perforation, and pathway muscle rupture. Counterpulsation reduces pulmonary artery pressure and increases cardiac output. It also has been seen to decrease the regurgitant V waves seen in mitral insufficiency.

3. **True.** Commonly accepted indications for intraaortic balloon pump utilization include unstable angina, and centers that utilize counterpulsation liberally for the treatment of unstable angina report surgical mortality rates approaching those for chronic stable angina (in a range of 2–5%). One of the most useful indications for intraaortic balloon pump counterpulsation is to aid in weaning those patients from cardiopulmonary bypass who have suffered from perioperative myocardial injury. A myocardial dysfunction is often reversible if the patient's circulation can be assisted for 24 to 48 hours. The preoperative use of intraaortic counterpulsation has been advocated for certain high-risk patients: those with hemodynamically significant stenosis of the left main coronary artery and those with marked impairment of left ventricular function as indicated by an injection fraction of less than 0.35. Although these indications have been advocated by some groups, most centers use intraaortic balloon counterpulsation selectively, rather than routinely, in patients with left coronary stenosis or diminished ejection fractions. Counterpulsation has been used to provide mechanical support for patients in failure while awaiting cardiac transplantation. Many centers now use counterpulsation to control unstable angina prior to and during coronary angioplasty.

4. **B.** Although some centers have utilized intraaortic balloon pump counterpulsation to control ventricular arrhythmia, more potent antiarrhythmic drugs and better long-term survival rates have been seen in patients who subsequently undergo surgical revascularization before being weaned. These data suggest that the use of intraaortic balloon pump counterpulsation to control ventricular arrhythmia will be less frequent. Absolute contraindications include acute valvular insufficiency, aortic dissection, and severe aortoiliac disease. In the presence of significant aortic regurgitation, the augmented diastolic pressure is transmitted directly to the left ventricle, compounding the deleterious effects of a valvular insufficiency. Because of the need for anticoagulation during counterpulsation, gastrointestinal bleeding, thrombocytopenia, and other bleeding diatheses are relative contraindications for counterpulsation.

5. **D.** Cessation of counterpulsation involves two steps: weaning and intraaortic balloon pump removal. The intraaortic balloon pump console can provide counterpulsation ratios of 1:1, 1:2, and 1:3. In addition, some consoles permit weaning by a gradual reduction in balloon volume. The patient may be progressively weaned by reducing the assist ratio or the intraaortic balloon volume and checking the cardiac index and filling pressures at each level. Once the patient has been weaned to a 1:3 ratio and has been stable, the intraaortic balloon pump may be removed. The heparin infusion should be stopped 2 hours before removing the percutaneous intraaortic balloon. The prothombin and partial thromboplastin time should be near normal and the platelet count greater than 75,000 before percutaneous removal of an intraaortic balloon pump. During removal, arterial bleeding should be allowed for 1 to 2 seconds to flush any residual thrombus, and then the application of pressure firm enough to obliterate the femoral pulse for 45 minutes before the operator checks for bleeding should be utilized. Occasionally, local pressure will not control bleeding from the puncture site, and a hematoma occurs that requires surgical closure. Further, distal perfusion of the limb should be monitored to avoid complications of femoral artery thrombosis or distal embolization.

Chapter 10

1. **True.** When these conditions exist for more than a few hours, there is an 85 percent mortality. In addition to hemodynamic criteria, other conditions must also exist to make a candidate for a ventricular assist device. There must be no surgically corrective lesions, and metabolic abnormalities should be absent. Other conditions that must exist prior to left ventricular assist device placement include optimizing preload and placement of an intraaortic balloon counterpulsation device. Additionally, it is assumed that the heart possesses some degree of possibility for future recovery, which will allow for removal of the device.

2. **B.** Infections responding to antibiotic therapy should not absolutely preclude mechanical ventricular support. Contraindications at this time include massive myocardial infarction, bleeding disorders, or active bleeding from the gastrointestinal tract or central nervous system. Other contraindications include the presence of a chronic debilitating disease such as metastatic cancer, severe pulmonary hypertension, severe peripheral vascular diseases, and neurologic impairment. Although the presence of chronic renal failure has served as a deterrent, it is considered a relative contraindication at this time. The presence of single-organ dysfunction should not preclude placement of a ventricular assist device.

3. **E.** Early signs of potential success and indications for left ventricular assist device weaning include less than 75 hours of pump support, no evidence of postoperative myocardial infarction by ECG or physiologic criteria, some evidence of left ventricular recovery, mild or absent right ventricular failure, control of bleeding diathesis, and maintenance of renal function.

Chapter 11

1. **True.** The pleural space is a closed serous sac surrounded by two layers: the parietal pleura and the visceral pleura. The lung fills all but approximately 10 ml of the hemithorax in the normal physiologic state.

2. **False.** Although 500 ml of fluid may enter the pleural space each day under normal conditions, less than 3 ml of fluid is normally present within the space at any given time. This normal equilibrium may be disrupted by increased fluid entry due to alterations in hydrostatic or oncotic pressures or by changes in the parietal pleura itself such as in an inflammatory situation. A derangement in lymphatic drainage, such as seen with lymphatic destruction, may also produce fluid accumulation.

3. **D.** Accumulation of blood in the pleural space, or hemothorax, may be classified into two broad categories: spontaneous and traumatic. A hemothorax may also occur secondary to attempted thoracentesis or chest tube placement. In trauma, a pulmonary parenchymal source of hemorrhage is often self-limiting due to the low pressure of the pulmonary vascular system. However, if a systemic source of arterial bleeding is present from intercostal internal mammary or subclavian arteries, or even the aorta or heart, the bleeding may be potentially life threatening. Placement of a large-bore chest tube (36 to 40 Fr.) not only assists in ventilation but also helps assess the need for immediate thoracotomy. In general, indications for open thoracotomy include initial blood loss of 1 to 1.5 liters, greater than 500 ml of blood loss in the first hour, greater than 200 ml per hour after 2 to 4 hours, or greater than 100 ml per hour after 6 to 8 hours, or in an unstable patient not responding to volume resuscitation.

4. **C.** The primary causes of chylothorax are trauma (including iatrogenic from surgery), malignancy, congenital, and miscellaneous, such as filariasis invasion or subclavian vein obstruction. Surgical procedures most often implicated in iatrogenic injury include those where mobilization of the aortic arch is performed or an esophageal resection. The appearance of chyle in the pleural space may be delayed 7 to 10 days after injury, especially if dietary restrictions are employed postoperatively. The fluid may collect in the posterior mediastinum before rupturing into the pleural space, sometimes on the right side. In a nontraumatic setting, malignancy must always be suspected. Leaks occur secondary to direct invasion of the thoracic duct or from obstruction by external compression or tumor embolus. Sarcoma, lymphoma, and primary lung carcinomas are most frequently implicated. Treatment consists of tube drainage and aggressive maintenance of fluid and nutritional status. Hyperalimentation and intestinal rest are recommended to limit flow through the duct. Approximately 50 percent will resolve spontaneously. A minimum of 2 weeks' observation is usually recommended. If this management fails, open thoracotomy is recommended to ligate the duct and close the fistula, with identification of the site aided by preoperative oral administration of cream or olive oil or by injection of Evan's blue dye.

5. **True.** In chest tube insertion, proper patient positioning and verification of the proper side and location for the chest tube placement must be accomplished before beginning the procedure. After the subcutaneous tunnel is created, the intercostal muscles have been divided, and the parietal pleura is entered, a finger must be inserted into the pleural space to explore the anatomy, confirming proper location and lack of pleural adhesions. The position of the diaphragm can be deceiving, and intrahepatic or intrasplenic chest tube placement in blind fashion can be fatal. Further, bluntly dissecting dense adhesions will tear the pulmonary parenchyma and may initiate troublesome bleeding.

Chapter 13

1. **False.** Patients with bacterial pneumonia should be treated with an effective narrow-spectrum antibiotic. The selection of the drug should be based on the identification of the cause of the organism. Although blood, pleural fluid, open thoracotomy, and percutaneous needle aspiration are all generally accepted, physicians most frequently rely on results of lower respiratory tract secretions or sputum.

2. **C.** A routine sputum culture is one in which the specimen has been expectorated into a container, transported to the laboratory after a variable period of time, and placed on a culture medium without undergoing dilution or homogenization. Contamination of expectorated sputum samples by aerobic pharyngeal organisms occurs readily, so the bacteriologic flora of the expectorated sputum sample may not reflect the nature of true bronchial flora. To improve the results of routinely processed expectorated sputum samples, special manipulations, including mouse inoculation and anaerobic incubation for pneumococci, have been tried. Homogenization of sputum has been advocated. In spite of these manipulations, lower respiratory tract infections, as diagnosed by transthoracic aspirations, have become sterile in some studies after initiation of proper antibiotic therapy while the expectorated sputum cultures from the same patients have continued to grow large concentrations of *S. aureus* and facultative gram-negative bacilli.

3. **False.** Murry and Washington concluded that when an imperial portion of expectorated sputum had less than 10 squamous epithelial cells per low-power field, it was as accreted as transthoracic aspirated cultures performed at their institution. Their results also showed that the best expectorated sputum sample was not necessarily the one with the greatest number of white blood cells, but the one with the fewest squamous epithelial cells.

4. **False.** Transtracheal aspiration, although the standard by which multiple studies are compared, is not routinely employed in the adult patient.

5. **False.** The protective brush method of sampling lower respiratory tract secretions involves a closed brush system within a bronchoscope, whereas bronchoalveolar lavage samples a larger and more representative amount of lower respiratory tract secretions than protected brush catheterization and provides a large enough sample to do smears for rapid identification as well as culture. The role of bronchoalveolar lavage with quantitative bacteriology has been less well defined than protected brush specimens. In some studies, when expectorated sputum has been negative, bronchoalveolar lavage has been useful in diagnosing *Legionella* pneumonia by culture and *Mycobacterium tuberculosis* infection.

Chapter 14

1. **D.** Regarding thoracentesis and a bloody effusion, grossly bloody effusions with a red cell count of 5000 to 10,000 cells per cubic millimeter must be present for fluid to appear pink colored. Those effusions containing greater than 100,000 red blood cells per cubic millimeter are consistent with trauma, malignancy, or pulmonary infarction. To distinguish a traumatic thoracentesis

from a preexisting hemothorax, several observations may be helpful. A preexisting hemothorax will have been defribinated so it will not form a clot on standing. Further, a traumatic thoracentesis is suggested when pleural and blood hematocrit values match.

2. **D.** Malignancies can produce pleural effusions by two basic mechanisms: implantation of malignant cells on the pleura or impairment of lymphatic drainage secondary to tumor obstruction. The most common tumors that cause pleural effusions are lung cancer, breast cancer, and lymphoma. Pleural fluid cytology should be performed for an exudative effusion of unknown etiology; between 100 and 200 ml of fluid is required. Heparin should be added to the container to prevent clotting of the fluid. In addition to malignancy, cytologic examination can diagnose rheumatoid pleuritis where there is a presence of slender elongated macrophages, giant round multinucleated macrophages, and an amorphous granular background material.

Chapter 16

1. **False.** The transport of critically ill patients to the operating room for elective and semielective tracheotomy is not without potential complications. As many as 33 percent of intensive care unit patients moved to other departments of the hospital for diagnostic tests and surgery will have significant and possibly dangerous physiologic changes. This is especially true of patients who are on specialized ventilatory support where that ventilator must either travel with the patient or may not be available in the other setting. Tracheotomy can be performed at the bedside in one of two ways: (1) by having the operating room personnel bring the sterile supplies to the intensive care unit and having the procedure performed as a surgical procedure, and (2) as a percutaneous bronchoscopic-assisted technique.

2. **False.** The tracheotomy tube has a cuff that is similar to the endotracheal tube cuff. This cuff is a low-pressure, high-volume cuff that is designed to minimize the chance of tracheal stenosis.

3. **B.** Late hemorrhage after tracheotomy is usually due to bleeding granulation tissue or some minor cause; however, it was previously reported that 50 percent of all tracheotomy bleeding, for more than 48 hours after the procedure, was due to rupture of the innominate artery caused by erosion of the tracheotomy tube. Although less common since the advent of the low-pressure cuff, tracheal–innominate artery fistulas still occur within the first month after tracheotomy. Infection and other factors, such as position of the tube, contribute to this potential complication. The innominate artery rises to the level of the sixth ring, anterior to the trachea, so low stomas can create close proximity of the tube or cuff to the innominate artery.

4. **False.** The cricothyroid space is 7 to 9 mm in its vertical dimension, which is smaller than the outside diameter of most tracheotomy tubes. The No. 6, or small Shiley, has an outside diameter of 10 mm.

5. **C.** The advantages of percutaneous guidewire dilatational elective tracheotomy, most often reported by Ciaglia in the literature reports, include no need for operating room, a faster overall time than standard tracheotomy, relatively less expense, and decreased dissection. However, it is not a technique for

emergency cricothyroidotomy, nor should it be performed in completely blind fashion. It is currently recommended in the literature that upper airway endoscopy may help to identify intratracheal placement of the needle and J-guidewire along with selection of the proper intratracheal ring membrane.

Chapter 17

1. **B.** Extracorporeal life support is a critical care technique that has made significant technologic advances in recent years. Extracorporeal life support is standard therapy for neonatal respiratory failure. Key factors to success in pediatric, infant, and adult populations is early intervention prior to the appearance of irreversible organ damage. The early trials in the 1970s comparing ECMO to conventional mechanical ventilation showed no survival advantage for ECMO; however, these trials were severely flawed in design. To date, almost 10,000 patients have been treated with extracorporeal life support at 90 centers across the United States and overseas.

Chapter 18

1. **C.** The absolute indications for dialysis in the intensive care unit are volume overload refractory to diuretic therapy; hyperkalemia not responsive to conservative therapy; uremic complications such as pericarditis, bleeding diathesis, or encephalopathy; and specific drug overdose amenable to dialysis. Relative indications include acidosis, hyperacidemia, hypermagnesemia, hyperurosemia, and obligate excess fluid intake from management such as antibiotic administration.

2. **True.** An important underrecognized risk of dialysis is the delay in recovery of renal function that may occur after institution of dialysis for acute renal failure. After an acute insult, it may take several weeks for acutely injured tissue to be repaired or replaced. Potential complications from dialysis include repeated bouts of relative hypotension, which could impair renal blood flow, and complement-mediated reactions to dialysis.

3. **A.** The movement of solute from blood to the dialysate can be accomplished by either diffusive or convective transport. Diffusive transport is achieved by concentration-dependent movement of the solute across the semipermeable membrane, whereas convective transport is based on ultrafiltration or is a flow-dependent phenomenon. Smaller-molecular-weight solutes, such as urea and potassium, have high diffusive clearances, whereas larger molecules, such as vitamin B_{12}, depend primarily on ultrafiltration for clearance.

Chapter 19

1. **C.** Lower gastrointestinal endoscopy can be performed for acute lower gastrointestinal bleeding. This procedure is technically difficult in the intensive care unit setting and in the unprepped bowel. For these reasons, and due to its relative lack of sensitivity in this setting, erythrocyte scanning, angiography, or both are indicated for diagnosis. Endoscopic colonic decompression is advocated for patients in the intensive care unit. Uncontrolled series suggest that when the diameter of the right colon exceeds 12 cm, perforation is imminent,

and decompression is indicated. The placement of nasogastric suction, rectal tube placement, and position changes should be initiated prior to attempts of endoscopic decompression. Placement of a decompression tube into the colon is recommended, since relapse is common.

Chapter 21

1. **C.** Aspiration pneumonia is the most common complication in the utilization of balloon tamponade for control of variceal hemorrhage. Incidence ranges from 0 to 12 percent. Acute laryngeal obstruction is the most severe complication. Migration of the tube is the cause of this potentially fatal complication and occurs when the gastric balloon is not inflated properly after adequate positioning in the stomach or when extensive traction of greater than 1.5 kg is used. Mucosal ulceration of the gastroesophageal junction is common and is directly related to prolonged traction time of greater than 36 hours.

Chapter 22

1. **True.** Precipitation of proteins when exposed to an acid pH may be an important factor leading to the clogging of formulas. Additionally, medications are a frequent cause of clogging, as is inadequate interval and volume of flushing between administrations of enteral feeding. Several maneuvers are used for clearing clogged feeding tubes. These include irrigation with warm saline, with carbonated liquid, with cranberry juice, or with an enzyme solution. Additionally, pancrease, which is a mixture of lipase, amylase, and protease, dissolved in a sodium bicarbonate solution, has been found to be useful. This mixture is instilled into the tube with a syringe and clamped for 30 minutes to allow enzymatic degradation of precipitated enteral feedings.

Chapter 23

1. **True.** Hemapheresis involves separation of the patient's whole blood into the components, removal of a specific component, and reinfusion of the remaining blood. Blood components of different specific gravities are usually separated by centrifugation. The plasma can also be separated from whole blood by a parallel plate membrane plasma exchange system of filtration.

2. **B.** The following are indications for treatment with therapeutic plasma exchange in the intensive care unit setting: acute Guillain-Barré syndrome, myasthenia gravis, thrombotic thrombocytopenic purpura, autoimmune hemolytic anemia, rapidly progressive glomerulonephritis, drug overdose, and poisoning. These conditions are due to plasma-mediated antibodies and complement consideration.

Chapter 25

1. **C.** Cerebral ischemia, defined as cerebral oxygen delivery insufficient to meet metabolic needs, can result from reduction from any of the three components: cerebral blood flow, hemoglobin concentration, and arterial hemoglobin

saturation. The brain constitutes only 2 percent of the body weight, receives 15 percent of cardiac output, and accounts for 20 percent of total oxygen consumption. Certain regions of the brain, such as the cerebellum, basal ganglia, CA-1 layer of the hippocampus, and arterial boundary zones between the major branches of intracranial vessels (watershed areas), appear to be selectively vulnerable to ischemic injury.

2. **False.** The jugular venous bulb is a sensitive and specific site for measurement of cerebral oxygen consumption. Retrograde cannulation of the jugular bulb is a low-risk, technically simple procedure. The internal jugular vein can be located via external anatomic landmarks, and the catheter is directed toward the mastoid, over which lies the jugular venous bulb. Continuous monitoring of the venous saturation is feasible using commercially available oximetry catheters.

Chapter 27

1. **B.** Bursitis, tendonitis, and cellulitis may all mimic true joint arthritis. Prior to performing arthrocentesis, physical examination must be performed to be certain that the joint is inflamed and that an effusion is present. If a large effusion is suspected, one should perform a patellar tap. Arthrocentesis is also used for therapeutic purposes.

2. **False.** The viscosity of synovial fluid is a measure of the hyaluronic acid content of the fluid. Hyaluronic acid is one of the major substances in the synovial fluid that gives it its viscous quality. Enzymes such as hyaluronidase are released in inflammatory conditions, thus destroying hyaluronic acid in other proteinaceous material. This produces a thinner, less viscous fluid.

Chapter 28

1. **True.** Investigators have noticed that a return of consciousness can take minutes following termination of up to 8 hours of propofol infusion even though the elimination of propofol is 5 hours. This suggests that the initial fall in drug concentration following termination of the infusion is a function of redistribution more than elimination half-life.

2. **C.** The practice of administering small doses of naloxone (0.04 mg) to patients to reverse respiratory depression of narcotic administration is inadvisable in the ICU setting. There are many anecdotal reports indicating that naloxone has significant side effects on cardiovascular function, with or without prior narcotic administration. Naloxone levels also decline rapidly, whereas narcotic levels may be persistently elevated for a longer time. Recurring respiratory depression therefore remains a distinct possibility in the unintubated patient, with potential morbidity and even mortality.

3. **True.** Recent data suggest that reversal of opiods with an opioid combination agonist-antagonist such as nalbuphine may be safer than naloxone. Antagonists with some intrinsic analgesic properties result in a more gradual reversal than naloxone. It is important to note that a mixed agonist-antagonist can either increase or decrease opioid effect, depending on the dose administered, the particular agonist already in the bloodstream, and the amount of drug to be reversed.

4. **False.** Barbiturates are used to facilitate endotracheal intubation, and they reduce cerebral oxygen utilization. However, cardiovascular side effects include hypotension with possible cardiac arrest, myocardial depression, and an increase in venous capacitance. Etomidate has the same beneficial effect on cerebral oxygen kinetics as barbiturates, yet is virtually devoid of cardiovascular side effects.

5. **A.** Midazolam provides more complete anterograde amnesia than diazepam or lorazepam and produces less pain on intravenous injection than diazepam or lorazepam. Midazolam is highly protein-bound, approaching 95 percent to albumin, and has a comparatively short half-life of 2 hours versus 36 hours for diazepam and 12 hours for lorazepam. However, the half-life can be notably prolonged in ICU patients, obese patients, and elderly patients and in about 5 percent of normal patients for unknown reasons.

6. **False.** Depending on the level of discomfort of the procedure and the requirements of the ICU setting, a combination of analgesia and sedation is critical. Analgesic agents such as alfentanil, sufentanil, and ketamine and sedative agents such as propofol and midazolam are utilized in combination in the ICU setting and are effective in combination. It should be emphasized that sedative agents without analgesic agents are to be avoided for any procedures in the ICU setting. Sedative agents alone may be appropriate for ventilator weaning and anxiety, where there are no pain considerations.

Chapter 29

1. **D.** Intramucosal pH monitoring is used to monitor changes in tissue pH in response to changes in **local** oxygen delivery and metabolism. These trends can be utilized to identify organ tissue dysfunction and predict multiple organ failure in some studies. The technique measures PCO_2 and pH in saline within a gas-permeable balloon placed in the lumen of a hollow viscus. The most common site monitored in the intensive care unit setting is the stomach.

Chapter 31

1. **False.** The presence of infection with any fluid accumulation in the abdomen is almost always an absolute indication for drainage.

2. **False.** The aftercare of catheter insertion requires frequent flushing starting a few hours after insertion. Normal saline is injected every 4 hours to flush the catheter and prevent clogging of the side holes. After 24 hours, the purpose of flushing is to agitate dependent debris in the collection so that sediment can eventually be aspirated into the catheter.

3. **False.** Cholestasis is a common condition in the intensive care unit setting and actually occurs in most patients. Distention of the gallbladder is a common finding. In the patient with sepsis of unknown source, cholecystostomy is indicated in the presence of a distended gallbladder and especially with findings of pericholecystic fluid or thickened gallbladder wall by ultrasound.

II. Cardiovascular Problems in the Intensive Care Unit

32. Cardiopulmonary Resuscitation

1. True or False. High-impulse cardiopulmonary resuscitation (CPR) maximizes stroke volume and coronary blood flow with chest compressions of moderate force and brief duration.

2. True or False. The majority of infants and children who require resuscitation in an intensive care unit setting have had a primary myocardial dysrhythmia or other pump failure as the cause of their need for CPR.

3. True or False. The proper use of defibrillator devices in the intensive care unit setting requires special attention to selection of proper energy levels.

4. Select the best answer.

   A. The administration of calcium can be through use of its two available salts: calcium chloride and calcium gluconate.
   B. Each form of calcium is degraded in the plasma, and each provides the same bioavailability of calcium.
   C. Calcium chloride salt provides the least direct source of calcium ion and produces the slowest effect.
   D. Calcium gluconate salt is unstable. Calcium gluceptate and gluconate salts require renal degradation to release the free calcium ion.

33. Critical Aortic Stenosis and Hypertrophic Cardiomyopathy

1. True or False. The most common symptom occurring in left ventricular outflow obstruction is angina pectoris.

2. True or False. An auscultatory finding that is common to all forms of left ventricular outflow obstruction is the systolic (crescendo-decrescendo type) murmur.

3. True or False. The chest radiograph in patients with left ventricular outflow obstruction shows a dilated heart silhouette in the majority of patients.

4. Select the best answer.

A. Cardiac catheterization has the principal objective of corroborating Doppler findings in the setting of severe aortic stenosis.
B. Cardiac catheterization for coronary arteriography is no longer mandatory prior to surgical intervention given the sensitivity of Doppler echocardiography.
C. An accurate measure of cardiac output by the Fick method or dye dilution technique can be performed when measuring the gradient across a diseased valve.
D. A grading of 50 mm Hg or more is found in normal individuals.

34. Critical Care of Pericardial Disease

1. True or False. Acute pericarditis may be asymptomatic but is usually *symptomatic* with a pleuritic chest component. Frequently, there is sudden onset of symptoms.

2. True or False. Pericardial friction rubs have traditionally been described as having a "to-and-fro" description, although the classic pericardial rub has three components.

3. True or False. There are three potential ECG stages recognizable in the evolution of pericarditis.

4. Select the best answer.

A. The optimal treatment of pericarditis is indomethacin over a 2- to 3-day period.
B. Initial and optimal treatment of pericarditis is to begin with ibuprofen, 60 mg PO q6h.
C. Effective initial treatment of pericarditis can lead to relief of pain within 15 minutes.
D. Azathioprine (Imuran) should never be used for treatment of pericarditis.
E. Steroid therapy in high doses is often indicated in treatment of pericarditis.

5. Select the best answer.

A. Any pericardial effusion greater in volume than 250 ml will cause symptomatic compromise of myocardial function.
B. The configuration of the cardiac silhouette on x-ray easily distinguishes between cardiomegaly, large pericardial cyst, and pericardial effusion.
C. Rapid accumulation of as little as 200 ml of intrapericardial fluid can cause acute hemodynamic compromise and circulatory collapse.
D. If pericardial fluid is of an inflammatory nature, it is unlikely that a pericardial rub will be audible.

6. Select the best answer.

A. It is not imperative to differentiate between extrapericardial and intracardiac aspirated samples during pericardiocentesis.

B. Intrapericardial blood will clot more readily than intracardiac blood or intravascular blood.
C. Echocardiography may be used to monitor the progress of pericardiocentesis and may be used to directly visualize the needle as it progresses into the effusion.
D. Failure of pericardiocentesis to deliver fluid from the pericardium rules out pericardial effusion.

35. Sudden Cardiac Death

1. True or False. Sudden cardiac death occurs in 400,000 patients per year in the United States.

2. True or False. Cardiac causes of ventricular tachycardia and ventricular fibrillation in the absence of acute myocardial infarction include prior myocardial infarction, cardiomyopathies, and electrical disorders.

3. Select the best answer.

A. Prevention has no role in the treatment of sudden cardiac death.
B. Amiodarone and sotalol are effective agents in the treatment of known ventricular arrhythmias.
C. Implantable cardioverter-defibrillator devices have become obsolete in the management of ventricular fibrillation.
D. Individualized therapy is not indicated in patients with known dysrhythmias.

36. Dissection of the Aorta

1. True or False. Aortic dissection is much more common than acute myocardial infarction.

2. True or False. The process of aortic dissection begins with an intimal tear.

3. True or False. Hypertension is the most important disease associated with the development of aortic dissection.

4. True or False. The original classification of DeBakey divides aortic dissection into five types.

5. Select the best answer.

A. The electrocardiogram is very useful in diagnosing acute aortic dissection.
B. The most common plain chest radiograph finding (seen in more than 80% of patients with aortic dissection) is widening of the superior mediastinum.
C. Echocardiography is not useful in the diagnosis of aortic dissection.
D. The chief limitation of computed tomography scanning to diagnose aortic dissection is limited visualization of the descending aorta.

6. Select the best answer. Regarding acute aortic dissection:

A. Untreated acute aortic dissection has a nearly uniformly fatal outcome.
B. The first surgical correction of aortic dissection was accomplished in 1965 by DeBakey.
C. Maintenance of a high mean arterial blood pressure is critical in the treatment of acute aortic dissection.
D. The utilization of adequate beta-blockade is contraindicated in conjunction with the use of sodium nitroprusside in the medical management of acute aortic dissection.

37. Acute Aortic Insufficiency

1. True or False. Acute aortic insufficiency is generally the result of myocardial infarction.

2. True or False. It is uncommon for acute bacterial endocarditis to be caused by *Staphylococcus aureus*.

3. True or False. Large valvular vegetations of the aortic valve are consistent with fungal endocarditis.

4. Select the best answer. Regarding acute infective endocarditis with aortic insufficiency:

A. It is common for an infection of the aortic valve to affect a previously normal valve.
B. Infective endocarditis of an aortic valve rarely involves an anatomically bicuspid aortic valve.
C. Usually there is no significant aortic stenosis or aortic insufficiency prior to the onset of infective endocarditis.
D. Infective endocarditis resulting in acute severe aortic insufficiency rarely causes life-threatening cardiac complications.

5. Select the answer that is **false**. Regarding acute endocarditis of the aortic valve:

A. Patients with a congenital bicuspid aortic valve are at increased risk for aortic valve endocarditis.
B. A bicuspid aortic valve is associated with turbulent flow.
C. A bicuspid aortic valve is commonly symptomatic and, if not symptomatic, is usually noted by routine physical examination in childhood.
D. Antibiotic prophylaxis is indicated for dental or other surgical procedures in patients with known bicuspid aortic valve.

6. Select the best answer. Hemodynamic findings associated with acute severe aortic sufficiency include

A. Decreased arterial pulse pressure.
B. Equilibration of left ventricular end-diastolic and aortic diastolic pressures.
C. Marked decrease in left ventricular end-diastolic pressure.
D. Decreased pulmonary artery wedge pressure.

38. Acute Mitral Regurgitation

1. True or False. Life-threatening acute mitral regurgitation caused by papillary muscle rupture in the setting of myocardial infarction occurs in less than 1 percent of patients suffering from acute myocardial infarction.

2. True or False. The presence of moderately severe or severe mitral regurgitation in the setting of acute myocardial infarction is associated with a higher mortality rate than that seen in patients suffering from acute myocardial infarction who have no evidence of mitral regurgitation.

3. True or False. The anterolateral papillary muscle is more vulnerable to ischemia than the posteromedial papillary muscle.

4. Select the best answer. Regarding intensive care unit management of mitral regurgitation:

A. Afterload reduction is imperative in the management of mitral regurgitation.
B. The intraaortic balloon pump is not indicated in cases of severe mitral regurgitation.
C. Inotropic support with high-dose dopamine is very effective in the management of mitral regurgitation.
D. Pulmonary artery catheterization should only be used in severe cases of mitral regurgitation.

39. Syncope

1. True or False. Syncope is classified into cardiovascular and noncardiovascular.

2. True or False. Syncope due to obstructive disorders of the heart typically occurs during exercise.

3. True or False. Hypertrophic cardiomyopathy is an important cause of syncope, and any young patient who has complained of syncope should have a work-up.

4. Select the best answer.

A. Tachycardia rarely results in syncope.
B. Pulmonary hypertension may lead to recurrent syncope.
C. Pulmonary embolism is a rare cause of syncope.
D. Acute myocardial ischemia rarely presents with syncope.

5. Select the best answer. Regarding the sick sinus syndrome:

A. The sick sinus syndrome is characterized by impaired sinoatrial impulse formation or propagation.
B. Sinus node dysfunction is frequently masked by low concentration of drugs such as digoxin, beta-blockers, and calcium channel blockers.
C. A decreased sensitivity to endogenous adenosine appears closely related to the development of the sick sinus syndrome.
D. Patients with this syndrome who manifest syncope usually require surgical correction of this syndrome.

40. Systemic Embolism

1. True or False. Embolism to the systemic circulation nearly always originates as a thrombus within the left heart.

2. True or False. Systemic emboli do not originate in the venous circulation.

3. Select the best answer. Regarding the source of systemic emboli:

   A. Atrial fibrillation is a rare cause of systemic embolization.
   B. Coronary artery disease with left ventricular dysfunction is a rare cause of systemic embolization.
   C. Valvular heart disease is a common cause of systemic embolization.
   D. Coronary artery disease and valvular heart disease are most likely to be complicated by systemic embolism when low ejection fraction and normal sinus rhythm are present.

4. Select the best answer. Regarding arterial emboli:

   A. The upper extremities are the location where most of the noncerebral emboli lodge.
   B. It is important to differentiate between arterial thrombosis superimposed on atherosclerotic disease of the lower extremities and systemic embolization to the lower extremities.
   C. Embolic arterial occlusion to the lower extremities is rarely life threatening.
   D. The Fogarty catheter has markedly reduced the high mortality of patients who suffer embolization to the lower extremities.
   E. The limb salvage rate with or without embolectomy is poorly related to the severity of ischemia on presentation.

5. Select the best answer. Regarding the treatment for suspected systemic embolism:

   A. Intravenous heparin is contraindicated due to the need for operative intervention.
   B. For acute systemic embolism to the lower extremities, embolectomy represents initial therapy.
   C. Patients with systemic embolism are rarely subject to recurrent embolization.
   D. Chronic atrial fibrillation and acute myocardial infarction together account for less than 50 percent of all cases of systemic embolism.

41. Supraventricular Tachycardias

1. True or False. A supraventricular tachycardia cannot by definition have the atrioventricular (A-V) junction participate in generation of the arrhythmia.

2. True or False. The three general mechanisms that account for the generation of supraventricular tachyarrhythmias are increased automaticity, reentry, and suppression of triggered activity.

3. True or False. A telemetry reading is of no value in the diagnosis of a tachyarrhythmia. A 12-lead electrocardiogram (ECG) is the only way in which proper diagnosis can be made.

4. True or False. Treatment of a supraventricular tachycardia is geared toward treatment of the myocardial dysfunction.

5. Select the best answer. Regarding adenosine in the treatment of supraventricular tachycardias:

   A. Adenosine is an exogenous nucleoside that causes adenosine receptor stimulation with a resultant hyperpolarization of cells.
   B. Adenosine is given by slow intravenous infusion.
   C. Injection of adenosine results in symptoms of dyspnea, flushing, and chest discomfort felt to be mediated by hypersensitivity reaction.
   D. Adenosine has a rapid metabolism, and its effects resolve within several seconds.

6. Select the best answer. Regarding the use of cardiac glycosides (digoxin) in the treatment of supraventricular tachycardia:

   A. The mechanism of action is conduction slowing and increased refractoriness of SA and A-V nodes through hypersensitization of the carotid baroreceptor.
   B. Digoxin is administered by the intravenous route only. Its onset of action is usually within 10 minutes.
   C. Oral absorption is completely predictable.
   D. Digoxin is excreted primarily by the liver, and therefore the maintenance dose must be adjusted in patients with hepatic failure.

7. Select the best answer. Regarding digoxin toxicity:

   A. Digoxin toxicity is uncommon given its broad therapeutic window. Toxic levels of digoxin rarely lead to arrhythmias.
   B. If digoxin administration leads to an arrhythmia, it is a solitary type.
   C. The increased vagal tone from digoxin toxicity can produce sinus bradycardia or A-V block.
   D. The therapy for digoxin toxicity is immediate intravenous administration of digoxin-specific Fab antibody fragments.

8. Select the best answer. Regarding atrial fibrillation:

   A. Atrial fibrillation is a reentrant arrhythmia with multiple wavelets of depolarization traveling in random sequence.
   B. On electrocardiography, the atrial depolarizations are irregular and discharge at a rate of 130 to 150 beats per minute.
   C. The ventricular response is irregular, with a variable rate depending on the conduction time through the SA node.
   D. In untreated patients with normal A-V node function, the rate is usually 80 to 90 beats per minute.

9. Select the best answer. Regarding atrial fibrillation on clinical examination:

   A. The intensity of the peripheral pulse, although irregularly irregular, is constant.
   B. Physical examination should be directed at finding a possible cause such as valvular disease, pericardial friction rub, or hyperthyroidism.

C. Echocardiography is not helpful in new onset of atrial fibrillation and should be reserved for chronic atrial fibrillation to rule out thrombus.
D. Transthoracic echocardiography is superior to transesophageal echocardiography for visualization of intracardiac thrombi.

10. Select the best answer. Regarding atrial flutter:

A. Atrial flutter usually exists in patients without underlying structural heart disease.
B. Atrial flutter is an unstable rhythm.
C. The atrial conduction rate during flutter is usually the same as atrial fibrillation.
D. There is a lack of constancy to the conducted atrial beats.

11. True or False. Regarding the acute and chronic management of atrial fibrillation and atrial flutter, there is more of a risk of thromboembolism with atrial flutter than with atrial fibrillation.

Answers

Chapter 32

1. **True.** Mayer et al. reported data from an experimental model in a dog suggesting that stroke volume and coronary blood flow were maximized with chest compressions of moderate force and brief duration with an increase in the rate of compression to 150 per minute. The cardiac output continued to increase with increased rate.

2. **False.** The majority of infants and children who require resuscitation have had a primary respiratory arrest. Cardiac arrest results from the ensuing hypoxia and acidosis. The focus of pediatric resuscitation should therefore be airway maintenance and ventilation. In children, the cessation of cardiac activity is usually the manifestation of prolonged hypoxia.

3. **True.** The selection of proper energy levels for defibrillation in the intensive care unit setting lessens myocardial damage and the induction of arrhythmias that are brought about by an unnecessarily high delivery of energy. Furthermore, inadequate energies will not terminate an arrhythmia.

4. **D.** The gluconate salt is unstable. Administration of calcium may be by any of its three available salts: calcium chloride, calcium gluceptate, and calcium gluconate. The gluconate is unstable. Chloride salt provides the most direct source of calcium and produces the most rapid effect. The gluceptate and gluconate salts require hepatic degradation to release free calcium ion. Calcium chloride is highly irritating to the tissues and must be injected into a large vein.

Chapter 33

1. **True.** Angina pectoris is the most commonly encountered symptom associated with outflow obstruction. In the absence of epicardial coronary disease, myocardial ischemia is presumed to be due to exaggerated oxygen requirements caused by left ventricular hypertrophy.

2. **True.** The crescendo-decrescendo systolic ejection murmur is common to all forms of left ventricular outflow obstruction. This murmur is often accompanied by a palpable thrill. The intensity of the murmur is related poorly to the severity of stenosis. The duration of the murmur is a better index of severity of obstruction.

3. **False.** In most patients, the heart is not dilated, and the cardiothoracic ratio will be normal on a posteroanterior chest film (*See* Chest Roentgenogram.)

4. **C.** Cardiac catheterization is warranted in any patient suspected of having severe symptomatic aortic stenosis. Catheterization has two principal objectives: to corroborate Doppler findings and to define significant coronary artery stenosis. Coronary arteriography is mandatory prior to surgery in older individuals who have a high incidence of coronary artery disease. An accurate measure of cardiac output by either the Fick method or dye dilution technique should be performed with gradient measurement across a diseased valve. The cross-sectional valve area can then be estimated. A mean systolic gradient of 50 mm Hg or more is consistent with severe aortic stenosis. In such severe cases, the calculated valve area will usually be less than 0.8 cm^2. However, as cardiac output drops due to systolic pump dysfunction, mean systolic gradients less than 50 mm Hg can be recorded with critical stenosis.

Chapter 34

1. **True.** Acute pericarditis may be asymptomatic, but more often there is central chest pain, usually very sharp, often with a pleuritic component. There may be a sensation of pressure. The onset is often sudden and may interrupt sleep.

2. **True.** The pericardial rub or friction sound is pathognomonic in pericarditis. A fully developed rub has three components: an atrial rub, a ventricular systolic rub, and an early diastolic rub. The diastolic rub follows the second heart sound, is usually the faintest of the three components, and often is not audible. This accounts for the "to-and-fro" description of the pericardial friction rub.

3. **False.** There are four potential ECG stages.

   Stage I. An atypical ECG is diagnostic of pericarditis. Concave S–T segment changes are seen with elevation in most leads, particularly leads I, II, aVL, aVF, and V_3 through V_6.

   Stage II. This evolutionary stage shows all S–T junctions returning to baseline.

   Stage III. Widespread T wave inversions appear that are not distinguishable from those of diffuse myocardial injury or myocarditis.

   Stage IV. The T waves return to their prepericarditic condition. The entire ECG evolution occurs in days or weeks. Usually, transition from stage III is relatively slow, while stage I revolves into stage II relatively quickly. Some patients continue with some degree of T wave inversion for long periods of time.

4. **C.** The initial optimal treatment of pericarditis is to begin with ibuprofen, 600 mg PO q6h, which will often give relief of pain within 15 minutes to 2

hours. The dose can then be reduced to 400 mg or increased to 800 mg. Should this fail, aspirin or indomethacin may be used. Symptomatic pericarditis occasionally calls for drastic treatment, such as phenylbutazone. Corticosteroid therapy should be employed at the lowest effective dose only, with appropriate tapering, and should be avoided if at all possible because patients may become steroid dependent. Although pericardiectomy may be resorted to in an extreme case of treatment failure, it may not be successful in relieving pain and must be considered a final therapeutic maneuver.

5. **C.** The pericardium is a nondistensible membrane encircling the heart, wherein as little as 200 ml of fluid accumulation in an acute setting may cause hemodynamic collapse. Conversely, rather large effusions may not clinically embarrass the heart as long as the rate of exudation is slow enough to prevent the pericardium from stretching. The configuration of the cardiac silhouette cannot distinguish between cardiomegaly, large pericardial cyst, and pericardial effusions. This must be done by contrast x-ray, radioisotope scanning, computed tomography (CT scan), or most often, echocardiography. (*See* Cardiac Tamponade.)

6. **C.** In pericardiocentesis, the pericardiocentesis needle is inserted in the left xiphocostal angle perpendicular to the skin and the 0.5 to 1.0 cm below the costal margin. The hub of the needle is depressed, and the needle is advanced toward the left shoulder. If bloody fluid is withdrawn, it is important to know quickly whether the needle has penetrated the heart. A microhematocrit apparatus should be available. Furthermore, any blood drained should be observed for coagulation because intrapericardial blood will not clot because the mechanical action of the heart tends to defibrinate the blood. Echocardiography, especially two-dimensional, can also be used to monitor the needle and its progress, and under direct vision, the needle can be seen to enter the pericardial effusion and the efficacy of the aspiration documented directly. Failure of pericardiocentesis to deliver fluid does not rule out pericardial effusion or hemorrhage.

Chapter 35

1. **True.** Sudden cardiac death occurs in 400,000 patients per year in the United States, accounting for approximately 50 percent of all cardiovascular mortality. Sudden cardiac death is defined as loss of consciousness within 1 hour of the onset of symptoms in an individual who has known or unknown preexisting heart disease.

2. **True.** Cardiac causes of ventricular tachycardia and ventricular fibrillation in the absence of acute myocardial infarction include prior myocardial infarction and cardiomyopathies, including idiopathic dilated, valvular, hypertrophic, arrhythmogenic right ventricular dysplasia, congenital heart disease, and infiltrative diseases. Electrical disorders can also cause ventricular tachycardia and ventricular fibrillation and include long Q–T syndrome, preexcitation syndromes (e.g., Wolff-Parkinson-White), conduction disorders, and primary idiopathic ventricular fibrillation.

3. B. Recent data with the drug sotalol from the ESVEM Trial and amiodarone from other trials had suggested these drugs may prevent future arrhythmic events in patients with known ventricular arrhythmias. There are ongoing trials comparing amiodarone and implantable cardioverter-defibrillator devices for protection against sudden cardiac death in survivors of sudden cardiac death and in patients at risk for sudden cardiac death. Several noncontrolled, nonrandomized studies in patients who have received implantable devices appear to demonstrate that the devices can decrease the recurrence of sudden cardiac death to 1 percent or less per year. The overall approach to patients at risk or having sustained a sudden cardiac arrest can be divided into several phases:

a. Adequate prevention of coronary artery disease in those at high risk.
b. Early cardiopulmonary resuscitation and advanced cardiac life support on the scene.
c. Stabilization, appropriate individualized therapy, and evaluation of such therapy, which may involve anti-ischemic therapy, coronary artery bypass grafting, arrhythmia surgery, specific antiarrhythmic therapy, beta-blockers, and finally implantation of the implantable cardioconverter-defibrillator device.

Chapter 36

1. False. The severe chest pain associated with aortic dissection usually leads to a mistaken initial diagnosis of acute myocardial infarction. However, acute aortic dissection is much less common than acute myocardial infarction. Estimates indicate that 1 in 10,000 patients admitted to the hospital have aortic dissection.

2. True. It is generally accepted that the process of aortic dissection begins with an intimal tear, with most reported series of aortic dissection indicating that less than 5 percent of patients suffering from acute dissection do not have an identifiable intimal tear at autopsy.

3. True. Hypertension is by far the most important disease associated with development of aortic dissection. Clinical evidence or a history of hypertension was present in 92 percent of 463 autopsy cases reviewed in Hurst's classic article. After hypertension, congenitally malformed aortic valves are the most common pathologic state predisposing to aortic dissection. Other conditions associated with aortic dissection include Marfan's syndrome, Ehlers-Danlos syndrome, pregnancy, coarctation of the aorta, aortic stenosis, Turner's syndrome, and relapsing polychondritis.

4. False. The original classification of DeBakey that is still used divides aortic dissection into three types:

a. Type I dissection begins in the ascending aorta and extends distally to the arch and descending aorta.
b. Type II dissection begins in and is limited to the ascending aorta.
c. Type III dissection begins in and is limited to the descending aorta.

Daley et al. in 1970 changed the classification to involve those cases involving the ascending aorta (type A) and those in whom the dissection was limited to the descending aorta (type B). Dissection is considered acute if it is less than 2 weeks in duration or chronic if it is greater than 2 weeks.

5. **B.** The most common plain chest radiograph finding, seen in more than 80 percent of patients with aortic dissection, is widening of the superior mediastinum. This finding is nonspecific and may be seen in hypertension, aortic aneurysm, and aging. Electrocardiography is more useful in ruling out myocardial infarction in the setting of acute onset of chest pains. Echocardiography is especially useful if it is multiplane, transesophageal echocardiography, which allows for visualization of the ascending aorta, aortic arch, and descending aorta. Computed tomography can be useful, but its chief limitation would be an inability to visualize aortic valve disruption and aortic valvular insufficiency and an inability to adequately visualize the *ascending* aorta.

6. **A.** Untreated acute aortic dissection has an extremely rapid, usually fatal clinical course. In Jamieson's series, the time from presentation to death was less than 24 hours in 72 percent of untreated patients. In 1955, DeBakey published results of the first surgical correction of aortic dissection. Initial management of patients with suspected acute aortic dissection includes establishing venous access and continuous blood pressure monitoring. Despite adequate blood pressure lowering, nitroprusside increases myocardial contractility and thereby may *cause* progression of dissection. To avoid this, adequate beta-blockade is essential and should be initiated prior to infusing sodium nitroprusside. Intravenous propranolol, labetalol, or esmolol, due to its short half-life, may be administered to achieve beta-blockade. The goals of medical therapy are to stop the spread of intramural hematoma and to prevent rupture. Immediate surgery is recommended in all ascending aortic dissections in the absence of contraindications. Patients with uncomplicated dissection limited to the descending aorta should be managed with intensive parenteral drug therapy for 48 to 72 hours, after which they should be treated with an oral regimen or other antihypertensive medications. Even if asymptomatic, patients who develop evidence of expansion, complications, or continued dissection should immediately undergo surgery.

Chapter 37

1. **False.** Acute aortic insufficiency is usually the result of infective endocarditis, dissection of the ascending aorta, trauma, or spontaneous rupture of the valve itself.

2. **False.** Acute bacterial endocarditis is commonly the result of *S. aureus*. It often produces necrosis and perforation and/or detachment of one or more aortic valve leaflets. Infection of the aortic annulus with necrosis and abcess formation can cause weakening and progressive dilation of the aortic root so that the aortic valve leaflets fail to coapt properly during diastole. This leads to aortic insufficiency.

3. **True.** Large valvular vegetations may prevent proper diastolic coaptation of the aortic valve leaflets. Although present in staphylococcal endocarditis, such bulky vegetations are more characteristic of fungal endocarditis caused by aspergillosis, histoplasmosis, or other such fungal species.

4. **C.** Most commonly, acute endocarditis infections resulting in aortic insufficiency involve an anatomically bicuspid aortic valve. Acute endocarditis with an organism of sufficient severity to cause valve destruction can infect a previ-

ously normal valve. This is more common in narcotic addicts who use intravenous drugs. Usually there is no significant aortic stenosis or aortic insufficiency prior to the onset of infective endocarditis. Infective endocarditis resulting in acute severe aortic insufficiency may cause several life-threatening cardiac complications.

5. **C.** Patients with a congenitally bicuspid aortic valve are at an increased risk for aortic valve endocarditis. This bicuspid valve is associated with turbulent flow, and this may contribute to the increased incidence of endocarditis. The valve lesion is commonly asymptomatic and may escape detection into adulthood. The asymptomatic nature of a congenital bicuspid aortic valve means that antibiotic prophylaxis may not have been prescribed for dental or other procedures throughout the patient's life.

6. **B.** Hemodynamic findings associated with acute severe aortic insufficiency include slightly increased arterial pulse pressure, equilibration of left ventricular and aortic pressures, and marked elevation in left ventricular end-diastolic pressure. Other hemodynamic findings in aortic insufficiency are indicative of left ventricular failure. It is important to distinguish between acute and chronic aortic insufficiency.

Chapter 38

1. **False.** In the prethrombolytic era, life-threatening acute myocardial infarction with mitral regurgitation was estimated to occur in 1 percent of acute myocardial infarctions. More recently, an analysis at Duke University Medical Center of 1480 patients undergoing acute cardiac catheterization within 6 hours of myocardial infarction reported a 17.9 percent incidence of mitral regurgitation, with a 3.4 percent incidence of moderately severe or severe mitral regurgitation.

2. **True.** The presence of moderately severe or severe mitral regurgitation is associated with a higher mortality rate (24% at 30 days, 42% at 6 months, and 52% at 1 year). When the presence of mitral regurgitation is added to the regression model, it approaches statistical significance as an independent predictor of mortality following acute myocardial infarction.

3. **False.** The pathophysiology of papillary muscle rupture and mitral regurgitation depends on the amount of tissue infarcted. The papillary muscles are supplied by the most distal portions of the coronary arterial tree, and therefore they are vulnerable to transient ischemia and infarction as well as trauma and catastrophic acute coronary artery occlusion. Because the entire blood supply of the papillary musculature comes from the posterior descending artery, the posteromedial papillary muscle is more vulnerable to ischemia than the anterolateral papillary muscle. In a recent report by Sharma et al. of 50 consecutive patients presenting with severe ischemic mitral regurgitation, 14 of 15 patients requiring surgery for valve repair or replacement had pathologic documentation of posteromedial papillary muscle dysfunction. (*See* Anatomy.)

4. **A.** The mainstays of medical therapy in mitral regurgitation are vasodilating drugs and the intraaortic balloon pump. Afterload reducing agents such as nitroprusside, hydralazine, and angiotensin-converting enzyme inhibitors im-

prove hemodynamics in acute mitral regurgitation by lowering systemic vascular resistance and impedance to left ventricular ejection, with resultant decrease in left ventricular volume. These agents also decrease the size of the regurgitant mitral valve orifice. In cases of mitral regurgitation, systemic arterial pressures and pulmonary arterial pressures should be continuously monitored with an indwelling arterial catheter and pulmonary arterial catheter. In patients who have low systemic arterial pressures, the judicious use of inotropic agents such as dopamine or dobutamine can be useful. High-dose dopamine, however, carries the disadvantage of elevating systemic vascular resistance and may therefore increase mitral regurgitation and myocardial ischemia. Patients with low systemic arterial pressures are probably best managed with a combination of vasodilator drugs and intraaortic balloon pump therapy. (*See* Treatment.)

Chapter 39

1. **True.** Syncope can be classified into cardiovascular and noncardiovascular. Cardiovascular syncope accounts for 85 percent or more of cases of syncope. Cardiovascular syncope may further be divided into neurally mediated and neurally independent mechanisms.

2. **True.** Syncope due to obstructive disorders of the heart typically occurs during exercise. This is due to the fact that limited cardiac output is unable to meet the increased oxygen demand and overcome peripheral vasodilation. Syncope is one of the classic presenting signs of aortic stenosis and usually suggests that valve replacement is required due to critical reduction in valvular cross-sectional area.

3. **True.** Hypertrophic cardiomyopathy is a particularly important cause of syncope to consider. Its physical signs may be subtle, and the disorder frequently involves young patients and athletes. The work-up of syncope in a young patient is particularly important to consider, since many patients with hypertrophic cardiomyopathy and syncope have an increased risk of sudden death.

4. **B.** Pulmonary hypertension with acute arterial spasm and marked increase in left ventricular preload may lead to recurrent syncope and sudden death. Any form of tachycardia including sinus tachycardia can lead to a sudden fall in cardiac output. Pulmonary emboli can also present with syncope; however, in animal studies, it is found that over half of the pulmonary artery vasculature must be occluded to cause hemodynamic compromise. Acute myocardial ischemia can also present with syncope from various mechanisms such as global ischemia, ventricular arrhythmia, conduction system disease, or mechanical complication.

5. **A.** The sick sinus syndrome is characterized by impaired sinoatrial impulse formation or propagation manifesting as sinus pause or sinus arrest resulting in syncope. If this syndrome is accompanied by a supraventricular tachyarrhythmia, most commonly atrial fibrillation, the term *bradycardia-tachycardia syndrome* is used. Sinus node dysfunction is frequently unmasked by a relatively low concentration of drugs such as digoxin, beta-blockers, and calcium channel blockers. Essentially all patients with syncope secondary to sick sinus syndrome require a permanent pacemaker implantation. Some patients respond to the use of theophylline, which is an adenosine antagonist.

Chapter 40

1. **True.** Embolism to the systemic circulation nearly always originates as a thrombus within the left heart. In a large series in the literature of 1575 patients with systemic emboli, it was found that 89 percent of emboli originated as thrombi within the heart. Other sources include a diseased aorta, with or without aneurysm, and paradoxical venous source.

2. **False.** Systemic embolization may occur with its source in the venous circulation. This is termed paradoxical embolism. It may occur in patients with an intracardiac defect, such as an atrial or ventricular septal defect, patent ductus arteriosus, or pulmonary arteriovenous fistula. The vast majority of cases of paradoxical embolism occur in patients who have a patent foramen ovale.

3. **C.** Valvular heart disease is a common cause of systemic embolization. The three most frequent disorders that cause thrombi in the left heart that may predispose to systemic embolization are atrial fibrillation, coronary artery disease with infarction, and valvular heart disease including patients who have prosthetic heart valves. Of these disorders, atrial fibrillation is most commonly associated with systemic embolism. In patients with coronary artery disease and valvular heart disease, systemic embolization is most likely associated with atrial fibrillation.

4. **B.** The principal differential diagnosis of arterial embolism to the lower extremities is (a) arterial thrombosis superimposed on atherosclerotic disease and (b) arterial embolization. Of all arterial emboli that enter the circulation, the vast majority lodge in the lower extremities. Embolic occlusion of arteries in the lower extremities may lead to irreversible ischemia with tissue necrosis. This tissue necrosis can lead to acidosis, myonecrosis, hypokalemia, and possible renal failure. Embolectomy is performed by utilizing local anesthesia and the Fogarty thrombectomy catheter. The high mortality of patients who suffer emboli to the lower extremities and undergo embolectomy has not significantly changed since introduction of the Fogarty catheter in 1963. Although mortality is the same, the limb salvage rate with or without embolectomy is clearly related to the severity of ischemia on presentation. Thrombectomy may lead to the systemic release of toxic material from the involved limb on reperfusion if the degree of ischemia is irreversible.

5. **B.** Embolectomy is the initial treatment for suspected systemic embolization to the lower extremities. Once the diagnosis of systemic embolism is suspected, therapy with intravenous heparin should be initiated. Patients with systemic embolization are subject to recurrent embolism, with all series showing a low recurrence rate in patients who are anticoagulated. In the majority of patients, the underlying condition predisposing to systemic embolization will be evident on baseline evaluation. Chronic atrial fibrillation and acute myocardial infarction account for 70 to 80 percent of all cases of systemic embolism.

Chapter 41

1. **False.** A tachycardia is considered to be supraventricular in origin if the atrium or A-V junction participates in the arrhythmia either as the origin of the abnormal impulse or as an essential part of a reentry circuit.

2. **False.** There are three general mechanisms that account for the generation of supraventricular tachyarrhythmias. The first mechanism is increased automaticity. The sinus node is normally the dominant pacemaker because it has faster phase 4 depolarization than the other tissues of the heart. An increased automaticity tachyarrhythmia can be generated when another area of myocardium exhibits an enhanced rate of spontaneous depolarization. An example of this occurs in a patient with high catecholamine levels. This causes parts of the atrium other than the sinoatrial (SA) node to have a more rapid discharge rate than the SA node and allows that focus to become the dominant pacemaker.

   The second mechanism is reentry. In contrast to increased automaticity, there is no problem with impulse formation but rather a problem with abnormal conduction.

   The third mechanism is triggered activity. Triggered activity occurs as a result of a preceding impulse or series of impulses. This is in contrast to automaticity, which occurs spontaneously. The impulse that initiates triggered activity is an afterdepolarization and is classified as either early or late. An example of this is digoxin toxicity.

3. **False.** A direct recording of the arrhythmia is the most important initial information for diagnosis. In a patient who is hemodynamically stable, a 12-lead ECG is optimal. However, if the arrhythmia is of a transient nature, the patient is hemodynamically unstable, or the 12-lead ECG is not readily available, a telemetry tracing can be utilized to gather valuable information. The P waves can be identified, and their morphology, regularity, rate, and relationship to the QRS or ventricular depolarization should be noted. The size of the QRS complex is also suggested on telemetry.

4. **False.** The treatment of a supraventricular tachycardia is geared toward identifying and treating the underlying cause. In general, the primary treatment of arrhythmias produced by enhanced automaticity is to remove the stimulus or treat the underlying process. The ectopic automaticity can sometimes be diminished by agents which slow depolarization. Additionally, the ventricular rate can be controlled using agents to increase the degree of A-V block. Arrhythmias utilizing reentry circuits that involve the SA or A-V nodes may terminate in response to agents that change the refractoriness or slow conduction in these regions.

5. **D.** Adenosine is an *endogenous* nucleoside that causes adenosine receptor stimulation, which results in hyperpolarization of cells. It is administered for therapy of supraventricular tachycardias by intravenous bolus. The injection is often associated with symptoms of dyspnea and flushing. The symptom of chest discomfort is thought to be meditated by adenosine receptors. The symptoms last for 15 to 20 seconds, and the effect of the drug itself lasts for only seconds.

6. **A.** Cardiac glycosides have been used in the treatment of supraventricular tachycardias for many years. These drugs cause conduction slowing and increased refractoriness of the SA and A-V nodes mainly in an indirect fashion by hypersensitization of the carotid baroreceptors. Digoxin may be given orally or intravenously. Its onset of action after an intravenous dose is 30 minutes to 1 hour. It must be loaded regardless of route of administration. Digoxin is excreted primarily by the kidneys, and therefore the maintenance dose must be adjusted in patients with renal failure.

7. C. Digoxin toxicity is not uncommon because the drug has a narrow therapeutic window. Signs of toxicity include fatigue, nausea, visual disturbances, and confusion. Digoxin toxicity can also lead to multiple types of arrhythmia. They arise primarily from the increased vagal tone and can lead to sinus bradycardia or A-V block. This can lead to increased atrial and ventricular excitability, resulting in premature atrial and ventricular beats, ectopic atrial tachycardia, ventricular tachycardia, or ventricular fibrillation. Digoxin toxicity should be considered when a supraventricular tachycardia does not respond to increasing doses of digoxin. Therapy for a patient with digoxin toxicity depends on the arrhythmia and the underlying clinical condition. Often stopping the digitalis and correcting any underlying hypokalemia are sufficient treatment. A temporary pacemaker may be required, and digoxin-specific Fab antibody fragments can be used in life-threatening cases not responsive to conservative measures.

8. A. Atrial fibrillation is a reentrant arrhythmia with multiple wavelets of depolarization traveling in a random sequence. This results in disorganized atrial depolarization with ineffective atrial contraction. Electrographically, the atrial depolarizations are irregular at the rate of 400 to 600 beats per minute. The ventricular response is irregularly irregular, with a variable rate depending on conduction time through the A-V node. Usually in untreated patients, this rate is 120 to 180 beats per minute.

9. B. Physical examination in atrial fibrillation is directed at finding a possible cause of the atrial fibrillation such as murmurs indicative of valvular disease, a pericardial friction rub indicative of pericarditis, or signs of hyperthyroidism. The intensity of each peripheral pulse will vary, depending on ventricular filling time for the given beat. An echocardiogram should be performed on every patient with new onset of atrial fibrillation. Information on valvular function, left ventricular systolic and diastolic dysfunction, left atrial size, and presence or absence of thrombus can help guide treatment. Transesophageal echocardiography offers improved resolution and is superior to transthoracic echocardiography for visualization of chamber valves and atrial appendages. Thyroid function tests should also be performed. A sensitive thyroid stimulating hormone (TSH) assay is sufficient.

10. B. Atrial flutter is felt to be due to a reentry mechanism that occurs in patients with underlying structural heart disease in the setting of pulmonary embolism, pericarditis, ethanol abuse, or thyroid toxicosis. It is an unstable rhythm, reverting to sinus rhythm or degenerating into atrial fibrillation. The atrial rate during atrial flutter is 250 to 350 beats per minute. Usually a 2:1 block at the A-V node level results in a ventricular rate of 150 beats per minute. With a 2:1 A-V block, it can be difficult to distinguish atrial flutter from other regular narrow QRS complex supraventricular tachycardias. Vagal maneuvers or intravenous adenosine can be used to increase the degree of A-V block, thus unmasking the characteristic "sawtooth" flutter waves. They are normally inverted in the inferior leads on ECG.

11. False. Acute and chronic management strategies are similar in atrial flutter and atrial fibrillation except for the use of anticoagulation. Use of anticoagulation in atrial flutter is controversial. There is less of a risk of thromboembolism with atrial flutter than with atrial fibrillation.

III. Coronary Care

42. Acute Heart Failure

1. True or False. The mechanisms by which the heart may fail can be classified according to four categories: (1) Abnormalities of the heart valves, pericardium, endocardium, great vessels, and other structures; (2) Primary myocyte dysfunction; (3) Alterations in organization or signaling of cardioelectrical activity; and (4) Deranged response to sepsis and infection.

2. True or False. When confronted with cardiac failure, the body reacts through feedback compensatory responses occurring solely at the microscopic level.

3. True or False. On a cellular level, heart failure induces changes in energy production and utilization and in the structure and makeup of various cellular components as part of the compensatory mechanism.

4. True or False. The pulmonary artery catheter is no longer useful in the diagnosis of acute heart failure.

5. Select the best answer. Regarding computed tomography (CT scan):

   A. CT scan is limited by ineffective assessment of myocardial wall thickness.
   B. CT scan is effective in estimating left ventricular volumes and ejection fraction.
   C. CT scan is the most effective means of assessing myocardial perfusion.
   D. CT scan is effective and is more sensitive than other modalities in the assessment of aortic pathology, specifically proximal aortic dissection.

6. Select the best answer. Regarding magnetic resonance imaging (MRI):

   A. MRI is superior to all other modalities for diagnosis of myocardial pathology in areas of wall thickness, wall motion, regional perfusion, ejection fraction, and proximal coronary anatomy.
   B. The diagnosis of aortic dissection is more sensitive and specific when diagnosed by MRI than by CT scan.
   C. The main strength of MRI lies in areas other than the diagnosis of pericardial disease and effusion, cardiac masses, and aortic pathology.
   D. MRI has replaced other modalities in most medical centers for diagnosis of the etiology of acute cardiac failure.

7. Select the best answer. Regarding the management of hypertension:

   A. Systemic hypertension is a common disease in Western society and may be of primary or secondary form.

B. Hypertension places a pressure load on the right ventricle.
C. The increased wall stress in the right ventricle lowers myocardial oxygen requirements (MVO_2) and may perpetuate left ventricular dysfunction due to this lowered oxygen demand.
D. The magnitude of hypertension required to precipitate acute heart failure depends on the patient's cardiac function under stress.

8. Select the best answer. Regarding dysfunction of a prosthetic aortic valve:

A. In the intensive care unit, the syndrome of thrombosed prosthetic aortic valve with thromboemboli is relatively common.
B. Patients with dysfunction of a prosthetic aortic valve will present with chronic heart failure that has been present in progressive fashion over several months.
C. The diagnosis should be confirmed by arteriography.
D. When the diagnosis is made, immediate surgical repair is indicated.

9. Select the best answer. Regarding the diagnosis of pericardial tamponade:

A. The diagnosis of pericardial tamponade cannot be inferred through the history.
B. The diagnosis of pericardial tamponade should be suspected in patients who exhibit a physical examination consistent with increased blood pressure, bradycardia, pulsus paradoxus, jugular venous distention, and muffled heart sounds.
C. In pericardial tamponade, the chest x-ray classically shows an enlarged cardiac silhouette.
D. In pericardial tamponade, the electrocardiogram may demonstrate sinus bradycardia or atrial fibrillation with a slow ventricular response, increased voltage, or electrical alternans.
E. Echocardiography is only occasionally useful in the diagnosis and treatment of pericardial tamponade.

43. *Thrombotic Disorders of the Arterial and Venous Circulatory Systems*

1. Select the best answer. Regarding vascular thromboresistance:

A. The vascular endothelium is a bilayer of simple squamous cells approximately 0.5 mm in thickness that are joined by intercellular junctions.
B. Vascular endothelial cells are polygonal and are elongated in the long axis of the vessel (in the direction of blood flow).
C. The endothelium has four surfaces: the luminal or nonthrombogenic, subluminal, adhesive, and cohesive.
D. The luminal surface under normal circumstances is entirely nonthrombogenic due to its abundant electron-dense connective tissue.

2. True or False. Distal arterial embolization to the lower extremity, which occurs in approximately 1 million individuals yearly in the United States, is the most common arterial thrombotic event in clinical practice.

3. True or False. Hard collagenous material determines an arterial plaque's vulnerability to rupture.

4. True or False. The term *non-Q wave myocardial infarction* is reserved for those myocardial infarctions involving small portions of the left ventricle.

5. Select the best answer. Regarding heparin:

A. Heparin was discovered by McClain in 1816.
B. In 1939, Brinkhouse observed that the anticoagulant activity of heparin required a plasma cofactor.
C. Heparin accelerates the promotive activity between antithrombin III and several coagulation proteins including thrombin, factor XII, factor XI, factor X, and factor IX.
D. The inhibition of thrombin requires that thrombin binds to heparin alone.

6. Select the best answer. Regarding heparin:

A. Commercial heparin preparations are homogenous, with a molecular weight of 30,000 daltons.
B. Seventy percent of the heparin molecules bind to antithrombin III.
C. After intravenous injection, there is a rapid elimination phase followed by a more gradual disappearance, which is a combination of zero-order and first-order kinetics.
D. Heparin binds irreversibly to vascular endothelial cells.

7. Select the best answer. Regarding heparin clinicopharmacokinetics and pharmacodynamics:

A. The half-life of injected heparin is constant at 90 minutes.
B. Intravenous nitroglycerin given in high doses increases the anticoagulant activity of heparin.
C. The most common adverse effect of heparin is hemorrhage.
D. Other adverse effects associated with heparin use include thrombocytosis.

8. Select the best answer. Regarding low-molecular-weight heparin:

A. Low-molecular-weight heparin varies from 3200 to 6500 daltons in size.
B. Low-molecular-weight heparin is not related to standard heparin.
C. Low-molecular-weight heparin requires twice daily dosing.
D. The administration of low-molecular-weight heparin, although causing less incidence of thrombocytopenia, has a higher incidence of hemorrhagic complications compared with standard heparin fraction.

9. True or False. Hirudin is an anticoagulant derived from leech head extracts and is the most potent and specific thrombin inhibitor known.

10. Select the best answer. Regarding warfarin:

A. The activities of warfarin have been known for 150 years since its synthesis in 1839.
B. Warfarin is an oral anticoagulant preventing the synthesis of functional vitamin K–dependent coagulation factors.
C. Warfarin is fat soluble and is slowly, although predictably, absorbed from the gastrointestinal tract after oral administration.
D. The average half-life of warfarin and its racemic mixture is 72 hours.

11. True or False. Anticoagulant therapy with heparin can be interrupted for a surgical procedure. Heparin should be restarted 6 to 8 hours after the surgical procedure to allow for primary hemostasis.

12. Select the best answer. Regarding the complication of hemorrhage in the setting of anticoagulation:

A. For patients receiving warfarin, the international normalized ratio (INR) should be monitored, whereas patients receiving heparin should have the aPTT checked.
B. The platelet count should be checked at least once weekly in patients who are on intravenous heparin.
C. For hemorrhage in the setting of oral anticoagulation with warfarin, administration of vitamin K, 1 mg IV or 10 mg SQ, can reduce the INR within 4 hours.
D. Larger doses of vitamin K of 10 mg IV do not reduce the time to reversal of the INR.

44. Unstable Angina

1. True or False. Unstable angina is caused by thrombus formation on a complicated atherosclerotic plaque.

2. True or False. Unstable angina is classified as new onset or crescendo angina when chest pain occurs at rest or at a progressively lower threshold of exercise or when prolonged chest pain is poorly relieved with nitroglycerin.

3. Select the best answer. Regarding the differential diagnosis of chest pain:

A. Chest pain of cardiac origin should be considered after all other possible sources of pain have been considered and ruled out.
B. Chest pain from different causes may coexist in the same patient.
C. Noncardiac pain is most often pulmonary in origin.
D. The differential diagnosis for esophageal spasm is straightforward.

4. Select the best answer. Regarding the laboratory diagnosis of unstable angina:

A. Electrocardiography obtained during an episode of chest pain is less informative than an electrocardiogram obtained at rest.
B. Deep T wave inversions occurring during an episode of angina involving the anterior and lateral leads are characteristic of significant narrowing in the proximal right coronary artery.
C. Myocardial scintigraphy obtained during an episode of chest pain can detect transient myocardial ischemia.
D. Echocardiographic imaging should not be used during an episode of myocardial ischemia.

5. Select the best answer. Regarding thrombolytic therapy in unstable angina and myocardial infarction:

A. Clinical benefits of thrombolytic therapy have been well documented in the three largest trials completed to date.
B. Subset analysis of patients with non-Q wave myocardial infarction in the TIMI-3B and ISIS-2 trials as well as the GISSI-1 trial has not even documented a trend toward benefit.
C. The goal of treatment in Q wave myocardial infarction is to open the artery in question.

D. In unstable angina and non-Q wave myocardial infarction, the goal of therapy is to stent the occluded artery open to improve blood flow.

45. Complicated Myocardial Infarction

1. True or False. Following acute myocardial infarction (MI), a major cause of morbidity and mortality is recurrent ischemia and recurrent ischemic events.

2. True or False. Effective prevention of recurrent ischemic events has been shown to consist of three components: antiplatelet therapy, antithrombotic therapy, and beta-blockade.

3. True or False. The general protective measures used for treatment during recurrent ischemia consist of controlling heart rate, preventing coronary artery vasoconstriction and thrombosis, and ameliorating chest pain.

4. True or False. Patients who have Q-waves on ECG have been found to have similar peak enzyme levels and similar ejection fractions when compared to patients who do not have Q waves on ECG after MI.

5. Select the best answer. Regarding right ventricular infarctions:

A. The treatment of right ventricular MI is the same as the treatment for left ventricular MI.
B. The coincidence of right ventricular infarction in patients who suffer an inferior wall MI is low.
C. The simplest test to determine the presence of a right ventricular infarction is echocardiography.
D. The differential diagnosis for right ventricular infarction includes hypotension due to left ventricular infarction, pericardial tamponade, constrictive pericarditis, and pulmonary embolism.

6. Select the best answer. Regarding clinical manifestations and complications of right ventricular infarction:

A. Systemic hypotension is a frequent complication of right ventricular infarction.
B. The incidence of atrioventricular or sinoatrial nodal block is less than with left ventricular infarction.
C. The incidence of cardiogenic shock is considerably less than with left ventricular infarction.
D. The prognosis with right ventricular infarction is considerably better than with isolated left ventricular infarction.

7. Select the best answer. Regarding the management of patients with right ventricular infarction:

A. Initial management should include measures to decrease forward output of the right ventricle.
B. Volume limitation is the mainstay of therapy.
C. Dobutamine or dopamine should be utilized to increase right ventricular output.
D. Venous dilators such as nitrates should be utilized.

8. Select the best answer. Regarding left ventricular dysfunction:

A. The severity of MI relates directly to the area of myocardium that is damaged.
B. The most important determinant of prognosis after MI is the degree of left ventricular dysfunction.
C. Left ventricular function prior to acute MI is an insignificant determinant of prognosis.
D. After MI, presence of creatine kinase isoenzymes, presence or absence of Q waves on the ECG, and location of myocardial infarction do not have an ability to predict outcome.

9. Select the best answer. Regarding diastolic dysfunction:

A. Diastolic dysfunction occurs almost uniformly in patients with acute MI.
B. Diastolic dysfunction is a common cause of late congestive heart failure in the setting of MI.
C. The pathophysiology of diastolic dysfunction begins with increased myocardial wall compliance from ischemia and infarction.
D. The heart sound associated with diastolic dysfunction is usually an S_3.

10. Select the best answer. Regarding the treatment of diastolic dysfunction:

A. The use of diuretics in the treatment of diastolic dysfunction is contraindicated.
B. Intravenous nitroglycerin and nitroprusside are contraindicated.
C. Administration of a beta-blocker is contraindicated.
D. Prognosis with diastolic dysfunction is good when compared to patients with systolic dysfunction.

11. Select the best answer. Regarding cardiogenic shock:

A. Congestive heart failure from systolic dysfunction is the most serious complication following an acute MI.
B. Cardiogenic shock is related to diastolic dysfunction.
C. Afterload reduction is contraindicated in systolic dysfunction and cardiogenic shock.
D. Cyclic adenosine monophosphate agents are contraindicated in the treatment of cardiogenic shock.

12. Select the best answer. Regarding myocardial infarction:

A. Rupture of papillary muscles is common after acute MI.
B. Ventricular septal rupture occurring in the setting of a new inferior MI is associated with a mortality of approximately 20 percent.
C. The development of thromboembolism can occur in 5 to 10 percent of patients after acute MI.
D. The occurrence of pericardial irritation occurs in approximately 40 percent of patients with acute MI.

13. Select the best answer. Regarding supraventricular tachyarrhythmias during acute MI:

A. Supraventricular arrhythmias complicating MI are associated with decreased sympathetic tone.
B. Sinus tachycardia increases myocardial oxygen demand and can lead to infarct extension.

C. Atrial fibrillation and atrial flutter occur in 39 percent of patients with acute MI.
D. Regular narrow-complex paroxysmal supraventricular tachycardia occurs frequently during acute MI.

14. Select the best answer. Regarding intraventricular conduction blocks:

A. The blood supply to the distal conducting system makes conduction disturbances an infrequent complication of anterior wall MI.
B. Intraventricular conduction disturbances carry a low in-hospital mortality if recognized early.
C. Beta-blockade should be administered in high-risk patients with intraventricular conduction block pending placement of a temporary pacemaker.
D. Patients with a permanent bundle branch block and transient Mobitz II second-degree atrioventricular block may benefit from permanent pacemaker implantation.

46. Thrombolytic Therapy: A Coronary Care Unit Perspective

1. True or False. Thrombolytic therapy in the treatment of acute myocardial infarction has not been shown to reduce mortality.

2. True or False. Thrombolytic therapy in the setting of acute myocardial infarction is associated with improved left ventricular function.

3. True or False. Angiographic studies indicate that occluded coronary arteries may spontaneously reperfuse in a relatively small proportion of patients after acute myocardial infarction.

4. True or False. The major complication associated with the use of thrombolytic therapy is bleeding.

5. True or False. The recently completed GUSTO trial vindicated the open artery hypothesis.

6. True or False. The GUSTO trial established that salvage or rescue percutaneous transluminal coronary angioplasty (PTCA) is indicated as a mechanical method to achieve coronary reperfusion.

7. True or False. Patients presenting within the first 12 hours of symptom onset should be treated with thrombolytic therapy.

8. Select the best answer. Regarding contraindications for thrombolytic therapy:

A. Hypertension is not a contraindication to thrombolytic therapy.
B. Pregnancy is a contraindication to thrombolytic therapy.
C. Recent surgery or trauma is not a contraindication to thrombolytic therapy.
D. Reports indicate no increased rate of intracranial bleeding in patients with a history of hypertension or poorly controlled blood pressure when given thrombolytic therapy.

47. Secondary Prevention After Acute Myocardial Infarction: A Coronary Care Unit Perspective

1. True or False. Admission to a coronary care unit offers a unique opportunity to assist patients with smoking cessation, with higher success rates than with outpatients.

2. True or False. Magnesium and calcium have a synergistic effect at the cellular level and cause both systemic and coronary vasodilation.

3. True or False. One of the most powerful predictors of death after myocardial infarction is the extent of left ventricular systolic dysfunction.

4. True or False. Angiotensin-converting enzyme (ACE) inhibitors are preferred in the early postmyocardial infarction period as effective intervention.

5. True or False. Nitrates have hemodynamic and antiplatelet effects.

6. Select the best answer. Regarding calcium channel blockers:

   A. Nifedipine and the dihydropyridines have been shown to have consistent benefit in an acute or threatened myocardial infarction.
   B. Verapamil and diltiazem are considered to have adverse effects based on their potent peripheral vasodilatory properties.
   C. Verapamil and diltiazem have a more profound negative inotropic effect than the dihydropyridines.
   D. The benefit of administration of calcium channel blockers after MI is best seen in patients with A-V block.

48. Diagnostic Testing in the Coronary Care Unit

1. True or False. Electrocardiogram (ECG) changes of 1 mm or greater S–T segment elevation in a single lead establish the diagnosis of acute myocardial infarction.

2. True or False. The normal pericardium is evident on plain chest radiographs.

3. True or False. Thallium stress test imaging is useful for diagnosis but is of no utility in predicting morbidity in a preoperative setting.

4. Select the best answer. Regarding cardiac performance:

   A. Left ventricular ejection fraction is the only measurement radionuclide techniques are capable of performing.
   B. First-pass radionuclide studies measure the initial transit of radiotracer through the heart.

C. Equilibrium studies such as radionuclide ventriculogram or radionuclide angiogram relay on counts of tracer present within the ventricles during multiple cardiac cycles.
D. Right ventricular function is the most important noninvasive predictor of reinfarction and sudden death following myocardial infarction.
E. Ejection fraction is determined by dividing the difference in count rates at end systole and end diastole by the count rate at end systole.

49. Clinical Management of Cardiac Arrhythmias in the Coronary Care Unit

1. True or False. Impulse propagation within myocardial tissue is related to the axial and transverse resistances that are determined by the degree of intercellular coupling.

2. True or False. In the first 48 hours after myocardial infarction, the incidence of ventricular arrhythmias ranges from 10 to 12 percent.

3. Select the best answer. Regarding ventricular tachycardia:

A. Ventricular tachycardia is defined as six or more consecutive ventricular depolarizations at a rate of greater than 100 beats per minute.
B. Sustained ventricular tachycardia lasts for more than 30 seconds.
C. Unsustained ventricular tachycardia lasts from 3 beats to less than 30 seconds and terminates with treatment.
D. Ventricular tachycardia can be described as uniform or polymorphic.

4. Select the best answer. Regarding supraventricular tachycardias:

A. Persistent sinus tachycardia may suggest ischemia, heart failure, or hypotension.
B. Beta-blockade should be undertaken in all patients who suffer from an episode of supraventricular tachycardias.
C. The most frequently seen supraventricular tachycardia associated with unstable coronary syndromes is sinus tachycardia.
D. Atrial fibrillation and atrial flutter are infrequently seen in critical care unit patients.

5. Select the best answer. Regarding the management of tachyarrhythmias:

A. Supraventricular and ventricular tachyarrhythmias show the same basic physiologic mechanism and therefore have a common treatment pattern.
B. Supraventricular tachycardias are usually associated with hemodynamic compromise.
C. Ventricular tachyarrhythmias are frequently associated with hemodynamic compromise.
D. The diagnosis of supraventricular tachycardia usually shows a QRS complex that is distinct from the sinus rhythm.

50. *Mechanisms of Acute Myocardial Ischemia and Infarction*

1. True or False. With increasing myocardial oxygen demands, oxygen extraction and coronary blood flow can increase by levels of three- to fourfold.

2. True or False. Coronary arterial blood flow is determined by the pressure gradient between the aorta in diastole and the coronary sinus.

3. True or False. There is no known interaction between coronary artery thrombosis and coronary artery spasm.

4. True or False. Penetrating and blunt trauma can each cause myocardial infarction.

51. *Nonischemic Chest Pain*

1. True or False. In studies of acute myocardial infarction, the electrocardiogram (ECG) usually shows S–T segment and Q wave changes.

2. From the following, select potential noncardiac causes of chest pain:

A. Pulmonary hypertension.
B. Pneumonia.
C. Pneumothorax.
D. Herpes zoster.
E. All of the above.

52. *Evaluation and Management of Hypertension in the Intensive Care Unit*

1. True or False. The management of hypertension in the intensive care unit (ICU) setting usually involves one of four situations: hypertensive emergencies, chronic hypertension, new onset of hypertension, and hypertension unique to the perioperative setting.

2. True or False. The differentiation between hypertensive emergencies and urgencies is made on the basis of mean arterial pressure.

3. True or False. The treatment of malignant hypertension or emergent hypertension in the ICU setting should involve initiation of treatment prior to diagnosis of the underlying cause.

4. Select the best answer. Regarding the treatment of hypertensive crisis:

A. The goal of initial therapy is to return blood pressure to normal levels.

B. The lower limit of cerebral autoregulation will determine target therapies.
C. A reasonable target for blood pressure reduction is to decrease systolic blood pressure by 50 percent, taking into consideration the patient's medical history.
D. In most patients with hypertensive emergencies, the pathophysiologic abnormality is a decrease in systemic vascular resistance.

5. Select the best answer. Regarding therapy of chronic hypertension:

A. Rebound hypertension represents a sensitization to baseline levels of catecholamine secretion.
B. Adrenergic inhibitors such as beta-blockers and central agonists such as clonidine are commonly described in conjunction with rebound hypertension.
C. The likelihood of rebound hypertension is not linked to the previous dose of medication.
D. Patients with decreased adrenergic activity are at great risk for rebound hypertension.

6. Select the best answer. Regarding perioperative hypertension:

A. In the setting of postoperative care, blood pressure above 160/100 mm Hg in a previously normotensive patient or an increase of more than 30 mm Hg over preoperative levels requires treatment.
B. About 50 percent of patients with preoperative diagnosis of hypertension will have worsening perioperative blood pressure control.
C. Routine blood pressure therapy should be discontinued on the morning of surgery.
D. Oral therapy is indicated for control of perioperative hypertension.

7. Select the best answer. Regarding labetalol:

A. Labetalol is a racemic mixture of a selective beta-blocker and a selective alpha$_1$-antagonist.
B. Labetalol produces prompt reduction in peripheral vascular resistance and blood pressure.
C. Myocardial oxygen consumption is increased and coronary hemodynamics are improved in patients with coronary disease.
D. The side effects of labetalol administration are related to beta-blockade effects and are manifested by orthostatic hypotension.

8. True or False. Metabolism of nicardipine is by renal excretion of its active metabolites.

Answers

Chapter 42

1. False. There are several mechanisms by which the heart may fail. Heart failure is classified into acute and chronic categories. Acute heart failure is a more dramatic decompensation. Chronic heart failure allows for adaptation. There are three classifications by which the heart may fail:

A. Abnormalities of the heart valves, pericardium, endocardium, great vessels, and other structures that impair cardiac filling and emptying.
B. Pathologic situations of primary myocyte dysfunction.

C. Alterations in the organization or signaling of cardiac contraction (dysrhythmias).

2. **False.** As with any insult, when confronted with cardiac failure, the body reacts through programmed compensatory responses. These responses occur at both macroscopic and microscopic levels and vary according to the type, severity, and duration of the insult.

3. **True.** On a cellular level, heart failure induces changes in energy production and utilization and in the structure and makeup of various cellular components. One variable determining these responses is the duration of the insult. Chronic heart failure is associated with an increase in mitochondrial mass and increased respiratory activity. Alterations in calcium homeostasis, alteration in regulatory G proteins, and downregulation of adrenergic receptors are also seen in chronic heart failure. The extent of these alterations in *acute* heart failure is not known.

4. **False.** The pulmonary artery catheter is useful in the diagnosis of cardiac tamponade, pericardial constriction, left-to-right shunting, noncardiogenic shock, or noncardiogenic pulmonary edema and cardiogenic shock due to severe left ventricular dysfunction. The hemodynamic monitoring offered by pulmonary artery catheter is useful in four general categories:

   A. When the diagnosis of cardiogenic versus noncardiogenic pulmonary edema is unclear.
   B. In instances where knowledge of the patient's intravascular volume status is critical but not discernible by noninvasive means.
   C. For diagnostic purposes in cases of acute cardiac failure.
   D. To assess therapeutic efficacy of vasopressor therapy.

5. **D.** Computed tomography, including ultrafast CT and gated CT as well as cine CT, has been studied to determine its usefulness in cardiac diagnostics. Although effective in assessment of wall thickness, myocardial mass, left ventricular volumes, and ejection fraction, other tests are superior in these areas of diagnostics. In the setting of acute heart failure, the only valid indication for CT scan is assessment of acute aortic pathology, most specifically proximal aortic dissection.

6. **B.** MRI is rapidly evolving as an important tool for the diagnosis of cardiac pathology. Although wall thickness, wall motion, regional perfusion, ejection fraction, and proximal coronary anatomy can be assessed by MRI, other modalities are superior. Currently, the major indications for MRI are for the diagnosis of pericardial disease and effusion, cardiac masses, and aortic pathology. In a clinical situation of acute heart failure, MRI is felt to be superior to CT scan for the diagnosis of aortic dissection and for demonstration of an intraluminal aortic flap. Limitation of MRI as a diagnostic modality is related to the contraindication to magnetic objects. Thus, any patient with a metallic prosthesis, imbedded metallic foreign body, or intravenous infusion pumps cannot undergo MRI testing.

7. **A.** Systemic hypertension is a common disease in Western society and may be of primary or secondary form. Hypertension places a pressure load on the left ventricle, and when a mismatch occurs between the pressure load and developed wall stress, cardiac output may decrease. With this decrease, there is an increase in wall tension, and elevated left heart pressure and pulmonary edema may ensue. Most importantly, increased wall stress raises myocardial oxygen

requirements (MVO_2) and may perpetuate left ventricular dysfunction. Left ventricular dysfunction secondary to hypertension is more common in patients with decreased contractile or ischemic cardiac reserve. Therefore, the magnitude of hypertension required to precipitate acute heart failure depends on a patient's baseline cardiac function.

8. **D.** The syndrome of a thrombosed prosthetic aortic valve is very rare ($<$ 0.5% in 100 patient-years) and is nearly always associated with mechanical valves and suboptimal systemic anticoagulation. Patients present with acute heart failure and syncope as well as altered prosthetic heart sounds. The diagnosis should be immediately suspected and confirmed by an echocardiogram. Immediate surgical therapy is indicated.

9. **B.** The diagnosis of pericardial tamponade should be suspected by the history and is supported by the findings of decreased blood pressure, tachycardia, pulsus paradoxus, jugular venous distention, muffled heart sounds, and a chest x-ray showing an enlarged cardiac silhouette. Electrocardiography is useful for diagnosis and treatment of pericardial tamponade and may demonstrate sinus tachycardia or atrial fibrillation with rapid ventricular response, low voltage, or electrical alternans. Echocardiography is mandatory for diagnosis and treatment of pericardial tamponade. It must be emphasized that the diagnosis of pericardial tamponade is a clinical diagnosis. Rapid diagnosis and therapeutic pericardiocentesis are mandatory.

Chapter 43

1. **B.** The vascular endothelium is essential for normal vessel responsiveness and thromboresistance. In most vertebrates, vascular endothelial cells form a single layer, with the cells 0.1 to 0.5 mm in thickness. The cells are polygonal and are elongated in the long axis of the vessel in the direction of blood flow. The endothelial layer has three surfaces: nonthrombogenic or luminal, adhesive or subluminal, and cohesive or abluminal. The luminal surface is nonthrombogenic due to its being devoid of electron-dense connective tissue. (*See* Vascular Thromboresistance.)

2. **False.** Myocardial infarction (MI) occurs in 1.25 million individuals yearly in the United States. This is the most commonly observed arterial thrombotic event in clinical practice.

3. **False.** Although dense collagenous sclerosis contributes a voluminous amount to a coronary arterial plaque, the lipid-rich component or atheromatous portion determines a plaque's vulnerability to rupture. (*See* Vascular Thrombosis.)

4. **False.** *Non-Q wave myocardial infarction* is the term that is utilized for myocardial infarctions that have no Q waves on electrocardiogram. This finding is associated with *nontransmural* myocardial infarction. (*See* Pathology of Thrombotic Events.)

5. **B.** Heparin is the mostly widely tested and clinically used anticoagulant. It is an acidic mucopolysaccharide discovered by McClain in 1916. In 1939, Brinkhouse observed that the anticoagulant activity of heparin required a plasma cofactor, later given the name antithrombin III. Heparin accelerates an inhibitory interaction between antithrombin III and several coagulation proteins in-

cluding thrombin, factor XII, factor XI, factor X, and factor IX. Inhibition of thrombin requires both antithrombin III and the enzyme thrombin itself to bind the heparin. In contrast, inhibition of factor X_a requires only that heparin bind antithrombin III.

6. **C.** The pharmacokinetics of heparin are complex. After intravenous injection, there is a rapid elimination phase followed by a more gradual disappearance, which is best explained by a combination of zero-order and first-order kinetics. Commercial heparin preparations are *heterogenous*, with molecular weights ranging from 3000 to 30,000 daltons. One-third of heparin molecules bind to antithrombin III. The remainder are essentially inactive. Heparin binds *reversibly* to vascular endothelial cells.

7. **C.** The most common complication of heparin administration is hemorrhage. The incidence of hemorrhage is influenced by total dose, anticoagulant response, method of administration, and patient-related factors including age and body weight. The anticoagulant response increases disproportionately in both intensity and duration with increasing dose. The half-life varies from 30 minutes following a 2000-unit bolus injection to 120 minutes following a 15,000-unit bolus injection. Intravenous nitroglycerin given in high doses can decrease the anticoagulant activity of heparin. Other adverse side effects associated with heparin use include thrombocytopenia with or without thrombosis.

8. **A.** Low-molecular-weight heparin is prepared from standard heparin by fractionation, enzymatic degradation, or chemical modification. Its mean molecular weight varies from 3200 to 6500 daltons. It contains high antifactor X_a activity and lower antithrombin activity. As a result, both the intrinsic and extrinsic coagulation pathways are inhibited. Low-molecular-weight heparin is almost completely absorbed following subcutaneous administration, allowing for once a day dosing without monitoring of prothrombin or partial thromboplastin times. Initial reports suggested less of an incidence of bleeding complications. Currently, low-molecular-weight heparin is felt to be at least as safe and effective as standard or unfractionated heparin and is more convenient from its once a day dosing standpoint, subcutaneous administration, and lack of need for monitoring of coagulation profile.

9. **True.** Hirudin is derived from leech head extracts. The active agent was isolated in the 1950s. Hirudin is from the leech *Hirudo medicinalis* and is the most potent and specific thrombin inhibitor known. It is a single peptide of 65 amino acid residues and does not require antithrombin III to exert its anticoagulant effects. There are two specific binding sites, and comprehensive experimental studies including the TIMI V, TIMI IX, and GUSTO II trials utilized this agent in myocardial infarction.

10. **B.** In 1939, warfarin was synthesized by Dr. Kyle Paul Link, who was investigating a rare hemorrhagic disease in cattle caused by spoiled sweet cloves. Vitamin K is an essential cofactor for the carboxylation of coagulation factors II, VII, IX, and X, enabling them to bind negatively charged phospholipid surfaces in the presence of calcium. Warfarin inhibits this critical step. Warfarin is highly water soluble and is rapidly absorbed from the gastrointestinal tract after oral administration, with peak absorption occurring in 60 to 90 minutes. The average half-life of warfarin in its racemic mixture is 35 to 40 hours.

11. **False.** Among patients in an intensive care unit receiving intravenous heparin, the interruption of heparin may be necessary for procedures. Intravenous heparin can be discontinued 2 to 4 hours before the scheduled procedure and then can be restarted postoperatively when hemostasis has been achieved. Often heparin can be restarted without a bolus at a relatively low infusion rate of 400 to 500 units per hour to maintain the activated partial thromboplastin time (aPTT) at the upper limits of normal. The infusion is then increased when clinically feasible. Patients at high risk for thromboembolism present a clinical challenge, where in most instances heparin is not interrupted.

12. **A.** For patients receiving heparin, the aPTT should be monitored, while the INR should be monitored for patients on warfarin. The platelet count should be assessed daily in patients on heparin. When a patient is on heparin and bleeding is noted, the site of bleeding must be identified and appropriate measures taken. This may include simply observing while continuing antithrombotic therapy, it may involve stopping the heparin infusion, or neutralizing residual heparin with protamine sulfate may be required. The anticoagulation effect of warfarin can be reversed by replacing vitamin K–dependent coagulation factors. Administration of vitamin K, 0.5 to 1 mg IV or 10 mg SQ, can reduce the INR within 12 to 24 hours. A larger dose of 10 mg IV can reduce the INR within 6 hours. Caution is recommended with high dose of intravenous vitamin K. More rapid reversal can be achieved with fresh frozen plasma administration.

Chapter 44

1. **True.** Unstable angina is a well-defined clinical entity with specific causes, pathophysiologic mechanisms, symptoms, laboratory findings, and treatment. In the mid-1980s, thrombus formation on a complicated atherosclerotic plaque was recognized as the cause of unstable angina.

2. **True.** The essential diagnostic feature of unstable angina is recognition that the symptoms are becoming more severe and departing from the usual pattern of angina for a given patient. Unstable angina is routinely classified as new onset or crescendo angina with chest pain occurring at rest or at a progressively lower threshold of exercise or prolonged chest pain poorly relieved with nitroglycerin. (*See* Diagnosis.)

3. **B.** Pain of cardiac origin must first be suspected and differentiated from noncardiac pain. Noncardiac pain may be of various causes, and these different causes may coexist in the same patient. Most often noncardiac pain is of musculosketetal origin, but it can also be from pulmonary or esophageal sources. The differential diagnosis for esophageal type pain is difficult, as is the differentiation between symptoms of gastroesophageal reflux and cardiac pain. (*See* Differential Diagnosis.)

4. **C.** Myocardial scintigraphy obtained during an episode of chest pain can detect transient myocardial ischemia with high sensitivity. However, the electrocardiogram remains the most useful tool for documentation of myocardial ischemia due to its availability in all medical centers and its relative sensitivity. The presence of ST–T wave changes on an admission electrocardiogram aids in the diagnosis of unstable angina. However, an electrocardiogram obtained during an episode of chest pain is far more informative. The ST–T changes can be

used to evaluate the location and severity of the ischemic process. Deep T wave inversions involving the anterior and lateral leads are characteristic of significant narrowing in the proximal left anterior descending coronary artery. Echocardiography can be useful in documenting the presence of transient wall motion abnormalities during an episode of myocardial ischemia, suggesting the areas at risk for infarction.

5. **C.** The goal of treatment in Q wave myocardial infarction is to open the artery in question. The goal of therapy in unstable angina and non-Q wave myocardial infarction is to prevent blood clot progression and thrombotic occlusion. Aspirin and heparin are useful in this regard. Clinical benefits have been inconsistently seen with thrombolytic therapy. The three largest trials reported an increased risk of fatal and nonfatal myocardial infarction with thrombolysis, suggesting its use could be harmful. These studies have tested recombinant tissue plasminogen activator, anisoylated plasminogen streptokinase activator complex, and urokinase. Subset analysis of patients with non-Q wave myocardial infarction in the TIMI-3B, GISSI-1, and ISIS-2 trials have not documented a benefit. Thrombolytic agents dissolve clot but have procoagulant effects by activating platelet factor 4 and also by increasing plasminogen activator inhibitor activity. (*See* Thrombolytic Therapy.)

Chapter 45

1. **True.** Following acute MI, recurrent ischemic events are a major cause of subsequent mortality and morbidity. The pathophysiology of recurrent ischemia may be due to (a) an unstable coronary plaque or thrombus that reoccludes the artery, or (b) a stable, persistently critically stenotic lesion that may lead to further ischemia with stress or increased oxygen demand by the myocardium.

2. **False.** The management of recurrent ischemic events falls into two categories: (a) prevention and treatment of the acute event, and (b) antithrombotic therapy and beta-blockade. The first component of antithrombotic therapy is aspirin and heparin. Warfarin is also utilized after the acute phase. Current interest in antithrombotic therapy focuses on the combination of warfarin and low-dose aspirin. Regarding beta-blockade and the setting of a myocardial infarction, studies have shown that early intravenous beta-blockade with metoprolol followed by oral beta-blockade should be used in all patients without contraindications such as bradycardia, atrioventricular block, hypotension, pulmonary edema, or history of bronchospasm. (*See* Recurrent Ischemia/Infarction.)

3. **True.** General therapeutic measures in ischemia consist of controlling heart rate and blood pressure, preventing coronary vasoconstriction and coronary thrombosis, and ameliorating ischemic pain. This consists of administration of sublingual or intravenous nitroglycerin, use of intravenous beta-blockade, use of calcium channel blockers, administration of intravenous heparin, and administration of aspirin, morphine, or analgesics to relieve ischemic pain. An electrocardiogram (ECG) should always be performed to identify the presence of S–T segment elevation during this therapy. (*See* Recurrent Ischemia/Infarction.)

4. **False.** The ECG is the most widely used tool in the evaluation of patients with acute MI, and the presence or absence of Q waves provides valuable information regarding the extent of the infarction as well as an indication of the patient's prognosis. The patients with Q wave infarctions have been found to

have higher peak creatine kinase and lower ejection fractions than those without Q waves. Furthermore, at autopsy, patients with Q wave infarctions were found to have larger infarctions.

5. D. While much attention is paid to the left ventricle during acute MI, consideration of right ventricular infarction is critical. The incidence of right ventricular infarction is quite high. Between 35 and 50 percent of patients with inferior MI have associated right ventricular infarction. The treatment for right ventricular infarction is different from the treatment of left ventricular infarction. The simplest test to investigate the presence of a right ventricular infarction utilizes the *right* precordial ECG leads. Other modalities include a thallium or sestamibi perfusion scan, coronary arteriography, echocardiography, or hemodynamic measurements with a pulmonary artery catheter. The presence of an elevated right atrial pressure equal or nearly equal to pulmonary capillary wedge pressure indicates the presence of right ventricular dysfunction. Thus, the differential diagnosis for right ventricular infarction includes hypotension due to left ventricular infarction, pericardial tamponade, constrictive pericarditis, and pulmonary embolism.

6. A. Right ventricular infarction carries a high morbidity and mortality when associated with left ventricular infarction. Systemic hypotension is a major complication of right ventricular infarction in which poor right ventricular output leads to decreased filling of the left ventricle. The second major complication is atrioventricular and/or sinoatrial nodal block. Nodal dysfunction occurs in 10 to 15 percent of patients with inferior wall MI but is seen in nearly 25 percent of patients with right ventricular infarction. The need for temporary pacing parallels the incidence of complete atrioventricular block, as does the occurrence of ventricular fibrillation, ventricular tachycardia, and cardiogenic shock.

7. C. The initial treatment of right ventricular infarction involves early reperfusion therapy. Measures should be used to increase forward output of the right ventricle. Volume expansion is the mainstay of therapy. If acute volume loading does not correct the hemodynamic disturbance, a pulmonary artery catheter should be utilized to direct inotropic therapy. This therapy can include dopamine, dobutamine, and phosphodiesterase inhibitors such as milrinone. In contrast to left-sided heart failure, venous vasodilators such as nitrates should be avoided because they will decrease right ventricular filling pressures and hence decrease right ventricular output. If hemodynamically significant sinus bradycardia or atrioventricular block develops, temporary ventricular pacing or A-V pacing may be necessary.

8. B. The most important determinant of prognosis after MI is the degree of left ventricular dysfunction. The severity of MI relates directly to the amount of myocardium that is damaged. Many factors influence residual ventricular function, including left ventricular function prior to the acute MI, infarct size, presence or absence of Q waves on the ECG, and location of the MI. An Ml with an anterior location has been noted to have the worst prognosis.

9. A. Diastolic dysfunction occurs almost uniformly in patients with acute MI. It becomes clinically significant in up to one-third of patients and is the most common cause of early congestive heart failure. The pathophysiology of diastolic dysfunction begins with increased wall stiffness from ischemia and infarction. This decreased left ventricular compliance results in clinical signs of elevated pulmonary venous congestion such as shortness of breath, dyspnea, orthopnea, rales on physical examination, or pulmonary vascular redistribution on chest x-ray. The heart sound associated with diastolic dysfunction is usually an S_4, which indicates decreased compliance of the left ventricle. Systolic function may be entirely normal in these patients.

10. D. The treatment of diastolic dysfunction includes diuresis and treatment of ischemia. Furosemide is commonly used as a diuretic, although it is important to guard against overdiuresis. Intravenous nitroglycerin and nitroprusside are widely used. Nitroglycerin is the vasodilator most active in producing venous dilation, whereas nitroprusside is a balanced vasodilator. Administration of a beta-blocker may be invaluable in patients whose pulmonary congestion is due to isolated diastolic dysfunction, since these agents will reduce ischemia and improve left ventricular compliance. Left ventricular systolic function is often preserved in patients with isolated diastolic dysfunction, rendering a prognosis that is relatively good compared to those patients with systolic dysfunction.

11. A. Congestive heart failure on the basis of systolic dysfunction is the most serious complication following an acute MI. The most malignant end of the spectrum of congestive heart failure after an acute MI is cardiogenic shock. Hemodynamic characteristics of cardiogenic shock include an elevated pulmonary capillary wedge pressure and reduced cardiac index. The initial treatment goals are to ensure adequate oxygenation and to maintain systolic blood pressure. Preload and afterload reduction and inotropic support may be necessary for patients with marked systolic dysfunction and cardiogenic shock. Dopamine and dobutamine are often utilized as agents in this setting. In addition to these agents, phosphodiesterase inhibitors such as milrinone and amrinone can be used to increase intracellular cyclic adenosine monophosphate by reducing its metabolism. This improves contractility and causes vasodilation. Since the beta-agonists and phosphodiesterase inhibitors act by different pathways, their beneficial effects in this setting are additive when proper attention is paid to volume status.

12. C. The development of thromboembolism is a recognized complication of acute MI and can occur in 5 to 10 percent of patients. Both arterial and venous emboli can occur with left ventricular mural thrombi. Ventricular septal rupture occurring in the setting of an inferior MI is associated with a mortality of 75 percent, while infarction and rupture of the papillary muscles are relatively infrequent following MI. The occurrence of pericardial irritation occurs in approximately one-quarter of patients with acute MI, and it usually begins 2 to 4 days following MI. Three types of presentation are seen: an asymptomatic pericardial effusion, an early symptomatic pericarditis with or without effusion, and late pericarditis.

13. B. The occurrence of refractory sinus tachycardia in the setting of MI increases myocardial oxygen demand and can lead to infarct extension. Supraventricular arrhythmias complicating acute MI are frequently associated with increased sympathetic tone. Ongoing ischemia, hypoxia, pain, fever, pericarditis, and anxiety may all play a role. Atrial fibrillation and atrial flutter occur in up to 16 percent of cases of acute MI. Regular narrow-complex paroxysmal supraventricular tachycardia occurs infrequently during acute MI. The most common are atrioventricular nodal reentrant tachycardia and atrioventricular reentrant tachycardia by an accessory pathway. Vagal maneuvers may be effective in terminating episodes. Adenosine is the drug of choice in the non-MI setting, but few data exist about the use of this drug during the course of an acute MI.

14. D. Patients who develop complete heart block as a result of acute MI should receive a permanent pacemaker prior to discharge. Because of the blood supply to the distal conducting system, intraventricular conduction disturbances frequently accompany anterior wall MI. This usually reflects a large infarction and carries a high in-hospital mortality. Beta-blockers should be avoided in high-risk patients with complete heart block unless placement of a temporary pacemaker is undertaken.

Chapter 46

1. False. When administered to select patients with acute myocardial infarction, thrombolytic therapy reduces infarct mortality. This has been demonstrated for streptokinase administered alone as well as streptokinase administered with aspirin. Mortality reduction has also been demonstrated with other thrombolytic agents including anisoylated plasminogen streptokinase activator complex (APSAC) as well as recombinant tissue plasminogen activator (t-PA).

2. True. In addition to its positive influence on mortality, thrombolytic therapy limits infarct size and is associated with improved left ventricular function. This occurs both globally and regionally at the infarct zone. Improved left ventricular function has been demonstrated to occur following treatment with streptokinase and t-PA.

3. True. Pioneering work in 1980 by DeWood identified the presence of total coronary occlusion in 87 percent of acute myocardial infarction patients evaluated within 4 hours of onset of symptoms. In patients studied 6 to 12 hours after onset of symptoms, the frequency of occlusion was 68 percent, and in those presenting between 12 and 24 hours after onset, the occlusion rate was 65 percent. This has led to the focus of reperfusion therapy by pharmacolgic or mechanical means.

4. True. The major complication associated with the use of thrombolytic therapy is bleeding. The rates of hemorrhage reported in major thrombolytic trials have varied. The rates generally parallel those from the TIMI-II trial, where 4.2 percent of 1400 patients had major bleeding events and 8.7 percent of patients had minor bleeding events. The most serious complication of thrombolytic therapy is intracranial bleeding, and there appears to be an increased rate of intracranial bleeding in patients who are elderly, are hypertensive, or have had previous cerebrovascular events.

5. True. Great debate exists about whether the ability to open more arteries confers benefit in regard to measurable clinical outcomes such as mortality reduction and preservation of left ventricular function. The open artery hypothesis suggests that outcome is better with those agents that have higher reperfusion rates. The GUSTO trial comparing accelerated IV t-PA with IV heparin, IV t-PA and streptokinase with IV heparin, IV streptokinase with subcutaneous heparin, and IV streptokinase with IV heparin suggested that recombinant t-PA was a superior agent in terms of mortality reduction. The large difference in cost between streptokinase and t-PA is an important issue that must be factored into the decision regarding choice of agent for thrombolytic therapy.

6. **False.** The data are quite conclusive, showing that there is no need for routine cardiac catheterization and subsequent PTCA in patients treated with thrombolytic therapy who do not have recurrent symptoms of angina or ischemia during exercise stress testing.

7. **False.** Based on multiple trials, there is strong agreement that otherwise eligible patients presenting within the first 6 hours of symptom onset should be treated with thrombolytic therapy. Data supporting treatment beyond 6 hours have been mixed. However, the Late Assessment of Thrombolytic Efficacy (LATE) trial was designed to evaluate the benefit of thrombolytic therapy given beyond the first 6 hours. Results indicate lower mortality for the group treated with t-PA up to 12 hours from symptom onset. Based on this study, there is consideration from the literature to extend the window for thrombolytic therapy to 12 hours.

8. **B.** The absolute contraindications for thrombolytic therapy include incidences where active bleeding or potential hemorrhage exists. Therefore, patients with aortic dissection, ongoing internal bleeding, recent intracranial surgery, intracranial neoplasm, head trauma, or history of hemorrhagic stroke should not be treated with thrombolytic therapy. Similarly, sustained uncontrolled hypertension is also an absolute contraindication to thrombolytic therapy. Blood pressure greater than 200/120 mm Hg is an absolute contraindication. Other contraindications include pregnancy, recent surgery, or trauma. Also, previous allergic reaction to streptokinase or APSAC suggests contraindication to use of those agents. However, patients who show reaction to recent treatment with APSAC or streptokinase can be treated with t-PA or urokinase.

Chapter 47

1. **True.** There is evidence that an organized approach to assist those who wish to quit smoking after admission to the coronary care unit offers a unique opportunity for success. Cessation rates of 40 to 70 percent are seen. Many patients cite the advice of their physicians as the most important factor in the decision to quit smoking.

2. **False.** Magnesium has several effects on the myocardium that may be protective following a myocardial infarction. Magnesium antagonizes the effect of calcium at the cellular level and causes both systemic and coronary vasodilation. Platelet aggregation and adhesion may be reduced. Magnesium also suppresses some types of ventricular arrhythmias and may limit ischemic injury to the myocardium following reperfusion.

3. **True.** One of the most powerful predictors of death after myocardial infarction is the extent of left ventricular systolic dysfunction. Ejection fraction is commonly utilized to measure left ventricular performance. The 1-year mortality rises precipitously as the left ventricular ejection fraction falls below 40 percent. A more powerful predictor of death is the extent of left ventricular dilation as seen on echocardiography or cardiac catheterization.

4. **False.** Trials suggest that ACE inhibitors are a safe but only modestly effective intervention in the unrestricted myocardial infarction population. ACE inhibitors are preferred in patients with extensive myocardial infarction, heart

failure, or left ventricular dysfunction and have the most impact when continued long term.

5. **True.** Nitrates have been used for more than a century in the treatment of angina. Hemodynamic benefits include a reduction in preload and ventricular filling pressure, and coronary vasodilatation. Recent evidence supports an antiplatelet effect as well.

6. **C.** Cellular calcium overload has been identified as a final common pathway of cellular injury in myocardial infarction. The observation led to the widespread administration of calcium channel blockers to reduce infarction size, decrease mortality, and reduce reinfarction. The available agents are grouped according to chemical structure. Generally nifedipine and dihydropyridines have been found to have an overall lack of benefit, and in some instances, there has been evidence of harm in studies after acute myocardial infarction. The leading hypothesis to explain the adverse effects of dihydropyridines is that their potent peripheral vasodilatory action reduces coronary perfusion pressure and triggers reflex catecholamine release. Verapamil and diltiazem, on the other hand, tend to depress atrioventricular nodal conduction and sinus node activity to a greater degree and are considered rate slowing. At recommended doses, most investigators have also found a more potent negative inotropic effect.

Chapter 48

1. **False.** The ECG is of critical importance for early confirmation of acute myocardial infarction. When a patient presents with typical chest pain and characteristic ECG changes of 1 mm or greater S–T segment elevation in two or more contiguous leads, the diagnosis of acute myocardial infarction is established. (*See* Electrocardiography.)

2. **False.** The normal pericardium is seldom evident on plain chest radiographs. A pericardial stripe greater than 2 mm along the inferior heart border seen on the lateral projection suggests pericardial effusion.

3. **False.** In addition to its diagnostic utility, thallium stress test imaging is helpful in determining prognosis from coronary artery disease in unselected patients, patients with recent myocardial infarction, or patients undergoing preoperative evaluation for vascular surgery. Thallium is a cationic potassium analog whose myocardial uptake is dependent on cell membrane integrity and is proportional to blood flow. Thallium scintigraphy after infusion of dipyridamole has been shown to have independent and significant prognostic utility in unselected patients referred for diagnostic work-up.

4. **B.** Right and left ventricular ejection fractions and regional wall motion may be safely and reproducibly determined noninvasively by radionuclide techniques. First-pass radionuclide studies measure the initial transit of radiotracer through the heart, while equilibrium studies such as the gated blood pool scan (MUGA), radionuclide ventriculogram, and radionuclide angiogram rely on counts of tracer within the intravascular space during multiple cardiac cycles. Left ventricular function is the most important noninvasive predictor of reinfarction and sudden death following myocardial infarction. The ejection fraction is determined by dividing the difference in count rates at end diastole and end systole by the count rate at end diastole ($EF = [ED - ES] / ED$).

Chapter 49

1. **True.** It has been shown that in ischemic border zones around scar tissue in the myocardium, islets of injured cells, interspersed with normal cells, produce fragmented and slowed electrical impulses during diastole. These slowly conducting electrical impulses are then able to reenter and reactivate excitable tissue, initiating a reentrant beat. An important determinant of impulse propagation within myocardial tissue is the axial and transverse resistances that are determined by the degree of intercellular coupling. The higher the degree of coupling between cells, the lower the resistance to current flow and the faster the conduction velocity. Uncoupling of cells and slowing of conduction occur with ischemia, acidosis, and calcium overload.

2. **False.** In the first 48 hours after myocardial infarction, the incidence of ventricular arrhythmias ranges from 34 to 100 percent. Ventricular arrhythmias tend to be associated with larger infarcts, congestive heart failure, and previous or new conduction disturbances.

3. **D.** Ventricular tachycardia is defined as three or more consecutive ventricular depolarizations at a rate of greater than 100 beats per minute. Sustained ventricular tachycardia lasts for more than 30 seconds, while unsustained ventricular tachycardia lasts from 3 beats to less than 30 seconds and terminates spontaneously. Ventricular tachycardia can further be distinguished as uniform or of constant morphology or polymorphic.

4. **C.** The most frequent tachycardia associated with unstable coronary syndromes is sinus tachycardia. This is usually an appropriate physiologic response related to pain, anxiety, metabolites of tissue injury, and medications. The presence of sinus tachycardia can indicate persistent ischemia, impending heart failure, and hypotension due to pump failure. Treatment of the primary disorder is recommended as well as treatment of the sinus tachycardia with beta-blocking agents to decrease myocardial oxygen consumption. Beta-blockade should only be undertaken in patients without signs of congestive heart failure or bronchospasm.

5. **C.** Although supraventricular and ventricular tachyarrhythmias derive from the same physiologic mechanism, management of these tachyarrhythmias may vary considerably. Supraventricular arrhythmias are usually not associated with hemodynamic compromise and rarely require emergent intervention. On the other hand, ventricular arrhythmias may lead to hemodynamic compromise and death and may require emergent intervention. Appropriate management of a patient with tachyarrhythmia requires accurate identification of the arrhythmia and its underlying mechanism. The diagnosis of supraventricular tachycardia is almost always certain when the QRS complex of the tachycardia is identical to that of the sinus rhythm. Proper identification of the mechanism underlying a wide QRS tachycardia may be very difficult.

Chapter 50

1. **False.** With increasing myocardial oxygen demands, oxygen consumption may increase three- to fourfold. Myocardial oxygen extraction cannot increase substantially. Therefore, coronary blood flow must increase to meet the demands placed on the heart.

2. **True.** Coronary arterial blood flow is determined by the pressure gradient between the aorta in diastole and the coronary sinus. This relationship is influenced by atherosclerotic narrowings and elevations in left ventricular and diastolic pressure and right atrial pressure. Coronary blood flow is maintained when the mean arterial pressure exceeds 65 mm Hg.

3. **False.** An interaction between coronary thrombosis and coronary spasm is possible, especially in conditions such as Prinzmetal's variant angina. Diseased coronary artery endothelium may exhibit impaired production of endogenous plasminogen activator such as t-PA when a thrombic potential of diseased endothelium is combined with coronary stasis. This can lead to a vicious cycle, resulting in ischemia or frank necrosis.

4. **True.** Both penetrating and blunt trauma can cause myocardial infarction. Penetrating trauma such as stab or gunshot wounds can cause coronary laceration or pericardial tamponade. Blunt trauma can cause myocardial infarction even in the absence of preexisting atherosclerotic disease. This infarction is possibly related to intimal coronary tear, coronary artery rupture, myocardial contusion, or a combination of those factors.

Chapter 51

1. **False.** Only 13 percent of patients with acute myocardial infarction have S–T segment elevation and Q waves on their presenting ECG. In one study of acute myocardial infarction, 62 percent of patients discharged from the emergency ward had a normal ECG upon careful review. Serial ECGs, however, are abnormal in 80 to 90 percent of cases of acute myocardial infarction.

2. **E.** Pulmonary causes of chest pain include pulmonary hypertension, pleuritic chest pain from pleural effusion, pneumonia, pneumothorax, and pulmonary embolism. Vascular causes of chest pain include aortic dissection and aortic aneurysm. Herpes zoster (shingles) can affect the anterior chest and mimic angina pectoris. However, the pain is dermatomal and does not cross the midline. Pleurodynia is associated with Coxsackie B infection and causes pleuritic chest pain. Usually there is a viral prodrome. The discomfort experienced among patients with pulmonary hypertension may be identical to that described for typical angina. The pain may be caused by underlying right ventricular ischemia or dilatation of the pulmonary arteries. Underlying causes include pulmonary embolism, primary pulmonary hypertension, severe chronic obstructive pulmonary disease, mitral stenosis, and severe long-standing left ventricular failure. When infectious pneumonia extends from the pulmonary parenchyma to the pleural surface, pleuritic pain may occur. For each of these causes of noncardiac chest pain, there is usually little diagnostic confusion, since the accompanying history, physical findings, ECG, chest x-ray, and pulmonary artery catheterization are helpful in diagnosis. Occasionally, the diagnosis of pulmonary embolism may require pulmonary artery catheterization and ventilation perfusion scanning to confirm the diagnosis.

Chapter 52

1. **True.** The management of hypertension in the ICU usually involves one of four situations: hypertensive emergencies, also known as hypertensive crisis;

chronic hypertension treatment in patients unable to continue with their usual oral regimens; the new onset of short-lived transient hypertension; and hypertension related to the perioperative setting.

2. **False.** The differentiation between a hypertensive urgency and emergency is based on the presence of target end damage. According to this definition, hypertensive emergency refers to blood pressure elevation associated with ongoing target end damage. Pathologic changes found in the vessels within affected organs include fibrinoid necrosis and myointimal proliferation.

3. **False.** A brief history and physical examination should be initiated to assess the degree of target organ damage and rule out secondary causes of hypertension. Important historical data include symptoms attributable to changes in target organ perfusion and function. The history should include inquiries about prior hypertension, other diseases, neurologic symptoms, cardiac symptoms, or urinary symptoms. This history may be obtained from the patient but also should be obtained from family members and the medical record. The evaluation should involve intraarterial monitoring if necessary. Ophthalmologic examination should follow, with examination for hemorrhages, exudates, and papilledema. Auscultation of the lungs and heart includes determination of the presence of rales and S_3. Laboratory evaluation should include electrolytes for hypokalemia and acidosis; blood urea nitrogen and creatinine for assessment of renal function; complete blood count with differential for anemia, sepsis, disseminated intravascular coagulation, or microangiopathic hemolytic anemia; and assessment of cardiac function with electrocardiogram, cardiac isoenzymes, chest x-ray, and possibly pulmonary artery catheterization. An important consideration in the choice of initial therapy is to use agents that will not complicate or interfere with further evaluation. Two examples are hypertension felt to be related to renal artery stenosis and hypertension possibly due to pheochromocytoma.

4. **B.** The goal of initial therapy is to terminate ongoing target organ damage, not to return blood pressure to normal levels. The lower limit of cerebral autoregulation will determine targets for initial therapy. In hypertensive and normotensive patients, this target is approximately 25 percent below the initial mean arterial pressure or a diastolic pressure between 100 and 110 mm Hg. Therefore, a reasonable target for blood pressure reduction is to decrease the mean arterial pressure by 20 to 25 percent. In most patients with hypertensive emergencies, the pathophysiologic abnormality is an increase in the systemic vascular resistance, not a change in cardiac output. It is the increase in systemic vascular resistance that overrides autoregulation within the end organs and leads to ischemia and organ damage.

5. **B.** Although any antihypertensive agent can be associated with rebound hypertension, adrenergic inhibitors such as beta-blocking agents or central agonists such as clonidine or methyldopa are most commonly described. Rebound hypertension represents the rapid return of catecholamine secretion previously suppressed by therapy. The likelihood of rebound hypertension is proportional to the dose of medication, and patients with more severe hypertension are at greater risk for rebound. If a patient is taking both beta-blockers and central agonists, the beta-blocker should be weaned and stopped first to avoid unopposed vasoconstriction. Rebound syndromes generally respond rapidly to reinstitution of initial therapy. In general, medications in the same class should be utilized.

6. B. The patient who arrives postoperatively in the ICU from surgery may often have transient hypertension. Elevated blood pressure can induce target organ damage, increase vascular suture breakdown, and risk bleeding. In the ICU setting, concern exists with blood pressure above 160/100 mm Hg in a previously normotensive patient or an increase of more than 30 mm Hg above preoperative levels in a known hypertensive patient. About 25 percent of patients will have worsening perioperative blood pressure with a known preoperative diagnosis of hypertension. Any routine blood pressure therapy should be continued up to the morning of surgery as regularly scheduled. Induction of anesthesia represents a challenge to circulatory stability. Pain, hypothermia with shivering, hypoxia, or reflex excitement after anesthesia can lead to changes in blood pressure requiring subtle minute-to-minute adjustment. Since hypertension in this setting is neither severe nor long lasting, small doses of intravenous antihypertensive medications are indicated. Sodium nitroprusside is effective in most situations. In a patient with fixed coronary lesions, nitroglycerin can be used to improve poststenotic collateral flow. Labetalol as minibolus or infusion therapy can provide longer duration of action.

Many postoperative patients develop intravascular volume expansion during the first 36 to 72 hours secondary to extravascular fluid mobilization and intraoperative fluid administration. An increase in blood pressure in this period may respond well to intravenous loop diuretics, such as furosemide, and to fluid restriction.

7. B. Labetalol is a racemic mixture of a nonselective beta-blocker and a selective alpha$_1$-antagonist. It produces prompt reduction in peripheral vascular resistance and in blood pressure. The beta-blockade component prevents reflex tachycardia or changes in cardiac output. Myocardial oxygen consumption is reduced and coronary hemodynamics are improved in patients with coronary artery disease. The disadvantages relate to several factors; usually the alpha-blocking effects are cited. The alpha-blocking effects can cause orthostatic hypotension. Other side effects are nausea, vomiting, flushing, and tingling. The ratio of beta-blocking effects to alpha-blocking is approximately 7:1. For this reason, any contraindication to use of beta-blockade also applies to the use of labetalol.

8. False. Nicardipine is a rapid-acting systemic and coronary artery vasodilator. It has minimal effects on cardiac conductivity or inotropy. Metabolism is by hepatic degradation with no active metabolites. There is no dose adjustment necessary in renal insufficiency. Its advantages include rapid onset, increasing potency, and ability to titrate to blood pressure levels. It has also been found to have renal protective effects.

IV. Pulmonary Problems in the Intensive Care Unit

54. Pulmonary Edema: Etiologies and Pathogenesis

1. Development of noncardiogenic edema is characterized by:

A. Interstitial oncotic pressure rises compared with changes seen in hydrostatic edema.
B. An increased reflection coefficient for protein in the Starling equation.
C. Changes in pulmonary venous pressure that do not affect extravascular lung water.
D. Protein content of alveolar fluid is low compared with findings during hydrostatic edema.

55. Acute Respiratory Distress Syndrome

1. Select the best answer. Improved survival in acute respiratory distress syndrome (ARDS) has been proved with which of the following interventions?

A. Intravenous high-dose corticosteroids.
B. Nebulized artificial surfactant.
C. Inhaled nitric oxide.
D. Intravenous *N*-acetylcysteine.
E. None of the above.

2. The alveolar capillary injury in ARDS

A. Always begins on the capillary side.
B. Results in a heterogenous distribution of pulmonary edema.
C. Is dependent on normal neutrophil numbers or function.
D. Does not disturb surfactant levels or function.
E. None of the above.

56. *Status Asthmaticus*

1. Administration of theophylline during an acute asthma exacerbation

A. Improves outcome during the emergency room treatment of asthma.
B. Is more effective than treatment with beta-adrenergic agonists.
C. Is associated with fewer side effects than treatment with beta-adrenergic agonists.
D. Accelerates bronchodilator efficacy in hospitalized asthmatics.

2. A 38-year-old woman with severe asthma was admitted to the intensive care unit after emergency room treatment of asthma with beta-adrenergic agonists and 125 mg of methylprednisolone IV. Despite frequent albuterol nebulization, she remained bronchospastic and developed a respiratory acidosis necessitating endobronchial intubation and mechanical ventilation. On settings of an FiO_2 of 0.4, volume assist/control rate of 16 liters per minute, tidal volume of 750 ml, and an applied positive end-expiratory pressure (PEEP) of 0, peak airway pressures were 62 cm H_2O, and an intrinsic PEEP of 14 cm H_2O was present. Arterial blood gases showed a pH of 7.30, a PO_2 of 72, and a PCO_2 of 52. The most appropriate management would be

A. To decrease the tidal volume to 600 ml per breath.
B. To increase the mandatory rate to 20 per minute.
C. To paralyze the patient with pancuronium.
D. To add 10 cm applied PEEP to facilitate weaning.

57. *Chronic Obstructive Pulmonary Disease*

1. A 68-year-old man with advanced chronic obstructive pulmonary disease is admitted with a 3-day history of fever, cough with purulent sputum, and worsening dyspnea. Chest x-ray reveals a right middle lobar and right lower lobar infiltrate. The respiratory rate is 25 per minute. Arterial blood gases on 4 liters of oxygen by nasal cannula show a PO_2 of 52 mm Hg, a PCO_2 of 55 mm Hg, and a pH of 7.35. Sputum Gram's stain reveals many neutrophils and predominantly small gram-negative diplococci. Pending cultures, the most appropriate antibiotic choice is

A. Erythromycin.
B. Cefuroxime.
C. Penicillin G.
D. Ampicillin.

58. Extrapulmonary Causes of Respiratory Failure

1. Factors associated with prolonged neuromuscular blockade or weakness after pancuronium use to facilitate mechanical ventilation include all the following except

   A. Concomitant renal failure.
   B. Corticosteroid use.
   C. Pseudocholinesterase deficiency.
   D. Excessive dose.

2. A 22-year-old woman was transferred to the intensive care unit (ICU) because of worsening shortness of breath and a vital capacity of 700 ml determined at the bedside. She had been admitted to the neurology service 48 hours earlier with a 3-day history of distal lower extremity hypesthesia followed by progressive ascending muscle paralysis. Electromyography confirmed a demyelinating polyradiculopathy, and a diagnosis of Guillain-Barré syndrome was made. In the ICU, her respiratory rate increased to 40 per minute, and arterial blood gases showed hypoventilation with a respiratory acidosis. She was intubated and mechanically ventilated. The most appropriate next treatment is

   A. Plasmapheresis.
   B. Corticosteroids.
   C. Azathioprine.
   D. Pyridostigmine.

59. Acute Respiratory Failure in Pregnancy

1. A 36-year-old multiparous patient underwent cesarean section at 35 weeks' gestation due to fetal distress. During delivery of the infant, the anesthesiologist noted a dropping blood pressure, hypoxemia, and oozing blood from an upper extremity IV site. Also, the obstetrician commented on increased bleeding in the operative field. Arterial blood gases on 100% oxygen showed a pH of 7.27, a PCO_2 of 32 mm Hg, and a PO_2 of 63 mm Hg. The hemoglobin level was 10.2 gm per deciliter. Prothrombin time was 16.2 seconds, and the partial thromboplastin time was 82 seconds. The platelet count was 42,000 per cubic millimeter. Which of the following statements is true?

   A. She has probably suffered a venous thromboembolism.
   B. She probably has noncardiogenic pulmonary edema.
   C. She has probably aspirated gastric contents.
   D. She has probably suffered an air embolism.

2. A 32-year-old woman was placed on bedrest during her seventh month of pregnancy. Three weeks later, she awoke with shortness of breath and left-sided pleuritic chest pain. Evaluation in the emergency room showed a normal blood pressure, although tachypnea and tachycardia were present. Fetal heart tones were present. Her lower extremities showed mild bilateral pretibial

edema. There was mild to moderate right calf tenderness. Chest x-ray showed minimal atelectasis at the left base. Arterial blood gases on room air showed a PO_2 of 68 mm Hg, a PCO_2 of 28 mm Hg, and a pH of 7.50. Duplex ultrasound suggested a nonocclusive clot in the right common femoral vein. Ventilation-perfusion (V/Q) lung scan showed two segmental mismatched defects in the left lung. Which of the following statements is true?

A. She should be treated with intravenous heparin, and warfarin can be started on day 2.
B. She should be considered for inferior vena cava filter placement.
C. Thrombolytic therapy is indicated because of proximal deep venous thrombosis.
D. She should be treated with intravenous heparin followed by subcutaneous heparin.

60. Pulmonary Embolism and Deep Vein Thrombosis

1. A 46-year-old woman was 7 days postoperative from drainage of a complicated pelvic abscess. She had developed noncardiogenic edema related to sepsis preoperatively and was gradually improving. Although her chest x-ray still showed bilateral pulmonary infiltrates and she remained ventilator dependent, she has had no other organ failures. During morning rounds, she was noted to be tachypneic and tachycardic. Her blood pressure was stable. A physical examination was remarkable for dependent crackles in both dependent lung zones, a regular tachycardia without murmurs, gallops, or rubs, and mild pedal edema bilaterally. Arterial blood gases showed a worsening hypoxemia and a respiratory alkalosis. Her chest x-ray was without change, showing diffuse bilateral pulmonary infiltrates. The electrocardiogram showed a sinus tachycardia with normal ST–T wave changes. The most appropriate diagnostic test would be

A. Pulmonary artery catheterization to detect pulmonary capillary wedge pressure.
B. Bilateral lower extremity duplex ultrasound.
C. Ventilation-perfusion (V/Q) lung scan.
D. Pulmonary arteriogram.
E. Abdominal computed tomography scan.

True or False. Regarding patients with acute pulmonary embolism:

2. The chest radiograph is usually normal.

3. New onset arterial fibrillation is the most common arrhythmia.

4. The $P(A\text{-}a)O_2$ may be normal.

5. Most will have high-probability lung scans.

6. Warfarin therapy should be titrated for an international normalized ratio (INR) of 2 to 3.

7. Thrombolytic therapy is indicated if the PO_2 is less than or equal to 50 mm Hg.

61. *Managing Hemoptysis*

1. A 26-year-old white man with advanced cystic fibrosis was hospitalized for worsening cough, fever, and sputum production. A chest x-ray showed bilateral, severe, upper lobe predominant bronchiectatic changes. He was treated with intravenous antipseudomonal antibiotics. On the second hospital day, he expectorated 500 ml of bright red blood and developed increased shortness of breath. Chest x-ray demonstrated increased opacification in both upper lobes. He was taken back to the intensive care unit (ICU) and intubated because of continued large-volume hemoptysis. Follow-up bronchoscopy showed diffuse bilateral blood staining of all major bronchi. A definite bleeding source could not be identified, but blood clots were present in the right upper lobe orifice. The next procedure should be

   A. Intubation of the left main stem bronchus.
   B. Exploratory thoracotomy and probably right upper lobectomy.
   C. Bronchial arteriography.
   D. Pulmonary angiography.
   E. Computed tomography (CT) scan of the chest.

63. *Near-Drowning*

1. Which of the following statements about near-drowning is true?

   A. Freshwater near-drowning/aspiration inactivates surfactant.
   B. Freshwater near-drowning/aspiration stimulates type II pneumocyte function.
   C. Seawater near-drowning/aspiration inactivates surfactant.
   D. Seawater near-drowning/aspiration often results in severe hemoconcentration.

2. Freshwater near-drowning episodes are usually characterized by

   A. Hypoxemia due to laryngospasm but no actual fluid aspiration.
   B. Severe hyponatremia.
   C. Radiographic pulmonary edema.
   D. Metabolic alkalosis.

64. *Pulmonary Hypertension*

1. The pulmonary artery occlusion pressure is likely to be significantly less than the pulmonary artery diastolic pressure in all the following clinical conditions except

   A. Left heart failure.

B. Primary pulmonary hypertension.
C. Pulmonary veno-occlusive disease.
D. Severe chronic obstructive lung disease.

65. *Pleural Disease in the Critically Ill Patient*

1. A 72-year-old man was seen in the emergency room 48 hours after endoscopic esophageal dilation. He complained of fever, shortness of breath, and substernal and left-sided pleuritic chest pain for the past 24 hours. The chest radiograph showed a left hydropneumothorax. Barium swallow documented a distal esophageal rupture with extravasation of contrast into the left pleural space and mediastinum. The most appropriate management is

A. Lube thoracostomy and parenteral antibiotics.
B. Thoracotomy, drainage, and esophageal repair.
C. Thoracentesis, NPO, and parenteral antibiotics.
D. Immediate upper gastrointestinal endoscopy for confirmation of diagnosis.

2. A 42-year-old man was hospitalized for severe pancreatitis. Over the first 48 hours of hospitalization, he developed worsening dyspnea and hypoxemia with diffuse bilateral pulmonary infiltrates. Pulmonary artery catheterization confirmed normal left ventricular filling pressures, and the patient was diagnosed as having acute respiratory distress syndrome. On FIO_2 of 0.50, positive end-expiratory pressure (PEEP) of 10 cm H_2O, pressure-controlled ventilation with pressure relief at 40 cm H_2O, rate of 18 per minute, and an inspiratory-expiratory (I:E) ratio of 1:1, his arterial blood gases showed a PO_2 of 68 mm Hg, a PCO_2 of 38 mm Hg, and a pH of 7.44. On morning rounds, examination revealed bilateral neck and anterior chest wall crepitations. There was no evidence of air trapping on pressure and flow graphics. Chest radiograph showed pneumomediastinum but no pneumothorax. Appropriate ventilator adjustments are

A. Decrease PEEP, increase I:E ratio.
B. Decrease pressure relief, decrease PEEP.
C. Increase rate, decrease PEEP.
D. Decrease rate, increase I:E ratio.

3. Despite making the appropriate adjustments in the patient in question 2 and decreasing peak and mean airway pressures, he developed sudden distress and hypotension, and a right tension pneumothorax was diagnosed. A chest tube was placed emergently and placed to 20 cm H_2O water suction. A large continuous air leak was presented and persisted without improvement for 5 days. Oxygenation did not change, and the acid-base balance remained stable. Despite the continued air leak, chest radiographs showed good lung reexpansion. The most appropriate management of the bronchopleural fistula would be

A. Thoracotomy with oversewing of the pleural defect.
B. Bleomycin pleurodesis.
C. To increase chest tube suction to 40 cm H_2O.
D. To continue present management.
E. Bronchoscopically directed occlusion of the offending bronchus.

66. Mechanical Ventilation: Initiation

1. In pressure-support mode of mechanical ventilation, the dependent variables include all the following except

A. Pressure.
B. Flow.
C. Volume.
D. Rate.

2. Positive end-expiratory pressure (PEEP) in subjects with noncardiogenic edema

A. Decreases intrapulmonary shunt.
B. Decreases extravascular lung water.
C. Decreases peak airway pressure.
D. Decreases mean airway pressure.

3. The application of extrinsic PEEP to a ventilator-dependent patient with chronic obstructive pulmonary disease with evidence of significant intrinsic or "auto PEEP"

A. Decreases alveolar overdistention.
B. Improves lung compliance.
C. Decreases peak airway pressure.
D. Facilitates inspiratory triggering.

67. Mechanical Ventilation: Weaning

1. The most common reason for failure to wean patients after prolonged (> 7 days) mechanical ventilation is

A. Inadequate respiratory drive.
B. Psychological difficulties.
C. Respiratory muscle fatigue.
D. Persistent lung or cardiovascular disease.

2. A 72-year-old man was intubated and mechanically ventilated for hypercapnic respiratory failure following a bronchitic exacerbation. After 4 days of mechanical ventilation, he was awake, alert, and afebrile. He was on pressure-support mode with 18 cm H_2O inspiratory pressure. He was breathing 18 times per minute with an average tidal volume of 450 ml. On 35% oxygen, his arterial blood gases showed a pH of 7.42, a PCO_2 of 58 mm Hg, and a PO_2 of 69 mm Hg. Morning bedside mechanics using a hand-held spirometer revealed a negative inspiratory force of 26 cm H_2O, respiratory rate of 26 per minute, and tidal volume of 350 ml. Vital capacity was attempted, but patient effort and cooperation were questionable. Which of the following statements is true?

A. This patient can probably be weaned and extubated.
B. This patient probably cannot be weaned and extubated at this time.
C. There is insufficient information provided to decide about weaning and extubation.

68. Air Embolism and Decompression Sickness

1. A 22-year-old amateur diver surfaces from a scuba dive to 40 feet. He immediately complains of chest pain and shortness of breath. True statements concerning this diver include all the following except

A. Immediate recompression is needed.
B. He should hold his breath while ascending.
C. Air embolism is possible.
D. Pneumothorax may occur.

69. Respiratory Adjunct Therapy

1. A 26-year-old woman was admitted in severe respiratory distress from status asthmaticus precipitated by a bronchitic infection. She was treated with continuous albuterol nebulization (5 mg/hr), methylprednisolone (125 mg IV every 6 hours), and aminophylline, but she required intubation and mechanical ventilation because of progressive hypercapnic respiratory failure after 6 hours of therapy. She remained difficult to ventilate, with severe bilateral bronchospasm. She developed a progressive respiratory and metabolic acidosis. Tidal volumes of 300 ml produced a peak airway pressure of 70 cm H_2O. On 40% oxygen, her arterial blood gas showed a pH of 7.14, PCO_2 of 66 mm Hg, and PO_2 of 66 mm Hg. Respiratory rate was 30 per minute and pulse rate 150 per minute. An appropriate intervention at this point would be

A. To increase methylprednisolone to 250 mg every 6 hours.
B. To increase continuous albuterol nebulization to 10 mg per hour.
C. Terbutaline, 0.5 mg subcutaneously every 6 hours.
D. To increase tidal volume to 600 ml.
E. To deliver a helium-oxygen mixture.

71. Acute Inhalation Injury

1. Carbon monoxide exposure and the formation of carboxyhemoglobin results in

A. Shift of the oxyhemoglobin dissociation curve to the left.
B. Increased total oxygen-carrying capacity in the blood.
C. Decreased affinity of hemoglobin for oxygen.
D. Increased oxidative metabolism at the cellular level.

2. Silo-fillers' disease results from significant exposure to nitrogen dioxide (NO_2) and is characterized by

A. Nasal and oral mucous membrane edema.
B. Pulmonary edema.
C. Eosinophilia.
D. Laryngeal edema.

3. Fatalities from smoke inhalation are most often due to

A. Pulmonary edema.
B. Heat injury to the lower airway.
C. Upper airway edema and obstruction.
D. Carbon monoxide poisoning.

72. Disorders of Temperature Control: Hypothermia

True or False. Regarding the shivering phase of hypothermia:

1. Oxygen consumption rises two to five times.

2. Cardiac output increases dramatically.

3. Severe lactic acidosis may develop.

4. Mixed venous oxygen saturation decreases.

True or False. Characteristic changes in pulmonary mechanics and gas exchange during hypothermia include

5. Increased minute ventilation during shivering.

6. Widened alveolar-axterial oxygen tension gradient ($P[A\text{-}a]O_2$).

7. Poor thoracic compliance.

8. Increased airway resistance.

9. Hypothermic effects on organ system function can be characterized as follows:

A. A decreased glomerular filtration rate, leading to concentrated urine and oliguria.
B. A leukocytosis that is common in severe hypothermia and not necessarily associated with infection.
C. Hypoglycemia is a common finding due to the associated liver dysfunction and exaggerated insulin action at the tissue level.
D. A common associated diagnosis is pancreatitis.

73. Disorders of Temperature Control: Hyperthermia

Matching:

1. Excessive thermogenesis due to muscle contraction.

A. Malignant hyperthermia.

2. Autosomal dominant pattern of inheritance.
3. Allergic reaction.
4. Rhabdomyolysis.
5. Dantrolene is effective.
6. Pancuronium is effective.
7. Bromocriptine is effective.
8. Extrapyramidal signs are common.

B. Neuroleptic malignant syndrome.
C. Both.
D. Neither.

74. Acquired Immunodeficiency Syndrome: Pulmonary Complications and Intensive Care

1. The most common pulmonary disease in patients with the acquired immunodeficiency syndrome (AIDS) is

   A. *Pneumocystis carinii* pneumonia (PCP).
   B. *Mycobacterium tuberculosis.*
   C. Bacterial pneumonia.
   D. *Mycobacterium avium-intracellulare.*

2. A 28-year-old HIV-positive man was hospitalized with 5 days of fever, minimally productive cough, and shortness of breath. Physical examination revealed bibasilar inspiratory crackles, and a chest x-ray showed bilateral interstitial infiltrates. Sputum induced by hypertonic saline was positive for *Pneumocystis* cysts on periodic acid–Schiff stain. He was started on parenteral trimethoprim-sulfamethoxazole (15 mg/kg/day trimethoprim component), but 24 hours later he was worse, with increased dyspnea and hypoxemia. His PO_2 was 52 mm Hg on a 70% face mask. His chest x-ray had progressive interstitial infiltrates. The most appropriate treatment is to add

   A. Prednisone.
   B. Parenteral pentamidine.
   C. Clarithromycin.
   D. Isoniazid, rifampin, ethambutol, and pyrazinamide.

75. Severe Upper Airway Infections

1. The most common cause of acute epiglottitis in adults is

   A. *Moraxella catarrhalis.*
   B. *Streptococcus pneumoniae.*

C. *Staphylococcus aureus.*
D. *Haemophilus influenzae.*

2. A 42-year-old man with advanced dental caries presented to the emergency room with a several-day history of fever, chills, mouth and neck pain, and dysphagia. Physical examination revealed swelling and tenderness over the lower right gingiva, with advanced caries and pyorrhea. There was diffuse submandibular swelling, erythema, and tenderness. The most appropriate empiric antibiotic regimen is

A. Penicillin and metronidazole.
B. Clindamycin and ceftazidime.
C. Nafcillin and gentamicin.
D. Vancomycin and sulfamethoxazole.

76. Acute Infectious Pneumonia

1. Risk factors for nosocomial pneumonia include all the following except

A. Endotracheal intubation.
B. Sucralfate use.
C. Nasogastric tubes.
D. Altered consciousness.

2. Bronchoalveolar lavage (BAL) and protected specimen brush specimens obtained bronchoscopically in a patient with suspected nosocomial pneumonia

A. Have poor sensitivity in the presence of concomitant antibiotic administration.
B. Cannot diagnose a nonbacterial cause of infection.
C. Discriminates between airway and parenchymal infection.
D. Results in decreased mortality.

3. Enteral feeding through a nasogastric tube

A. Results in increased clinical aspiration compared with small-bowel feeding.
B. Results in improved feeding efficiency compared with small-bowel feeding.
C. Should only be done in the supine position.
D. May predispose to nosocomial pneumonia.

4. Studies on selective decontamination of the digestive tract (SDD) in critically ill patients have shown

A. Decreased rates of lower respiratory tract infections in treated patients.
B. Lower in-hospital mortality rates in treated patients.
C. No evidence of emergence of resistant bacteria.
D. Decreased length of stay in the intensive care unit (ICU) in treated patients.

5. A 54-year-old male cigarette smoker presented to the emergency room with 72 hours of low-grade fever, fatigue, dyspnea, cough, and minimal yellow sputum production. He had intermittent bouts of bronchitis in the winter months, but he had no prior history of pneumonia. The physical examination was pertinent for tachypnea (32 per minute), fever of 38.4°C, and a regular tachycardia at 120 beats per minute. The chest examination revealed bibasilar crackles, left greater than right, and scattered expiratory wheezes. Pulse oximetry on room air was 84 percent. The white blood count was 12,400 per cubic millimeter with 80 percent neutrophils and 10 percent band forms. The chest radiograph showed bilateral, lower lobe, patchy infiltrates compatible with bronchopneumonia. Sputum Gram's stain showed few neutrophils and no predominant organism. The most appropriate initial antibiotic regimen is

A. Ampicillin-sulbactam.
B. Cefuroxime-erythromycin.
C. Ceftazidime-tobramycin.
D. Clindamycin-ceftazidime.

Answers

Chapter 54

1. **A.** Noncardiogenic edema results from increased pulmonary vascular permeability, and fluid that accumulates in the interstitial compartment reflects this increased protein concentration compared with hydrostatic edema where the endothelial surface is intact. Increased protein concentration raises oncotic pressure. A decrease in the reflection coefficient for protein in the Starling equation signifies increased pulmonary vascular permeability. Changes in the pulmonary venous pressure in the setting of increased pulmonary capillary permeability can result in dramatic shifts in extravascular lung water. Protein concentration in alveolar fluid reflects the fluid in the interstitium, which has increased protein in noncardiogenic edema compared with hydrostatic edema.

Chapter 55

1. **E.** None of these agents has demonstrated efficacy in reducing mortality in ARDS in randomized placebo-controlled trials. At present there is no specific treatment for the abnormal vascular permeability characteristic of ARDS.

2. **B.** Although the chest radiograph characteristically shows diffuse abnormalities, computed tomography scans of the chest in patients with ARDS show more heterogenous distribution of pulmonary edema to dependent lung zones, possibly due to the effect of hydrostatic forces. Injury to the alveolar capillary surface interface may begin on the vascular side (e.g., endotoxinemia) or the airway side (e.g., gastric acid aspiration). Although neutrophils are important in some animal models with ARDS, normal neutrophil number and function are not a prerequisite for ARDS in patients, presumably due to other tissue and circulating inflammatory and phagocytic cells and cytokines. The edema, inflammation, and hemorrhage in ARDS decrease and denature surfactant, resulting in worse alveolar collapse and shunt.

Chapter 56

1. **D.** Most studies support no clear role for theophylline administration in the emergency room treatment of acute asthma. Theophyllines do not affect the rate of improvement and eventual emergency room outcome (admission to the

hospital or discharge to home). They also are no more effective than is treatment with beta-adrenergic agonists alone and do not have any less toxicity. Adding theophylline to beta-adrenergic agonist and corticosteroid treatment of hospitalized patients may accelerate airway obstruction relief, decrease nocturnal symptoms, and enhance diaphragmatic contractility.

2. **A.** This patient has severe airway obstruction manifested by poor alveolar ventilation, high peak airway pressures, and severe gas trapping at end expiration. The most appropriate treatment is "controlled hypoventilation" to decrease peak airway pressure and gas trapping with resultant alveolar distention, thereby decreasing the risk of barotrauma while maintaining adequate oxygenation and acid-base balance. A reduction in tidal volume will decrease airway pressures and minute ventilation. Reduction in rate by change to intermittent mandatory ventilation at lower rates may also be necessary. Higher $FI0_2$ and supplemental sodium bicarbonate may be required to compensate for decreased alveolar ventilation. Introducing applied PEEP to a patient with severe air trapping and intrinsic PEEP may facilitate machine triggering by spontaneous ventilatory effort, but "weaning" is inappropriate at this point, and applied PEEP will likely increase peak airway pressures. Increasing minute ventilation will worsen the risk of barotrauma, and a lower PCO_2 is not necessary at this point. Paralysis may rarely be necessary in treating status asthmaticus. The combination of a neuromuscular blockade and corticosteroids associated with paralyzed neuromuscular weakness should be avoided in these patients whenever possible.

Chapter 57

1. **B.** Cefuroxime covers the most likely pathogens in this patient including pneumococcus, *Haemophilus influenzae* and *Moraxella catarrhalis.* Beta-lactamase production is common in hospital isolates of *H. influenzae* (15–30%) and in *M. catarrhalis* infection (70–80%). This Gram's stain is most suggestive of *M. catarrhalis.* Ampicillin is not an effective agent in beta-lactamase–producing strains, and penicillin and erythromycin will not adequately cover the gram-negative possibilities.

Chapter 58

1. **C.** Pseudocholinesterase deficiency prolongs the action of succinylcholine, the only commonly used depolarizing neuromuscular blocker. Pancuronium is a nondepolarizing neuromuscular blocker and is not degraded by pseudocholinesterase. Approximately 1 of 3000 persons is homozygous for pseudocholinesterase deficiency. Pancuronium and its metabolites are primarily renally excreted, and prolonged neuromuscular block has been associated with concomitant renal failure. Myopathy has also been associated with pancuronium use; this has been described most commonly in association with corticosteroid use. Excessive doses of neuromuscular blocker could also be responsible, since most reports identify patients who were not closely monitored with peripheral nerve stimulation as having an increased risk of excessive medication.

2. **A.** Plasma exchange in patients with Guillain-Barré syndrome accelerates recovery and decreases time on mechanical ventilation if done early in the

disease course. Intravenous immunoglobulin G may be just as effective. Corticosteroids and azathioprine have not been shown to be effective in Guillain-Barré syndrome. Pyridostigmine is an anticholinesterase that is useful in treating myasthenia gravis, which also responds acutely to plasmapheresis when patients present with an exacerbation. Pyridostigmine has no role in Guillain-Barré syndrome.

Chapter 59

1. **B.** The patient has likely suffered an amniotic fluid embolism, which characteristically occurs during labor and delivery or the early puerperium. The cause of hypoxemia is often noncardiogenic edema. Disseminated intravascular coagulation (DIC) is also characteristic and occurs in up to 50 percent of patients with amniotic fluid embolism. Multiparous patients and those undergoing cesarean section are at increased risk. Although thrombotic pulmonary embolism is possible, the associated findings suggestive of DIC make this less likely. The patient has no history of vomiting or aspiration, and this sudden change in her status would be unlikely to be due to aspiration without a more obvious or witnessed event. Clinically significant air embolism is possible during normal labor and delivery but very uncommon.

2. **D.** The V/Q scan shows a high probability for pulmonary embolism, and the duplex ultrasound is positive for a nonocclusive thrombus. One could make an argument over the necessity of the V/Q scan under these circumstances, but the radiation exposure is low. Warfarin crosses the placenta and is associated with increased risk of fetal hemorrhage and birth defects. It is contraindicated throughout pregnancy. Heparin is the drug of choice and should be given IV initially for 10 to 14 days followed by adjusted-dosed subcutaneous heparin to maintain the partial thromboplastin time at 1.5 to 2.5 times control. Inferior vena cava filter placement is not indicated unless anticoagulation fails. Thrombolytic drugs are not indicated for a hemodynamically stable patient with a nonocclusive thrombus.

Chapter 60

1. **B.** This patient is at high risk for deep venous thrombosis and pulmonary embolism, and the change in symptoms and subsequent test results are consistent with the latter diagnosis. A V/Q lung scan will be indeterminate given the chest x-ray findings, so a pulmonary arteriogram would almost certainly be necessary to document pulmonary embolism. However, positive noninvasive lower extremity studies specifying the presence of proximal lower extremity deep venous thrombosis will dictate similar treatment to document pulmonary embolism (i.e., systemic anticoagulation). Thus, this would be the most appropriate next step for this otherwise stable patient. If negative, pulmonary arteriogram would be indicated. Such would be the case if all proximal lower extremity clots have already embolized, or the source of the clot in the patient may be in the pelvis.

2. **False.** The chest radiograph in acute pulmonary embolus is usually abnormal, but the findings are nonspecific in the vast majority of patients and rarely diagnostic.

3. **False.** Sinus tachycardia is the most common arrhythmia in acute pulmonary embolus. New onset atrial fibrillation occurs in less than 5 percent of patients.

4. **True.** Most patients with acute pulmonary embolism are hypoxemic with a widened $P(A\text{-}a)O_2$, but occasional patients will have a normal PaO_2 and $P(A\text{-}a)O_2$.

5. **False.** Although most patients with a high-probability lung scan have a pulmonary embolus, most patients with pulmonary embolus do not have a high-probability scan. Low- and intermediate-probability scans are more common and cannot be dismissed.

6. **True.** Warfarin is the most commonly prescribed chronic therapy for venous thromboembolism, and the dosage should be titrated to an INR of 2 to 3 for maximal efficacy and safety.

7. **False.** Thrombolytic therapy hastens clot resolution acutely in most patients and may be indicated in those presenting with hemodynamic instability. Hypoxemia, unless severe or refractory, is not necessarily an indication for thrombolysis unless associated with hemodynamic instability.

Chapter 61

1. **C.** Massive hemoptysis in the patient is most likely secondary to bronchiectasis, and the source of the bleeding is probably from the bronchial arterial supply. Despite the nondiagnostic nature of the bronchoscopy, bronchial arteriography can likely localize the bleeding site if this bleeding continues. Embolization of a bleeding vessel will stop bleeding over 90 percent of the time. Even if a definitive bleeding site is not identified, empiric embolization of a large bronchial vessel may be successful. Because the bleeding is likely bronchial, pulmonary angiography would not be helpful. Thoracotomy and right upper lobectomy would not be appropriate in this patient who does not have preoperative localization, and it is unlikely that a CT scan would be helpful in this case. Selective intubation may be necessary in exsanguinating bleeding when localization is more definite, but it is not appropriate here.

Chapter 63

1. **A.** Experimentally, freshwater aspiration inactivates surfactant, leading to atelectasis, shunt, and hypoxemia. Fresh water also damages type II pneumocytes, leading to subsequent decreased surfactant production. Hypertonic sea water does not appear to directly inactivate or denature surfactant. Hemoconcentration and severe electrolyte disorders are uncommon in human seawater near-drowning due to limited volume of fluid actually aspirated.

2. **C.** Noncardiogenic edema is common after freshwater near-drowning. Laryngospasm as the cause of hypoxemia occurs in only 10 to 15 percent of near-drowning victims. Others aspirate fluid as the primary cause of hypoxemia. Severe hyponatremia and other electrolyte abnormalities are uncommon due to the limited amount of fluid aspirated. Metabolic acidosis is common post-resuscitation due to tissue hypoxia and cardiovascular abnormalities.

Chapter 64

1. A. In left heart failure, the pulmonary artery occlusion pressure and the pulmonary artery diastolic pressure will both be elevated. Assuming there is no significant pulmonary vascular disease, the gradient between the two pressures should be minimal. All the other diseases listed imply that the pulmonary artery diastolic pressure will be significantly higher than the pulmonary artery occlusion pressure. Even in pulmonary venoocclusive disease, the pulmonary artery occlusion pressure is usually normal, since the "wedged" catheter tip measures downstream pressures in larger veins, which are connected to vascular beds of obstructed vessels but not affected themselves.

Chapter 65

1. B. Esophageal rupture dictates immediate operative intervention. Less aggressive or delayed approaches are associated with increased mortality. Endoscopy is relatively contraindicated given the diagnostic radiographic study, and this procedure may further enlarge the esophageal defect, making surgical repair more difficult.

2. B. This patient shows manifestations of pressure (volume)–induced lung injury and is at high risk for pneumothorax. It is important to attempt to decrease airway pressure by whatever means possible and safe. Decreasing pressure relief and decreasing PEEP will decrease airway pressures but will also likely decrease minute ventilation by decreasing tidal volume. The patient's acid-base status can tolerate a mild to moderate respiratory acidosis, however, and this is preferable to the current situation. Increasing the I:E ratio will increase mean airway pressure and may result in air trapping, and the patient's oxygenation does not demand extreme measures to improve oxygenation at this time. There is no indication to increase rate at the current time, and air trapping could also result from increased rate.

3. D. The patient's oxygenation and acid-base status are stable, and his lung appears to be expanded. There is no urgent need to intervene operatively. Medication-induced pleurodesis is rarely effective in closing a bronchopleural fistula on mechanical ventilation. Increasing chest tube suction is not indicated and may make the fistula worse. Examples of successful bronchoscopically directed occlusion of a bronchus leading to a bronchopleural fistula have been reported, but the overall efficacy is uncertain, and the procedure is not appropriate at this time. If this patient's lung function improves and he can be successfully weaned from positive-pressure ventilation, his fistula may spontaneously close.

Chapter 66

1. A. Pressure-support is a pressure-limited breath triggered by patient effort. Airway pressure is preset, and flow, volume, and rate are dependent variables. Inspiratory flow in pressure-support ventilation is triggered off when it decreases to a certain level below the initial value.

2. A. PEEP decreases intrapulmonary shunt by recruiting previously atelectatic airless alveoli, which increases functional residual capacity and improves ventilation-perfusion matching. Peak and mean airway pressures rise when PEEP is applied to patients with acute respiratory distress syndrome. Extravascular lung water is redistributed in the lung by PEEP but not reduced.

3. **D.** Patients with severe intrinsic PEEP and subsequent dynamic hyperinflation and airway compression at end expiration must generate negative airway pressure sufficient to overcome this positive recoil pressure to trigger an inspiratory cycle during weaning. This could be extremely difficult for some patients and can dramatically increase the work of breathing. The application of extrinsic PEEP at 50 to 75 percent of measured intrinsic PEEP counterbalances the positive recoil pressure present at end expiration without significantly affecting expiratory flow-volume events and decreases the magnitude of negative pressure necessary to initiate inspiratory flow for patients making spontaneous efforts. This level of applied pressure will not necessarily alter alveolar distention or lung compliance. Peak airway pressure also may not change, but it will not fall. If airway pressure does rise significantly, the applied PEEP is probably in excess of the intrinsic PEEP and should be reduced.

Chapter 67

1. **C.** Respiratory muscle fatigue is the likely etiology of "failure to wean" patients after prolonged mechanical ventilation. Nutritional, metabolic, and electrolyte disturbances may all affect respiratory muscle function. Excessive work, superimposed illness affecting oxygen delivery or consumption by respiratory muscles, and associated cardiovascular disease will also impact muscle function. Careful attention to mechanical ventilatory support with gradual reduction in ventilator assistance while monitoring for signs of respiratory muscle fatigue in those patients is essential.

2. **A.** Based on this patient's f/TV ratio, spontaneous tidal volume, respiratory rate, and negative inspiratory force, he can probably be weaned and extubated rapidly.

Chapter 68

1. **B.** This diver is possibly suffering from lung volume expansion, often due to breath-holding during ascent. From 40 feet to the surface, lung volume will double if gas is not vented by exhalation during ascent. Symptoms of lung damage occur immediately at the surface. Gas can enter the pulmonary veins and cause systemic gas embolism. Other forms of pulmonary barotrauma may also occur. Immediate recompression may be lifesaving.

Chapter 69

1. **E.** Administration of a helium (40%)–oxygen (60%) mixture to a patient with severe airway obstruction may improve oxygenation and ventilation due to decreased airway turbulence. There is no evidence that a larger dose of methylprednisolone is more effective. Increasing beta-agonist dosage or drugs is relatively contraindicated due to the tachycardia. Supplemental bicarbonate may be appropriate if the patient becomes hemodynamically unstable trying to

maintain an arterial pH above 7.2. Increasing the tidal volume will increase airway pressure and place the patient at even more risk of barotrauma.

Chapter 71

1. **A.** The formation of carboxyhemoglobin results in increased affinity of the remaining sites for oxygen, shifting the oxyhemoglobin curve to the left. Total oxygen-carrying capacity is decreased, however, due to the higher affinity of carbon monoxide for the hemoglobin. Oxidative metabolism is decreased, partly related to the binding of carbon monoxide to cytochromes, interrupting the electron transport chain.

2. **B.** Noncardiogenic edema may develop several hours after significant NO_2 exposure. Poor water solubility of NO_2 results in few signs of upper airway or laryngeal edema or inflammation. Eosinophilia is not characteristic. The disease is caused by direct toxicity and not hypersensitivity.

3. **D.** Most smoke inhalation fatalities are related to severe carbon monoxide poisoning, sometimes associated with cyanide toxicity. Pulmonary edema may occur late, depending on the particular vapor exposure. Direct heat injury is usually confined to the upper airway and may occasionally cause significant problems with laryngeal edema and obstruction.

Chapter 72

1. **True.**

2. **False.**

3. **True.**

4. **True.**

The shivering phase of hypothermia usually occurs in the 35 to 30° C range. Physiologic changes include marked increases in heat production, oxygen consumption, and metabolic rate. Cardiac output changes very little, however. Increased consumption without concomitant increased carbon monoxide leads to a residual mixed venous oxygen and lactic acidosis.

5. **True.**

6. **False.**

7. **False.**

8. **False.**

Compliance, airway resistance, lung volume, and $P(A\text{-}a)O_2$ change little with hypothermia. Minute ventilation increases due to increased oxygen demand during shivering.

9. **D.** Despite decreased blood pressure and glomerular filtration rate, urine output is maintained in hypothermia ("cold diuresis") due to tubular defects in

reabsorption, resulting in diluted urine. Additional stimuli for this effect may be the triggering of volume receptors as the central volume is increased in response to peripheral vasoconstriction and possibly an insensitivity to antidiuretic hormone. The white blood cell count may be slightly elevated in mild hypothermia but is characteristically low at temperatures below 28°C, and absolute neutropenia may result. Mild hyperglycemia is a common finding due to decreased insulin release, peripheral insulin resistance, and increased counterregulatory hormones. Subclinical pancreatitis is common, perhaps partly related to alcohol ingestion in some patients.

Chapter 73

1. **C.**

2. **A.**

3. **D.**

4. **C.**

5. **C.**

6. **B.**

7. **B.**

8. **B.**

Malignant hyperthermia (MH) and neuroleptic malignant syndrome (NMS) are characterized by excessive thermogenesis due to uncontrolled muscle contraction. Rhabdomyolysis is common in both disorders. MH is caused by a calcium transport defect in skeletal muscle triggered by exposure to general anesthetics or succinylcholine and is inherited as an autosomal dominant trait with variable penetrance. NMS results from hypersensitivity of dopaminergic receptors in the hypothalamus as a result of agents designed to block dopamine receptors or the withdrawal of drugs with dopaminergic effects. Extrapyramidal reactions are common in NMS. Dantrolene is a direct muscle relaxant and is effective in both conditions. Bromocriptine increases central dopaminergic tone, which decreases the central drive, muscle rigidity, and thermogenesis. Pancuronium will relax muscle in NMS but not MH because of the postsynaptic etiology of the muscle rigidity in the latter syndrome.

Chapter 74

1. **C.** Prospective series identify bacterial pneumonia as the most common among this group. These pneumonias usually present in the typical fashion. Bronchitis may be found to be even more common if careful histories are taken. *M. tuberculosis* is becoming more common owing to increased numbers of injection drug users in the human immunodeficiency virus (HIV)–infected population and the problem of isoniazid resistance in some communities. *M. avium-intracellulare* rarely represents an important pulmonary pathogen in patients with AIDS.

2. **A.** Patients with severe PCP have shown improved symptoms, better oxygenation, and increased survival with the early addition of steroids to effective antimicrobial therapy. The usual starting dosage is equivalent to prednisone, 80 mg/kg/day tapered over 21 days. The beneficial effect is presumably secondary to diminished inflammatory response to killed organisms. There is no indication at this point to abandon first-line PCP treatment or to entertain alternative diagnoses.

Chapter 75

1. **D.** *H. influenzae* is the most common identifiable infectious cause of acute epiglottitis in adults.

2. **A.** This patient has a submandibular space infection as a complication of an odontogenic infection. He will require additional imaging studies such as a neck computed tomography scan to demonstrate the extent of infection and to search for any drainable abscess. These infections are usually polymicrobial, reflecting the common mouth flora of streptococcal and oral anaerobes. Some oral anaerobes show increasing resistance to penicillin, and a common oral gram-negative anaerobe, *Eikenella corrodens*, is also resistant to clindamycin. Penicillin G is the best drug to cover the aerobic streptococci, and metronidazole is the best agent for anaerobes. This patient is at low risk for enteric gram-negative rod or *S. aureus* infection; thus, an initial antibiotic selection aimed at this spectrum is unnecessary.

Chapter 76

1. **B.** Sucralfate use has not been associated with nosocomial pneumonia, although some studies have shown an increased pneumonia rate in association with H_2-antagonist and liquid antacid use. The other factors listed have been associated with nosocomial pneumonia in most studies. Other cited conditions include recent thoracic or abdominal surgery, head injury, shock, systemic antibiotic use, and duration of mechanical ventilation.

2. **A.** Concomitant antibiotic use in suspected pneumonia results in increased false-negative findings for any invasive diagnostic procedure. BAL can diagnose nonbacterial infectious diseases, most notably *Pneumocystis carinii* and cytomegalovirus. There is poor discrimination between airway and parenchymal infection by culture. No studies have shown an impact from bronchoscopy on the outcome of patients with suspected nosocomial pneumonia.

3. **D.** The nasogastric tube itself may result in some incompetence of the lower esophageal sphincter, and neutralization of gastric acid by feedings may result in increased gram-negative rod colonization. Whether gross aspiration is more common in gastric versus small-bowel feeding is unclear. Maintenance of proper positioning in the semierect posture and close monitoring of gastric volume are probably important factors. Problems with gastric atony in critically ill and postoperative patients make small-bowel feeding more efficient in many patients, with more consistent results in attaining nutritional goals.

4. **A.** Most studies have shown a decreased rate of pneumonia in patients treated with SDD, but not all. Despite this, convincing evidence of decreased

length of stay in the ICU or decreased overall mortality is lacking. Recent studies have documented increased resistant bacterial strains and a trend toward increased pneumonia from these organisms. There should be heightened concern over potential changes in hospital flora resistance if routine use of SDD is initiated in a significant number of ICU patients. Therefore, despite some positive trends in pneumonia incidence rates overall, more information is needed before this technique can be recommended.

5. B. This patient has a severe community-acquired pneumonia presenting with multilobar infiltrates and hypoxemia The clinical history and laboratory findings are nonspecific. There are no obvious risk factors for enteric gram-negative or anaerobic infection. Because of the illness severity, treatment should include a second-generation cephalosporin to cover *Haemophilus influenzae* and *Streptococcus pneumoniae* and erythromycin for the possibility of Legionella. Sputum cultures will likely be nondiagnostic based on the description of the inflammatory component seen.

V. Renal Problems in the Intensive Care Unit

78. Physiologic Concepts in the Management of Renal, Fluid, and Electrolyte Disorders in the Intensive Care Unit

1. Select the best answer. Regarding renal autoregulation:

A. The term *autoregulation* encompasses the maintenance of renal blood flow, glomerular filtration, and solute excretion.
B. Between mean arterial pressures of 60 mm Hg and 180 mm Hg, renal blood flow and glomerular filtration rate (GFR) are relatively constant.
C. Separate exogenous mechanisms regulate the autoregulation of blood flow and filtration in the kidney.
D. Diminished arterial pressure causes relaxation of the afferent arteriole and maintains glomerular blood flow.

2. True or False. Angiotensin II has different effects on renal blood flow, depending on the local and systemic concentrations.

3. Select the best answer. Regarding atrial natriuretic peptide (ANP):

A. Atrial natriuretic peptide is a single peptide isolated from cardiac myocytes.
B. When given systemically into the renal artery, ANP promotes renal vasodilatation.
C. When given intravenously into the renal artery, ANP promotes decreased GFR and a substantial increase in urinary sodium secretion.
D. ANP is not measurable in circulation.

4. True or False. Digoxin, dopamine, and glucocorticoids act as diuretic agents.

5. Select the best answer. Regarding diuretics:

A. Mannitol is a polysaccharide, freely filterable by the glomerulus, and like glucose, reabsorbable.
B. Acetazolamide activates the enzyme carbonic anhydrase, causing a loss of tubular hydrogen ion secretion.

C. Loop diuretics inhibit the action of sodium-potassium ATPase, enhancing sodium and chloride secretion.
D. Loop diuretics act to treat pulmonary congestion through a brisk diuresis.

79. Disorders of Plasma Sodium and Plasma Potassium

1. True or False. The syndrome of inappropriate antidiuretic hormone (ADH) secretion is characterized by plasma hypoosmolality with urinary osmolality above 100 to 150 mOsm per kilogram, normal adrenal, renal, and thyroid function, hyperkalemia, and normal acid-base balance.

2. Select the best answer. Regarding diabetes insipidus:

A. A glucose-induced osmotic diuresis is one form of diabetes insipidus.
B. Primary polydipsia, central diabetes insipidus, and nephrogenic diabetes insipidus cannot be differentiated on biochemical grounds.
C. Hypernatremia is common in diabetes insipidus and is a diagnostic criterion.
D. In central diabetes insipidus, both ADH release and thirst mechanisms may be impaired, leading to sodium concentrations that can exceed 160 mEq per liter.

3. True or False. Hyperkalemia occurs in up to one-half of patients treated with amphotericin B.

80. Metabolic Acidosis and Metabolic Alkalosis

1. True or False. The administration of sodium chloride is an effective treatment for chloride-resistant metabolic alkalosis after adequate repletion with potassium.

81. Acute Renal Failure in the Intensive Care Unit

1. True or False. The general management of acute renal failure involves utilization of definitive intensive care unit modes of therapy.

2. Select the best answer. Regarding hemodialysis:

A. Observations suggest an important interaction between initiation of dialysis and the maintenance of residual renal function.
B. Preserving residual renal function is of modest benefit only in the management of patients with advanced renal insufficiency.
C. Residual renal function is of minimal importance for clearance of larger solutes of greater than 500 daltons.
D. It is less important to preserve residual renal function for patients on peritoneal dialysis than it is for patients who are on hemodialysis.

Answers

Chapter 78

1. **D.** The term *autoregulation* encompasses the maintenance of renal blood flow and GFR over a wide range of arterial pressures between 80 mm Hg and 200 mm Hg. Separate mechanisms regulate blood flow and GFR, but both appear to be intrinsic to the kidney. Diminished arterial pressure causes relaxation of the afferent arteriole and maintenance of glomerular blood flow in this fashion.

2. **True.** Angiotensin II appears to selectively operate at the efferent sphincter or arteriole when locally produced. At higher circulating levels, sufficient to raise systemic blood pressure, angiotensin II also causes afferent vasoconstriction.

3. **B.** A series of peptides known collectively as atrial natriuretic peptide, isolated from cardiac myocytes, have been purified and sequenced. When given intravenously, or directly into the renal artery, ANP promotes mild renal vasodilatation, an increase in GFR, and a substantial increase in urinary sodium excretion. The substance is measurable in the circulation and appears to be released by atrial stretch or an increase in plasma volume.

4. **False.** Diuretics promote the excretion of water by acting along distinct nephron sites. Agents such as digoxin, dopamine, and glucocorticoids enhance glomerular filtration and increase urine flow but are pharmacologically distinct from diuretics.

5. **C.** In the thick portion of the ascending limb of the loop of Henle, sodium and potassium cross the luminal cell membrane with two chlorides. The loop diuretics inhibit this cotransport system, thereby enhancing sodium and chloride secretion. Mannitol is a polysaccharide, freely filterable by the glomerulus, but unlike glucose, it is not reabsorbable. Its osmotic activity thus constrains fluid absorption by the proximal nephron. Acetazolamide is secreted into the proximal nephron from the peritubular capillaries by a potent organic acid transport pathway. It inactivates the enzyme carbonic anhydrase, which catalyzes the conversion of carbon dioxide and water into bicarbonate. The loop diuretics stimulate renal prostaglandin synthesis, thereby increasing renal blood flow. The loop diuretics increase systemic venous capacitance, reduce cardiac preload, and lower left ventricular end-diastolic pressure within 5 minutes of intravenous administration. This effect precedes the diuretic effect and can occur in anephric patients. This suggests that the vasodilator effects of the loop diuretics may be responsible for their acute amelioration of pulmonary congestion.

Chapter 79

1. **False.** The syndrome of inappropriate ADH secretion is characterized by plasma hypoosmolality, urinary sodium concentration above 20 mEq per liter, normal adrenal, renal, and thyroid function, and **normal potassium** and acid-base balance.

2. **D.** Diabetes insipidus is a cause of hypernatremia that must be differentiated from other polyuric states. Specifically, in the absence of glucose-induced os-

motic diuresis in uncontrolled diabetes, the primary sources of true polyuria (> 3 liters/day) include primary polydipsia, central diabetes insipidus, and nephrogenic diabetes insipidus. Primary polydipsia is characterized by a primary increase of water intake. Thus a low plasma sodium concentration with a history of polyuria is usually indicative of primary polydipsia. A high-normal plasma sodium concentration suggests diabetes insipidus. Marked hypernatremia is uncommon with diabetes insipidus because the initial water loss stimulates the thirst mechanism. An exception to this rule occurs in patients with trauma or a central nervous system lesion that impairs both ADH release and thirst. In such patients, the plasma-sodium concentration can exceed 160 mEq per liter. Nephrogenic diabetes insipidus is characterized by normal ADH secretion but varying degrees of renal resistance to ADH.

3. **False.** **Hypokalemia** occurs in up to one-half of the patients treated with amphotericin B. Amphotericin B administration leads to an increase in membrane permeability that can promote potassium secretion from intracellular stores across the luminal membrane and into the tubular lumen. This has been shown to result from amphotericin interaction with membrane sterols.

Chapter 80

1. **True.** Individuals with a urinary chloride concentration greater than 15 mEq per liter are unlikely to respond to chloride-containing solutions such as physiologic saline. The associated chloride resorptive defect in severe hypokalemia is corrected with potassium chloride supplementation. Potassium treatment will convert the chloride-resistant alkalosis to one that is responsive to sodium chloride.

Chapter 81

1. **False.** The predialysis management of acute renal failure is applicable for any patient with acute renal failure and involves simple general considerations including fluid balance, acid-base and electrolyte management, avoidance of nephrotoxin, adjustment of renally excreted drugs, restriction of protein intake, adequate carbohydrate intake, and reduction of infectious risks.

2. **A.** The influence of dialysis on residual renal function is critical. Observations have suggested an important and potentially deleterious interaction between dialysis and residual renal function. Investigators have observed that patients with posttraumatic acute renal failure treated by hemodialysis had pathologically demonstrable fresh focal areas of tubular necrosis 3 to 4 weeks after the original hemodynamic insult. Further, hemodialysis is often associated with an acute decline in urine output. The preservation of residual renal function is of significant benefit in the management of patients with advanced renal insufficiency. Even a modest preservation of urine output simplifies management of patients' volume status. For the patient on hemodialysis, the effective residual renal function is even more important for the clearance of larger solutes of over 500 daltons. For patients treated by peritoneal dialysis, which is less efficient than hemodialysis, preservation of renal function is an even more important aid in management of volume status.

VI. Infectious Disease Problems in the Intensive Care Unit

84. Approach to Fever in the Intensive Care Patient

1. Which of the following conditions is unlikely to produce fever of a noninfectious nature?

A. Acute vasculitis.
B. Subarachnoid hemorrhage.
C. Acute alcohol withdrawal.
D. Myocardial infarction.
E. Pulmonary aspiration.

85. Use of Antimicrobials in the Treatment of Infection in the Critically Ill

1. Which of the following bacteria are covered by first-generation cephalosporins?

A. Enterococci.
B. *Listeria monocytogenes.*
C. Community-acquired *Escherichia coli* infections.
D. Methicillin-resistant *Staphylococcus aureus.*
E. *Staphylococcus epidermidis.*

2. Which of the following statements concerning cefoxitin is false?

A. It is less potent than first-generation cephalosporins against *S. aureus.*
B. It is active against most strains of *Proteus* and *E. coli.*
C. It is usually effective against anaerobes.
D. It is a good single-agent choice for enterococcal infections.
E. It is actually a cephamycin.

86. Prevention and Control of Nosocomial Infection in the Intensive Care Unit

1. Which of the following organisms is **not** commonly observed to be etiologic in nosocomial infections?

A. *Escherichia coli.*
B. Human immunodeficiency virus (HIV).
C. *Serratia marcescens*
D. Methicillin-resistant *Staphylococcus aureus.*
E. *Candida albicans.*

2. The patient factor that correlates most with the development of nosocomial infection includes:

A. Shock on admission.
B. The presence of invasive monitoring devices.
C. Immunosuppression.
D. Renal insufficiency.
E. All of the above.

3. Which of the following decreases the rate of bacterial transmission in nosocomial infections?

A. Intensive care unit design.
B. Handwashing.
C. Prophylactic antibiotics.
D. Laminar flow environments.
E. Negative-pressure patient rooms.

4. Which of the following are common etiologic agents in nosocomial pneumonias?

A. Gram-negative bacilli.
B. Polymicrobial bacterial populations.
C. *S. aureus.*
D. *Pseudomonas* species.
E. All of the above.

5. Which of the following is the most significant factor predisposing to the development of nosocomial pneumonia?

A. Antacid use.
B. Nasogastric intubation.
C. Endotracheal intubation.
D. Sucralfate use.
E. H_2-blocker use.

6. Which of the following measures is most effective at preventing the spread of *Clostridium difficile*?

A. Vinyl gloves.
B. Handwashing.
C. Prophylactic vancomycin.

D. Prophylactic metronidazole.
E. Avoiding clindamycin use.

87. *Central Nervous System Infections*

1. The most common organism responsible for bacterial meningitis among older children and young adults is

A. *Haemophilus influenzae.*
B. *Neisseria meningitidis.*
C. *Streptococcus pneumoniae.*
D. *Listeria monocytogenes.*
E. *Staphylococcus aureus.*

2. Which of the following statements concerning bacterial meningitis is true?

A. A normal cerebrospinal glucose level eliminates the possibility of bacterial meningitis.
B. Aztreonam is a reasonable choice for initial empiric therapy of bacterial meningitis.
C. Dexamethasone therapy is contraindicated in meningitis.
D. Patients with cerebrospinal fluid (CSF) shunts or intracranial pressure monitoring devices who develop meningitis should **always** have them removed to optimize the chances for cure.
E. Respiratory isolation is recommended for patients with meningococcal or *H. influenzae* meningitis.

3. The most reliable and definitive way to prove the presence of herpes simplex encephalitis (HSE) is

A. The detection of antibodies to herpes simplex virus in blood.
B. The detection of antibodies to herpes simplex virus in CSF.
C. Electroencephalography.
D. The demonstration of viral antigen or recovery of virus in brain tissue obtained at biopsy.
E. Computed tomography scan.

88. *Infective Endocarditis*

1. A 46-year-old male intravenous drug user presented with obtundation and fever. Physical examination revealed evidence of emaciation, the presence of splinter hemorrhages and petechiae on the plantar surface of the toes and the buccal mucosa, and a mitral regurgitant murmur. Laboratory data included the findings of a hemoglobin of 9.6 gm per deciliter and a serum creatinine of 2.3 mg per deciliter. Computed tomography of the brain was consistent with an acute infarction in the middle cerebral artery distribution. Blood cultures were repeatedly positive for *Streptococcus bovis*. Which of the following conditions should be considered in this patient?

A. Bacterial endocarditis.
B. Gastrointestinal malignancy.

C. Both.
D. Neither.

2. Which of the following organisms is most likely to infect a previously normal heart valve?

A. *Salmonella typhimurium.*
B. *Staphylococcus aureus.*
C. *Candida albicans.*
D. *Escherichia coli.*
E. Pneumococcus.

3. Bacterial endocarditis of which valve has the worst prognosis?

A. Tricuspid.
B. Pulmonary.
C. Mitral.
D. Aortic.

4. A patient with known bacterial endocarditis is found to have a painful, tender, purplish nodule on the pad of his right great toe. This finding is known as

A. A Janeway lesion.
B. A Roth spot.
C. An Osler's node.
D. A splinter hemorrhage.
E. Takayasu's arteritis.

5. Most cases of bacterial endocarditis require how many blood cultures for their detection?

A. One.
B. Two.
C. Three.
D. Four or more.

89. Infections Associated with Vascular Catheters

1. Which of the following agents has been shown to be most effective at preventing intravascular catheter-associated infections?

A. Skin disinfection with 70% alcohol.
B. Prophylactic administration of intravenous clindamycin.
C. Skin disinfection with 2% aqueous chlorhexidine.
D. Prophylactic administration of intravenous penicillin.
E. Skin disinfection with 10% povidone-iodine solution.

2. Which of the following conditions provides the greatest risk for the development of catheter-related sepsis?

A. Using gauze dressings instead of transparent dressings.
B. Failing to use an antiseptic ointment over the insertion site.
C. Changing the infusion set every 72 hours instead of every 24 hours.

D. Leaving the catheter in place for longer than 72 hours.
E. None of the above.

3. Which of the following statements concerning catheter-related infections is true?

A. Arterial catheters should only be suspected of being infected if they show signs of local inflammation.
B. Coagulase-negative staphylococci are the organisms most commonly associated with catheter-related infections.
C. *Candida* and *Malasezzia* species are uncommonly associated with infections of total parenteral nutrition catheters.
D. Excision of the vein should never be employed in cases of suppurative thrombophlebitis.
E. All cases of catheter-related sepsis should be treated with a 2-week course of the appropriate antibiotic for the organism(s) isolated.

90. Urinary Tract Infections

1. Which of the following statements concerning catheter-associated urinary tract infection (UTI) is false?

A. Removal of the catheter results in eradication of the infection in only 15 percent of patients.
B. Low bacterial colony counts in patients with urinary catheters will progress to high-grade bacteriuria in the majority of patients who do not receive suppressive antimicrobial therapy.
C. Polymicrobial bacteriuria occurs in over 15 percent of patients with catheter-related UTI.
D. Bacterial colony counts in the urine of less than 10^5 colony-forming units (CFU) per milliliter can allow the urinary tract to be safely disregarded as a potential source of active infection in the catheterized patient.
E. None of the above.

2. UTI associated with the use of indwelling urinary catheters in critically ill patients can best be prevented by

A. Effective meatal care with the application of antimicrobial povidone-iodine solution or topical polyantimicrobic ointments.
B. Avoiding catheterization where possible.
C. Using Silastic urinary catheters instead of latex catheters.
D. The use of systemic antimicrobial prophylaxis.
E. None of the above.

3. Which of the following statements concerning *Candida* infection of the urinary tract is true?

A. The isolation of *Candida* species from a sample of urine confirms the presence of invasive candidiasis and should be treated aggressively.
B. The finding of urinary casts made up of *Candida* elements indicates invasive upper tract candidiasis.
C. Bladder irrigation with 50 mg of amphotericin B in 1000 ml of sterile water is safe, effective, and nontoxic in eradicating *Candida* infections of the bladder.

D. Systemic amphotericin B should be avoided in treating patients who are found to have fungus balls within the urinary collecting system.
E. Fluconazole has been shown to be ineffective in the treatment of *Candida* cystitis.

91. Life-Threatening Community-Acquired Infections

1. The differential diagnosis of toxic shock syndrome should include all but which of the following conditions?

A. Rocky Mountain spotted fever.
B. Meningococcemia.
C. Acute pelvic inflammatory disease.
D. Streptococcal scarlet fever.
E. Rubeola.

2. Which of the following is specific treatment for Rocky Mountain spotted fever?

A. Penicillin.
B. Aztreonam.
C. Doxycycline.
D. Imipenem.
E. Ceftazidime.

3. The major host defense against invasive meningococcal infection is represented by

A. Basophil activity.
B. CD4 lymphocytes.
C. Eosinophils.
D. The complement system.
E. Antibody production.

92. Acute Infection in the Immunocompromised Host

1. Which of the following infections is associated with defects in cell-mediated immunity?

A. *Pneumocystis carinii.*
B. *Streptococcus pneumoniae.*
C. *Haemophilus influenzae.*
D. *Pseudomonas aeruginosa.*
E. *Neisseria meningiditis.*

2. In an immunocompromised patient, bacteremia without an obvious source is most likely arising from which of the following sources?

A. Intravenous catheters.

B. Foley catheter.
C. Gastrointestinal tract.
D. Lungs.
E. Surgical wound.

3. Which of the following is not an acceptable broad-spectrum antibiotic regimen for use in the neutropenic patient with a fever from an unknown source?

A. Ceftazidime and tobramycin.
B. Imipenem.
C. Aztreonam, tobramycin, and vancomycin.
D. Clindamycin and vancomycin.
E. Piperacillin and amikacin.

93. Acquired Immunodeficiency Syndrome

1. Which of the following is the target cell line for human immunodeficiency virus type one (HIV-l) infection?

A. Monocytes.
B. Gastrointestinal cells.
C. CD4 lymphocytes.
D. Neurons.
E. All of the above.

2. Pancreatitis may develop in patients with acquired immunodeficiency syndrome (AIDS) as a result of which of the following medications?

(1) Didanosine (dideoxyinosine, DDI).
(2) Zidovudine (azidothymidine, AZT).
(3) Zalcitabine (dideoxycytidine, DDC).
(4) Acyclovir.

A. 1, 2, and 3.
B. 1 and 3 only.
C. 2 and 4 only.
D. All of the above.
E. None of the above.

3. A 36-year-old man known to have AIDS presented with a headache and altered mental status. A computed tomography (CT) scan of the brain performed with contrast revealed the presence of a ring-enhancing lesion in the basal ganglia. Which of the following is the most appropriate next step?

A. A magnetic resonance image (MRI) of the brain should be obtained to determine if other lesions exist.
B. A lumbar puncture should be performed.
C. A neurosurgeon should be consulted for possible biopsy of the lesion.
D. Presumptive therapy for toxoplasmosis should be started.
E. Transvascular embolization under fluoroscopic guidance should be attempted.

94. Infectious Complications of Drug Abuse

1. Endocarditis developing as a consequence of intravenous drug abuse typically involves which heart valve?

A. Tricuspid.
B. Pulmonic.
C. Mitral.
D. Aortic.
E. All are affected in equal proportions.

2. The most common infectious cause for a drug user to require hospital admission is

A. Human immunodeficiency virus (HIV).
B. Hepatitis A.
C. Hepatitis B.
D. Hepatitis C.
E. *Candida*.

3. Which of the following is not a common pulmonary complication of intravenous drug abusers?

A. Acute pulmonary edema.
B. Unilateral bacterial pneumonia.
C. Septic pulmonary emboli.
D. Tuberculosis.
E. AIDS-related pulmonary infections.

95. Tuberculosis

1. Which of the following statements concerning the current status of tuberculosis in the United States is true?

A. The incidence of active cases of tuberculosis is rising.
B. The incidence of active cases of tuberculosis is declining.
C. The incidence of tuberculosis has been unaffected by the human immunodeficiency virus (HIV) epidemic.
D. The incidence of active cases of tuberculosis is stable.
E. The incidence of multidrug-resistant tuberculosis is stable.

2. Which of the following statements regarding tuberculosis of the central nervous system is true?

A. The finding of an elevated spinal fluid glucose concentration excludes the possibility of tuberculosis of the central nervous system.
B. Tuberculomas of the central nervous system are readily detected by computed tomography.
C. Tuberculomas of the central nervous system are rarely detected by magnetic resonance imaging.

D. The number of spinal taps does not increase the likelihood of obtaining a positive specimen for acid-fast bacilli.
E. None of the above.

3. Antibiotic agents that have activity against *Mycobacterium tuberculosis* include

A. Ciprofloxacin.
B. Gentamicin.
C. Rifampin.
D. Isoniazid.
E. All of the above.

96. Botulism

1. Which of the following conditions is necessary for the germination of *Clostridium botulinum* spores?

A. Low humidity.
B. High temperature (>39°C).
C. Anaerobic conditions.
D. A pH less than 4.0.
E. Oxygen.

2. Which of the following is the site of action of the *C. botulinum* toxin?

A. Cortical motor strip.
B. Medulla oblongata.
C. Spinal cord.
D. Autonomic ganglia.
E. Neuromuscular junction.

3. In a patient who has signs of botulism, the most sensitive indicator of the need for mechanical ventilation is

A. PaO_2.
B. Vital capacity.
C. Respiratory rate.
D. Dead space–to–tidal volume ratio.
E. Intrapulmonary shunt fraction.

97. Tetanus

1. Which of the following are the major complications of tetanus?
(1) Respiratory paralysis.
(2) Paralytic ileus.
(3) Cardiac arrhythmias.
(4) Hypocalcemia.

A. 1, 2, and 3.
B. 1 and 3 only.

C. 2 and 4 only.
D. All of the above.
E. None of the above.

2. Which of the following drugs is **not** often useful in the management of a patient with generalized tetanus?

A. Diazepam.
B. Meperidine.
C. Propranolol.
D. Baclofen.
E. Penicillin G.

3. Which of the following treatments is necessary in **all** cases of tetanus?

(1) Clindamycin.
(2) Human tetanus immune globulin.
(3) Flagyl.
(4) Tetanus toxoid.
(5) Penicillin.

A. 1, 2, and 3.
B. 1 and 3 only.
C. 2 and 4 only.
D. All of the above.
E. None of the above.

Answers

Chapter 84

1. E. Many noninfectious conditions can cause fever in intensive care unit patients, although acute bacterial infections are certainly the most common and serious causes of fever in critically ill patients. Many cardiovascular conditions can be associated with a noninfectious fever, such as acute vasculitis, dissection of an aortic aneurysm, mesenteric ischemia, deep venous thrombophlebitis, pulmonary embolism, or myocardial infarction. Also, hemorrhage into certain areas, such as the central nervous system, retroperitoneum, joint spaces, or lung, can cause temperature elevations. Certain metabolic conditions such as heat stroke, malignant hyperthermia, hyperthyroidism, adrenal insufficiency, and alcohol withdrawal can produce fevers. In alcohol withdrawal, it is important to exclude the possibility of pulmonary aspiration producing a fever from an infectious cause because of the frequent association of such aspiration with the syndrome of chronic alcoholism.

Chapter 85

1. C. First-generation cephalosporins are usually very effective against a number of gram-positive aerobes, with some notable exceptions. Methicillin-resistant strains of staphylococci, such as methicillin-resistant *S. aureus*, are usually also resistant to first-generation cephalosporins. Similarly, *S. epidermidis* is also frequently (roughly 50 percent of strains) resistant to methicillin and will share this resistance with first-generation cephalosporins. Importantly, enterococcus, despite its being a gram-positive aerobe (once having been considered a streptococcal organism), is resistant to first-generation cephalosporins. *L. monocytogenes* is usually resistant to first-generation cephalosporins. Many of the community-acquired gram-negative Enterobacteriaceae are sensitive to first-generation cephalosporins, including organisms like *E. coli, Proteus mirabilis*, and even *Klebsiella pneumoniae*, although many hospital-acquired infective isolates of Enterobacteriaceae are resistant to these agents.

2. **D.** Cefoxitin is a very popular cephamycin, although it is usually classified as a second-generation cephalosporin. It has broader activity against gram-negative aerobes than do the first-generation cephalosporins, although it is much less potent against gram-positive cocci such as *S. aureus*. Many of the gram-negative Enterobacteriaceae such as *E. coli, Proteus, Providencia*, and *Klebsiella* are covered by cefoxitin. It is usually very effective against anaerobes such as *Bacteroides fragilis*. As with virtually all the cephalosporin and cephalosporin-like antibiotics, cefoxitin has no independent activity against enterococcus, although it may potentiate an aminoglycoside's activity against that organism.

Chapter 86

1. **B.** While the microbiology of nosocomial infections can vary significantly from institution to institution, a pattern of the organisms commonly involved has emerged. Gram-negative organisms tend to predominate in most clinical series of nosocomial infections, with the most common of these being *E. coli, Klebsiella* species, *Enterobacter* species, and *Serratia* species. *Pseudomonas* species can also be observed, although less frequently. Gram-positive organisms are responsible for roughly one-fifth of the nosocomial infections, led by *S. aureus*. Additionally, methicillin-resistant strains are commonly found in critically ill patients. *Candida* species are the most common fungal infections seen and appear to be increasing in their importance over recent years. Although many critically ill patients may be infected with HIV, these infections are rarely nosocomial in nature. Universal precautions help to minimize the risk of transmission, although only if health care workers change gloves in between patient contacts. Moreover, the antibody screening that is now routine in blood banks minimizes the risks of infecting hospitalized patients with this virus.

2. **E.** A large multivariate analysis performed by Craven et al. of 1300 patients admitted to adult intensive care units at Boston City Hospital revealed the presence of invasive monitoring devices (e.g., urinary catheters, intracranial pressure monitors, arterial catheters, Swan-Ganz catheters) and patient factors (shock on admission, immunosuppression, and renal insufficiency) to be strongly correlated with the ultimate development of a nosocomial infection. The length of stay in the intensive care unit was another entity that was associated with nosocomial infection, independent of device utilization.

3. **B.** Various aspects of intensive care unit design have been attempted in an effort to reduce the bacterial transmission rate in nosocomial infections, including air filters, positive- and negative-pressure rooms, laminar flow environments, and individual room temperature and humidity controls. However, all of these have had an inconsistent effect on nosocomial infection rates On the other hand, handwashing by health care workers has clearly been shown to be effective at reducing bacterial transmission.

4. E. Currently, gram-negative bacilli account for 60 to 80 percent of nosocomial pneumonias; of these, *Pseudomonas* is the most common organism. Interestingly, polymicrobial infections are quite common. Among the gram-positive organisms, *S. aureus* is most commonly seen and is second overall to *Pseudomonas* organisms.

5. C. Several factors are associated with the onset of nosocomial pneumonia. Most of them interfere with the normal barriers protecting the upper respiratory tract from bacterial invasion. The most significant of these is endotracheal intubation. After only a few days of endotracheal intubation, the upper airways are colonized with bacteria, predominantly gram-negative rods. Agents such as antacids and H_2-blockers appear to increase bacterial growth in the upper gastrointestinal tract, thus providing a larger reservoir for potential aspiration into the airways, whereas sucralfate may be effective at combating such overgrowth by preserving stomach acidity while maintaining stress gastritis prophylaxis. Nasogastric tubes may predispose to the presence of sinusitis.

6. A. *C. difficile* is responsible for the condition of pseudomembranous colitis, which can be a very severe problem and is associated with increased morbidity and costs. The colitis is produced by exotoxins elaborated by the organism. While commonly associated with clindamycin use, nearly all antibiotics have been found to be capable of altering the colonic flora sufficiently to allow *C. difficile* to emerge. Oral vancomycin or oral metronidazole is an effective treatment for the condition, although prophylactic use with these agents fails to prevent infection. Interestingly, handwashing is not effective at removing the organism from the hands of health care workers who care for patients with pseudomembranous colitis; the majority of such personnel will have positive hand cultures. Only the use of vinyl gloves by health care personnel has been shown to be effective at limiting the spread of the organism from patient to patient.

Chapter 87

1. B. The most common bacterial etiology for meningitis among older children and young adults is *N. meningitidis*, being relatively uncommon in those older than 45. *H. influenzae* had been the most common cause of bacterial meningitis in young children between the ages of 3 months and 6 years until the introduction of new vaccines reduced the infantile incidence. Among adults, *S. pneumoniae* is the most common bacterial cause. *L. monocytogenes* is more common among neonates and in immunologically compromised individuals. *S. aureus* meningitis is less commonly observed, being seen primarily in those undergoing neurosurgery or sustaining head trauma.

2. E. While extremely low CSF glucose levels (e.g., <20 mg/dl) provide strong evidence for bacterial infection, a normal level does not exclude the possibility, as 13 to 40 percent of patients with bacterial meningitis will have normal CSF glucose levels. Aztreonam can achieve bactericidal concentrations in the presence of inflamed meninges; however, clinical experience with it in the management of meningitis is limited. Furthermore, it provides no coverage against *S. pneumoniae*, a frequent causative agent of bacterial meningitis. Therefore, aztreonam should not be used as an initial empiric agent for the treatment of meningitis. Dexamethasone may be useful in patients with very severe forms of bacterial meningitis in adults and potentially for all children with meningitis, where it has been shown to improve cerebral perfusion pressure and reduce the incidence of subsequent neurologic abnormalities. In general, patients who develop meningitis with CSF shunts or intracranial pressure monitoring devices in place should have such devices removed. On occasion, however, removal of these devices would severely adversely affect the patient's outcome, and treatment without removal, effective in nearly 30 percent of patients, could be attempted. Respiratory isolation until 24 hours after the initiation of antibiotic therapy is recommended for patients with bacterial meningitis due to *N. meningitidis* or *H. influenzae* because of their high contagious potential.

3. D. Confirming the diagnosis of HSE can be difficult, as much of the evidence is often indirect or difficult to consistently demonstrate. The most reliable and definitive method of establishing the diagnosis is through the demonstration of viral antigen or recovery of virus on biopsy of the brain. The detection of antibodies to herpes simplex in blood is unreliable for the diagnosis of HSE because seropositivity at the onset of the disease is 70 percent in both biopsy-positive and biopsy-negative cases. Even CSF antibody determination is imperfect, as this may be an insensitive technique during the first week of the illness. Anatomic techniques such as electroencephalography, computed tomography scans, and magnetic resonance imaging have been attempted to demonstrate the focus of the disease, although these are imperfectly sensitive and specific tests.

Chapter 88

1. C. The patient presents with classic signs of acute bacterial endocarditis. As a male and an intravenous drug user, the patient is in a high-risk category for the condition. The physical findings of a regurgitant murmur and evidence of embolization (petechiae, splinter hemorrhages, cerebral infarction, and impaired renal function) should provoke an evaluation of the heart valves as the source of the emboli. The distribution of the petechiae in bacterial endocarditis tends to be different from that seen in thrombocytopenia, with a greater predilection for the plantar surfaces of the toes and fingers and the buccal and conjunctival mucosa. The presence of fever and positive blood cultures make the diagnosis of bacterial endocarditis highly likely. The finding that *S. bovis* is the organism responsible should alert the physician to the possibility of a gastrointestinal malignancy because of the high association rate of this organism with benign and malignant gastrointestinal growths. The malignancy may actually be identified months to years after the bacteremic episode.

2. B. Bacterial endocarditis can be produced by any organism. However, most require some preexisting congenital or acquired heart valve abnormality to establish a nidus for the infectious process. Still, *S. aureus* is particularly virulent and appears to be able to infect even previously normal heart valves. *S. aureus* can account for up to half the cases of bacterial endocarditis in some series. Enteric gram-negative bacilli are frequently isolated from blood cultures in critically ill patients but are an infrequent cause of endocarditis, even in previously diseased valves. *Salmonella* species can be etiologic for endocarditis, but they appear to require damaged vascular endothelium to establish the infection. Pneumococci are relatively uncommon as causative agents for bacterial endocarditis. Endocarditis due to *Candida* species can be particularly hard to diagnose, as blood cultures may frequently be negative despite the presence of the disease.

3. **D.** While bacterial endocarditis of any valve is a serious problem, aortic valve infections have the worst prognosis. Aortic insufficiency is more poorly tolerated by the heart than insufficiencies of the other valves. With erosion of a sinus of Valsalva aneurysm into the pericardium or right atrium, pericardial tamponade or a large left-to-right shunt may develop. Invasion by the aortic abscess into the conducting system can produce a heart block. Vegetations on the aortic valve can also be easily dislodged into the coronary arteries, easily producing an infarction for the overstressed left ventricle.

4. **C.** Patients with bacterial endocarditis can present with a variety of clinical findings related to embolization of valvular vegetation material. The lesion described is an Osler's node. Janeway lesions are similar, although they are painless and commonly involve the palms and soles. Roth spots are a pale area within a retinal hemorrhage. Splinter hemorrhages are linear hemorrhages under the nail bed. Takayasu's arteritis is not specifically associated with endocarditis but is an arteritis that produces progressive thrombosis of the aortic arch and its branches.

5. **B.** Studies have demonstrated that 99.3 percent of all septic episodes will be detected by the first two blood cultures. Some rare cases can appear to be culture negative and should provoke the involvement of a clinical microbiologist for special growth conditions. Fungal forms can often be culture negative on multiple repeated samples, with only 50 percent of patients with *Candida* endocarditis being found positive.

Chapter 89

1. **C.** Several techniques have been employed in an effort to reduce the ultimate incidence of infections resulting from intravascular catheter insertion. In one study, chlorhexidine was shown to be more effective than alcohol or povidone-iodine at reducing the incidence of catheter-associated infection and bacteremia. This may be due to a greater persistence of the antiseptic effect that is known to exist with chlorhexidine. The prophylactic administration of intravenous antibiotics has not been definitively shown to be effective at preventing infections resulting from intravascular catheter use.

2. **D.** Proper maintenance of an indwelling intravascular catheter is an area where knowledge is still incomplete. Several factors have been evaluated as to their potential role in preventing or promoting catheter-related sepsis. Many institutions have employed transparent semipermeable polyurethane dressings instead of traditional gauze dressings. While they can allow for better monitoring of the insertion site's appearance, these transparent dressings may trap moisture and may actually be associated with increased infection rates over gauze dressings. Several antiseptic ointments have been evaluated with respect to their ability to minimize catheter infection rates, and their use is often considered a standard practice. However, the evidence of significant effectiveness by these ointments at reducing catheter-associated infections is not overwhelming. While the initial recommendations were to change the infusion sets associated with chronically indwelling catheters every 24 hours, subsequent studies have shown that in many circumstances, such sets can be left in place

for as long as 72 hours with no discernible impact on the rate of catheter-associated infections. Catheters that must remain in place for more than 72 hours carry the greatest risk of becoming infected, thus the recommendation that all peripheral intravascular catheters be changed every 72 hours. Centrally-placed catheters carry a greater risk from insertion; the relative risks of catheter placement versus those of catheter infection are not known with certainty, and thus no recommendations for routine rotation of central catheters currently exist.

3. B. In most series, coagulase-negative staphylococci are the organisms most commonly associated with catheter-related infections, although other organisms can certainly be isolated. In particular, *Candida* and *Malasezzia* species are the organisms most commonly associated with infections of total parenteral nutrition catheters. Many arterial catheters can be infected despite having a relatively innocuous clinical appearance. Excision of the vein has been advocated in patients with suppurative thrombophlebitis where gross purulence is present or sepsis persists despite adequate antibiotic treatment. Removal of the offending catheter is almost always necessary to eliminate the infection, although there is substantial controversy regarding the nature and duration of any accompanying antibiotic regimen.

Chapter 90

1. A. The major risk factor for UTI is the presence of an indwelling urinary catheter. Therefore, its removal can by itself eliminate the presence of a UTI in as many as 70 percent of patients so treated. Because of the persistent source of barrier violation provided by the catheter, initially low bacterial colony counts will progress to high-grade bacteriuria in a majority of patients unless suppressive antimicrobial therapy is employed. The presence of high-grade bacteriuria does not confirm the presence of bacterial infection, however. While greater than 10^5 CFU per milliliter of urine indicates that the urinary bladder is colonized with a significant number of bacteria and that active urinary tract infection is likely, a smaller number does not exclude the possibility in a catheterized patient. Polymicrobial bacteriuria can be seen in a significant number of patients with catheter-related UTI.

2. B. Because the urinary catheter represents the major risk factor toward the development of a catheter-related UTI, avoidance of catheterization whenever possible is the best means of preventing such infections. The use of condom catheters may be beneficial in many patients, although problems with their use (i.e., kinking, leakage, or penile maceration) may provide other problems, and they may not appreciably reduce the risk of UTI in many patients. Topical antimicrobial agents applied to the urethral meatus have not been shown to provide effective prophylaxis toward the development of catheter-associated UTI. Alternative catheter design or manufacture, such as with siliconized materials instead of latex, has not yet been shown to be effective at reducing the incidence of catheter-related UTI significantly. While systemic antimicrobial prophylaxis may reduce the incidence of symptomatic bacteriuria, especially in patients who are catheterized for only a short time, the subsequent development of widespread antibiotic resistance limits the utility of this preventative measure.

3. **B.** *Candida* species are normal inhabitants of the vaginal tract and therefore may merely be contaminants of a urine specimen. Moreover, *Candida* species frequently colonize the urinary tract without causing invasive infection. Therefore, the finding of *Candida* in a urine sample is not an indication of invasive candidiasis. However, the presence of urinary casts made up of *Candida* organisms does indicate invasive upper tract candidiasis. Similarly, fungus ball formation from *Candida* species is associated with ascending candidal infection and warrants systemic amphotericin B therapy. Bladder irrigation with amphotericin B should be with concentrations of 5 to 10 mg per liter of sterile water instilled for 60 to 90 minutes twice daily for 2 days, as higher concentrations have been shown to be toxic. Fluconazole is often effective in the treatment of *Candida* cystitis.

Chapter 91

1. **C.** Toxic shock syndrome presents as a dramatic and distinct syndrome that is similar to only a few other diseases. The primary clinical hallmarks of a fever, rash, orthostatic hypotension, and systemic signs of toxicity are mimicked by a few conditions. These include Rocky Mountain spotted fever, meningococcemia, streptococcal and staphylococcal scarlet fever, leptospirosis, rubeola, and rash-associated viral infections. Conditions such as acute pelvic inflammatory disease can produce severe illness, fever, and toxicity, although a rash is not a common finding, and evidence of pelvic inflammation should be detectable on physical examination. Therefore, it should not be included in the typical differential diagnosis of toxic shock syndrome.

2. **C.** The etiologic organism of Rocky Mountain spotted fever is *Rickettsia rickettsii*, an obligate intracellular bacterium. Lacking a typical bacterial cell wall, it is not affected by beta-lactam agents, such as penicillin, aztreonam, ceftazidime, or imipenem. Rather, specific treatment consists of tetracycline or doxycycline. Chloramphenicol is an alternative drug for those unable to take tetracyclines.

3. **D.** While all parts of the immune system are important barriers to infection, the complement system provides the major defense against meningococcal infection. The organism is opsonized primarily through attachment of C3 fragments. This incites the complement cascade to lyse the organism's membrane through the action of the membrane attack complex produced by complement components C5 through C9. Patients with complement deficiencies are at greater risk of developing meningococcal infection.

Chapter 92

1. **A.** Defects in cell-mediated immunity include abnormalities in T cells, such as cytotoxic killer T cells, and macrophages. Such defects are usually associated with infections due to viruses, protozoa, fungi, helminths, mycobacteria, and intracellular bacteria. *P. carinii* is a protozoan, commonly producing infections in patients with cell-mediated immunity such as is seen in those infected with HIV-1. Infection due to extracellular bacteria such as *S. pneumoniae, H. influenzae, N. meningiditis*, and *P. aeruginosa* may be seen in patients with altered humoral immunity (i.e., deficient B-cell lymphocyte function and antibody production).

2. **C.** While bacteremia can arise from any number of different sources, in many cases an obvious infection can be established. For example, the presence of white cells and bacteria in the urine or endotracheally acquired secretions can establish the urinary tract or the lungs, respectively, as a source for the bacteremia. However, in the immunocompromised patient, bacteremia without an obvious source is usually arising from the gastrointestinal tract. Chemotherapy and neutropenia appear capable of producing a breakdown in the normal intestinal mucosal barriers to bacterial invasion. Most of the breaches in the barrier may be clinically undetectable. Some that may be clinically apparent, however, include typhlitis, anorectal cellulitis or abscess formation, pseudomembranous colitis, and necrotizing colitis.

3. **D.** Because the neutropenic patient has little in the way of endogenous antibacterial defenses, antibiotic coverage must be sufficiently broad to cover all possible offending organisms when their precise identity and sensitivity are unknown. Of the combinations listed, only clindamycin and vancomycin stand out as being deficient because of that combination's lack of effective gram-negative coverage. All the other combinations (including imipenem by itself) represent a sufficient breadth of coverage for empiric antibiotic treatment of the febrile neutropenic patient.

Chapter 93

1. **E.** The cell line whose infection produces the majority of symptoms and mortality related to HIV-l infection is the CD4 lymphocyte, or T4 helper cells. However, HIV infection of monocytes, macrophages, gastrointestinal cells, and neurons can also occur. Many of these cellular infections produce significant symptomatology and morbidity, particularly neuronal involvement. HIV replicates by using the cellular replication machinery once it infects the host cell. Therefore, effective treatment of HIV infection will likely require use of agents that penetrate into the cells where the virus resides. Notably, because of neuronal infection, the treating agents should be able to penetrate the blood-brain barrier.

2. **B.** Pancreatitis has been reported as a consequence of DDI and DDC treatment in AIDS patients. Its presentation can range from a mild case of asymptomatic amylase elevation to a fulminant fatal case that develops with little to no warning. There is no appreciable association of the other listed antiviral treatment regimens with the development of pancreatitis.

3. **D.** The majority of intracranial mass lesions in AIDS patients are due to toxoplasmosis. The presence of a ring-enhancing lesion seen on a contrast study CT scan of the brain is typical of the findings for toxoplasmosis. MRI is of value only when the CT scan is negative in a patient in whom the clinical suspicion is high that an intracranial mass exists, since MRI will be able to show multiple lesions of diffuse cerebral toxoplasmosis involvement. Similarly, further diagnostic tests, such as biopsy and lumbar puncture, are unwarranted. Indeed, lumbar puncture is contraindicated in the presence of a mass effect because of the potential for downward herniation. Transvascular embolization would offer little therapeutic benefit. Rather, presumptive therapy for toxoplasmosis should be instituted. This should consist of pyrimethamine, 50 to 1000 mg PO once daily; sulfadiazine, 1.5 to 2.0 gm PO every 6 to 8 hours; and folinic acid, 10 to 20 mg per day. Response to therapy is usually rapid,

with over three-quarters of patients improved within a week. A brain biopsy may be warranted if the patient fails to respond to this initial approach.

Chapter 94

1. **A.** Endocarditis in a patient who abuses parenteral drugs is different from endocarditis in the nonaddict in that the underlying valve does not have to be diseased. Also, likely as a consequence of the frequent peripheral venous accesses that are made by these individuals, the tricuspid valve is more commonly involved, whereas left-sided valves are more commonly involved in nonaddicts. Because of the right-sided nature of tricuspid endocarditis, the typical stigmata of other forms of endocarditis, such as Osler's nodes, Janeway lesions, and Roth spots, are rarely observed. Rather, multiple patchy infiltrates can be seen on a chest radiograph, suggesting multiple pulmonary emboli more consistent with tricuspid disease. Left-sided endocarditis can be observed in the drug addict and may be present in addition to tricuspid endocarditis. Such patients often have a history of underlying heart disease.

2. **C.** Hepatitis B remains the principal pathogen responsible for hospital admissions among drug users in the United States. Estimates consider 60 to 80 percent of parenteral drug users to be infected with hepatitis B and 10 percent to be chronic carriers. Hepatitis C is also very prevalent among drug users, with some surveys finding up to 83 percent of drug users infected. Hepatitis A can also be observed. Intravenous drug use is the second most common risk behavior for HIV infection in the United States and accounts for 17 percent of acquired immunodeficiency disease syndrome (AIDS) cases. The prevalence of HIV infection among drug users varies with location, ranging from high rates of 60 percent in New York City and New Jersey to less than 5 percent in other regions. *Candida* infections can be observed in drug users to a lesser degree, with a form of disseminated candidiasis occurring exclusively in brown heroin abusers.

3. **E.** Several pulmonary complications can be seen frequently in intravenous drug abusers. Acute pulmonary edema is commonly seen as a result of drug injection, but it is not usually infectious in nature and clears within 24 to 48 hours. A unilateral bacterial pneumonia can develop as a result of exposure to pathogens in the community. Septic pulmonary emboli may arise as a result of bacterial endocarditis of the tricuspid valve, although they may occasionally develop as a result of mycotic aneurysms in the peripheral circulation. In a recent study of intravenous drug abusers, roughly 10 percent have been found to have tuberculosis. Strangely, however, AIDS-related pulmonary infections were not found to be common in that study.

Chapter 95

1. **A.** Until recently, the incidence of tuberculosis appeared to be getting so infrequent that the practice of routine screening for tuberculosis among health care workers was being increasingly questioned. However, the declining incidence of tuberculosis that had been apparent in previous decades ended in 1984. The major influences on this transition appear to be increased immigration into the United States, the HIV epidemic, and a deterioration in the health care delivery infrastructure marked by a drop in the funding of tuberculosis

control programs. Alarmingly, the rate of multidrug-resistant tuberculosis also appears to be increasing.

2. B. The central nervous system manifestations of tuberculosis include tuberculous meningitis and tuberculomas. Typical spinal fluid analysis reveals a lymphocytic pleocytosis, a low glucose concentration, and an elevated protein level. However, none of these parameters is absolute, as tuberculous meningitis can have either a polymorphonuclear predominance, an elevated glucose concentration, or a low protein concentration. Acid-fast bacilli can be detected in cerebrospinal fluid, although it appears that the likelihood of detection is increased if multiple spinal taps are performed (e.g., up to 87% with four spinal taps). Tuberculomas of the central nervous system can be readily detected with either computed tomography or magnetic resonance imaging.

3. E. Drugs commonly used in the treatment of tuberculosis include isoniazid, streptomycin, ethambutol, rifampin, and on occasion pyrazinamide. However, it is important to realize that several commonly used antibiotics also possess activity against *M. tuberculosis*. In addition to streptomycin, other aminoglycosides, such as gentamicin and amikacin, could ameliorate a course of tuberculosis. Fluoroquinolones, such as ciprofloxacin and ofloxacin, also possess antituberculous activity.

Chapter 96

1. C. The spores of *C. botulinum* are very heat resistant, able to survive boiling for hours. Yet their germination conditions require a favorable environment. An anaerobic environment is essential, as oxygen inhibits growth. Other conditions include adequate water and nutrients, a high pH (>4.6), a reasonable temperature (although very cold, nonfreezing temperatures can be tolerated), and a lack of inhibitory substances for growth.

2. E. The site of action of the potent neurotoxin produced by *C. botulinum* is the neuromuscular junction. The neurotoxin appears to inhibit the release of acetylcholine by the nerve cell at the cholinergic synapses. The toxin does not act centrally, nor does it act on adrenergic nerves. The toxin is distributed by the lymphatic and circulatory systems to the neuromuscular junctions. It is usually absorbed from the small intestine, although it may arise from *C. botulinum* growth within a wound.

3. B. Because botulism interferes with muscle activity, measurements of ventilatory muscle strength and activity are better suited to monitor the clinical progress of the disease. For this reason, the vital capacity is the most sensitive of the indices listed. When the vital capacity drops to 30 percent of the patient's predicted value, intubation and mechanical ventilation are prudent. The respiratory rate may also be sensitive for respiratory muscle fatigue, although it is less specific. The PaO_2 and intrapulmonary shunt determinations reflect the ability of the lung to function as a gas-exchanging organ. Because the lung is not the primary site of action of the toxin, gas exchange may be relatively unimpaired initially, although the patient's progressive hypoventilation may ultimately produce hypoxemia. The dead space fraction would not be expected to change in botulism without other complicating factors.

Chapter 97

1. **B.** The major complications of tetanus result from respiratory paralysis and excess sympathetic activity. Cardiac arrhythmias, such as sinus tachycardia and supraventricular tachycardia, are common. Because of respiratory failure and difficulties with airway protection, infections of the respiratory tract are also common.

2. **E.** Effective ventilatory support is key to the management of generalized tetanus. Sedatives such as diazepam are often useful to produce adequate sedation and prevent seizures. Pain from excessive contractures should be relieved with narcotic agents such as meperidine. Drugs such as baclofen administered intrathecally may reduce muscle contractures. Excess sympathetic activity should be managed with a beta blocker, such as propranolol. The use of antibiotics such as penicillin to specifically target the causative organism is usually of little value. Most often, there is a wound site of probable entry for the organism, and this area should be surgically opened, debrided, and cleansed as primary treatment against the infection itself Rarely, in cases where there is no obvious portal of entry for the organism, empiric penicillin administration may be employed, although there is no evidence that such an approach is effective.

3. **C.** Patients with tetanus should receive 500 units of human tetanus immune globulin intramuscularly as soon as the diagnosis of tetanus is made. Larger doses or repeated doses are of no value. Also, immunization with tetanus toxoid should be simultaneously started intramuscularly at another site. The use of antibiotics is of little value, as the most beneficial anti-infective therapy is that of effective debridement of the wound that served as the portal of entry for the organism.

VII. *Gastrointestinal and Hepatobiliary Problems in the Intensive Care Unit*

98. *Gastrointestinal Bleeding: Principles of Diagnosis and Management*

1. Which of the following statements regarding gastric lavage of the patient with upper gastrointestinal bleeding is true?

A. Gastrointestinal lavage via a nasogastric tube is often essential in getting an upper gastrointestinal hemorrhage to stop.
B. Gastric lavage with iced saline prolongs the bleeding time.
C. Gastric lavage is necessary for endoscopic visualization of the bleeding lesion.
D. The gastric vasoconstriction produced by ice water lavage helps to stop active bleeding.
E. None of the above.

2. Which of the following statements regarding inhibition of gastric acid production during acute upper gastrointestinal hemorrhage is true?

A. H_2-receptor antagonists can stop or prevent rebleeding.
B. The use of omeprazole can reduce transfusion requirements.
C. Therapy directed toward decreasing gastric acidity reduces the operative rates in patients with acute upper gastrointestinal hemorrhage.
D. Prescribing patterns suggest that H_2-receptor antagonists are administered primarily to stop bleeding rather than to treat peptic ulcer disease.
E. H_2-receptor antagonism is effective during acute upper gastrointestinal bleeding episodes because blood clots poorly in an acid medium.

3. Which of the following endoscopic findings carries the greatest risk for continued bleeding or rebleeding from gastric or duodenal ulcers?

A. Oozing.
B. Nonbleeding visible vessel.
C. Arterial bleeding.
D. Flat pigmented spot.
E. Adherent clot.

99. Stress Ulcer Syndrome

1. Endoscopic features that distinguish stress ulcers from chronic peptic ulcers include

A. Punched-out appearance.
B. Little surrounding inflammation.
C. Proximal location in the stomach.
D. Duodenal location is rare.
E. All of the above.

2. Which of the following conditions is currently debated as a potential complication of stress ulcer prophylaxis with H_2-receptor antagonists?

A. Urinary tract infections.
B. Acidosis.
C. Gram-negative nosocomial pneumonia.
D. Coagulopathy.
E. Alkalosis.

3. Which of the following choices is the best regimen to use in attempting to prevent stress gastritis?

A. Antacids.
B. H_2-receptor antagonists.
C. Sucralfate.
D. All of the above in combination.
E. None of the above.

100. Variceal Bleeding

1. What percentage of patients who present with acute upper gastrointestinal hemorrhage will have gastroesophageal varices as the source of their bleeding?

A. 10 percent.
B. 30 percent.
C. 50 percent.
D. 70 percent.
E. 90 percent.

2. Which of the following conditions are contraindications for the use of vasopressin in the management of a patient with acute gastroesophageal variceal bleeding?

(1) Severe peripheral vascular disease.
(2) Acute renal failure.
(3) Coronary artery disease.
(4) Diarrhea.
(5) Constipation.

A. 1, 2, and 3.
B. 1 and 3 only.

C. 2 and 4 only.
D. All of the above.
E. None of the above.

3. The initial management of the patient with acutely bleeding esophageal varices is best provided by which of the following therapeutic modalities?

A. Placement of a Sengstaken-Blakemore tube.
B. Distal splenorenal shunt.
C. Endoscopic sclerotherapy.
D. Placement of a Linton-Nachlas tube.
E. Performance of a Sugiura procedure.

101. Intestinal Pseudo-obstruction (Ileus)

1. In a patient with potential intestinal pseudo-obstruction, the most useful information that will provide a clue as to the presence of hollow visceral disease is

A. Whether nausea is present.
B. Whether diarrhea is present.
C. The frequency of urination.
D. Whether constipation is a problem.
E. Whether frequent belching occurs.

2. Which of the following intestinal segments returns motility most quickly postoperatively following a laparotomy?

A. Stomach.
B. Cecum.
C. Rectum.
D. Small intestine.
E. Colon.

3. Which of the following agents is most likely to improve intestinal motility in cases of paralytic ileus?

A. Naloxone.
B. Erythromycin.
C. Simethicone.
D. Penicillin.
E. Atropine.

102. Fulminant Colitis and Toxic Megacolon

1. Which of the following conditions provides the greatest risk factor for mortality in toxic megacolon?

A. Bleeding.

B. Ileus.
C. Diarrhea.
D. Fluid sequestration.
E. Perforation.

2. Reasons that may justify the use of corticosteroids in patients with toxic megacolon include the following:

(1) Parenteral corticosteroids or adrenocorticotropic hormone may abort the progressive dilation of the colon in patients with toxic megacolon.
(2) Most patients with toxic megacolon were receiving steroids before the condition developed, and augmented steroid dosing may be necessary for the additional stress.
(3) Steroids may reduce the mortality rate and the need for surgical intervention.
(4) Steroids help control the excessive metabolic response seen in toxic megacolon.
(5) None of the above.

A. 1, 2, and 3.
B. 1 and 3 only.
C. 2 and 4 only.
D. All of the above.
E. None of the above.

3. Which of the following are indications for emergent surgery in patients with toxic megacolon?

A. Perforation.
B. Septic shock.
C. Colon diameter greater than 12 cm.
D. All of the above.
E. None of the above.

103. Evaluation and Management of Liver Failure

1. Which of the following statements regarding fulminant hepatic failure (FHF) is true?

A. Higher survival rates have been quoted for patients with FHF secondary to hepatitis C.
B. The single most important predictor of outcome is the degree of encephalopathy.
C. Sepsis is rarely a cause of mortality following liver transplantation for FHF.
D. Survival rates for patients with FHF without transplantation are excellent.
E. Identification of the etiology of FHF is rarely important for clinical management.

2. In FHF, the most sensitive method for detecting the presence of elevated intracranial pressure is

A. The neurologic examination.

B. Computed tomography.
C. The grade of encephalopathy.
D. Routine clinical examination.
E. Intracranial pressure monitoring.

3. Select the best answer. Renal failure in FHF

A. Is a marker of a poor prognosis.
B. Occurs in only 25 percent of patients whose liver failure is due to acetaminophen toxicity.
C. Occurs in 60 percent of patients with FHF secondary to other causes.
D. Cannot be managed by continuous forms of dialysis.
E. Is rarely due to intravascular volume depletion.

104. Diarrhea

1. The most common nonhemorrhagic gastrointestinal complication seen in the intensive care unit is

A. Acalculous cholecystitis.
B. Diarrhea.
C. Hepatitis.
D. Constipation.
E. Intolerance of enteral feedings.

2. Which of the following drugs may promote the development of antibiotic-associated (pseudomembranous) colitis?

A. Clindamycin.
B. Metronidazole.
C. Ampicillin.
D. Vancomycin.
E. All of the above.

3. The most important early step in the management of patients with diarrhea of any type is

A. Prompt diagnostic sigmoidoscopy.
B. Empiric administration of oral vancomycin.
C. Empiric administration of oral metronidazole.
D. Discontinuation of enteral feedings.
E. Correction of fluid and electrolyte abnormalities.

105. Severe and Complicated Biliary Tract Disease

1. Which of the following studies are preferable in the initial evaluation of critically ill patients with suspected biliary tract disease?

(1) Endoscopic retrograde cholangiopancreatography.
(2) Hepatobiliary scan.
(3) Computed tomography.

(4) Abdominal ultrasound.
(5) Percutaneous transhepatic cholangiography.

A. 1, 2, and 3.
B. 1 and 3 only.
C. 2 and 4 only.
D. All of the above.
E. None of the above.

2. A 52-year-old man presented with the findings of fever, chills, jaundice, and right upper quadrant abdominal pain. His serum bilirubin level was 6.3 mg per deciliter, with 5.2 mg per deciliter being conjugated. A Tc^{99}-iminodiacetic acid (HIDA) scan demonstrated a lack of drainage into the small intestine, although a trickle of flow was detected on delayed films. Initial treatment should consist of

A. Oral lactulose and neomycin.
B. Intravenous fluid resuscitation and broad-spectrum antibiotics.
C. Monoclonal antibodies to endotoxin.
D. Cholestyramine.
E. Intravenous heparin.

3. After 6 hours of appropriate initial management, the patient described in question 2 remained febrile, with evidence of worsening renal and respiratory function. What should be done at this time?

A. A pulmonologist should be consulted to help manage the respiratory failure.
B. A nephrologist should be consulted regarding the possibility of impending acute renal failure.
C. Plans should be made for biliary lithotripsy.
D. The patient should undergo emergent biliary decompression.
E. A pulmonary artery balloon flotation catheter should be inserted to more effectively manage the resuscitative effort.

106. Complications of Gastrointestinal Procedures

1. Which of the following statements regarding conscious sedation is true?

A. Midazolam is more likely to produce cardiopulmonary complications than is diazepam.
B. Patients with chronic obstructive pulmonary disease are more likely to experience respiratory depression during endoscopy than are patients without such a condition.
C. The presence of the endoscope in the hypopharynx is the most significant factor contributing to hypoxemia during endoscopy.
D. Anaphylaxis to contrast exposure during endoscopic retrograde cholangiopancreatography is common.
E. Allergy to sedative or narcotic premedication during endoscopy is not infrequent.

2. For patients who may have sustained an overdose of benzodiazepines during conscious sedation for a procedure, an agent that can reverse the oversedation is

A. Lorazepam.
B. Naloxone.
C. Dextrose.
D. Flumazenil.
E. Atropine.

3. Which of the following findings after colonoscopic polypectomy mandate surgical management?

A. Localized abdominal pain.
B. Tachycardia.
C. Guarding.
D. Leukocytosis.
E. Free intraperitoneal air.

107. Hepatic Dysfunction

1. The most striking abnormality observed that distinguishes ischemic hepatitis from other forms of liver dysfunction seen in the critically ill is

A. A marked rise in serum bilirubin.
B. A marked rise in serum alkaline phosphatase.
C. A marked rise in serum aspartate aminotransferase (AST) and alanine aminotransferase (ALT).
D. A marked prolongation of the prothrombin time.
E. A marked rise in unconjugated bilirubin.

2. Which of the following statements regarding hepatic function during total parenteral nutrition (TPN) is true?

A. Abnormalities in liver function tests occur in roughly one-third of patients receiving TPN for 2 weeks or longer.
B. The most common abnormalities seen in liver function tests are coagulation abnormalities.
C. The pathophysiologic mechanisms underlying the hepatic effects of TPN are clearly related to the effects of gut rest on hormone secretion.
D. After 6 or more weeks of TPN, biliary sludge can form, with resultant acalculous cholecystitis or even cholelithiasis.
E. There is no benefit to enteral feeding if the patient is already receiving TPN.

3. It is currently believed that a key component in the liver dysfunction that is seen during sepsis and multiple organ failure is

A. An absolute or relative perfusion deficit.
B. Excessive ammonia production.
C. Administration of exogenous toxins.
D. Premature administration of TPN.
E. Excessive blood product administration.

Answers

Chapter 98

1. **B.** Although frequently used, the absolute value of nasogastric lavage has never been substantiated. In patients who fail to present with hematemesis or melena, a nasogastric tube may be helpful in confirming the presence of an upper gastrointestinal hemorrhage. While it may appear that nasogastric lavage would be helpful in clearing clots and thus facilitate visualization during endoscopy, many gastroenterologists do not think it necessary. Further, there is the possibility that the tube could produce suction artifacts that produce some confusion for the endoscopist. Contrary to common belief, iced saline lavage does not help slow upper gastrointestinal bleeding. Rather, iced saline lavage prolongs the bleeding time, increases the clotting time, and prolongs bleeding from ulcers compared to no lavage.

2. **D.** Although prescribing patterns for H_2-receptor antagonists suggest that these drugs are administered in an effort to stop acute upper gastrointestinal bleeding, there is little clinical or scientific evidence to support this practice. While it is true that blood clots poorly in an acid environment, it has not been shown that inhibition of acid production in the acutely bleeding ulcer patient slows the rate of bleeding, changes the transfusion requirements, or affects the operative or mortality rates. Potentially, this inability to see a beneficial effect from acid inhibition during an acute bleeding episode could be because the neutralizing effect of blood itself may diminish any further beneficial effect produced by drugs or antacids. Therapy toward reducing gastric acidity may be helpful in healing an ulcer, but it is difficult to demonstrate that such therapy stops bleeding or prevents rebleeding.

3. **C.** Several endoscopic findings can be associated with upper gastrointestinal bleeding from gastric or duodenal ulcers. Some, such as the presence of oozing, an adherent clot, a clean ulcer base, or a flat pigmented spot are associated with relatively low (<25%) incidences of continued bleeding or rebleeding. However, a visible blood vessel in the ulcer crater is associated with rebleeding 40 to 50 percent of the time, even though it may not be actively bleeding at the time of endoscopy. The endoscopic finding of active arterial bleeding is most highly associated with persistent or recurrent rebleeding, occurring in 90 percent of patients with the finding.

Chapter 99

1. **E.** Stress ulceration can have a typical endoscopic appearance that is quite distinct from that seen with chronic peptic ulcers. Because stress ulcers are usually in association with a more acutely stressful state, they do not have many of the stigmata of chronicity seen with chronic peptic ulceration. Thus, stress ulcers have more of a punched-out appearance, with little surrounding inflammation, edema, or induration. They tend to appear more in the proximal stomach, rather than in the distal antrum and duodenum, as is seen with peptic ulcer disease. Histologically, stress ulcers have minimal inflammatory cell infiltrate, in contrast to the marked inflammation seen with chronic peptic disease, which is consistent with the acutely ischemic nature of the stress gastritis process.

2. **C.** Although the issue is quite controversial, there is a strong concern raised that stress ulcer prophylaxis with H_2-receptor antagonists may predispose patients to develop gram-negative nosocomial pneumonias. The presence of an acid stomach appears to inhibit all organisms from growing in large concentrations. However, when the stomach pH is neutralized, it appears that gram-negative organisms have some survival advantage over gram-positive organisms. Furthermore, fungal growth appears to be more favored in a pH-neutral gastric environment. Several studies have indicated that stress ulcer prophylaxis with sucralfate may diminish the risk of developing pneumonia. On the other hand, at least one meta-analysis suggested that H_2-receptor antagonism may not increase the rate of pneumonia compared to patients receiving no stress ulcer prophylaxis (who presumably maintained an acid stomach). Thus, while the controversy continues, the use of agents that neutralize stomach acid may provide some disadvantages for patients who share any other risks for the development of nosocomial pneumonia, such as prolonged endotracheal intubation.

3. **E.** At the current time, no one method for preventing stress gastritis appears to have any advantage over any other. Furthermore, combinations of agents appear to provide no appreciable added benefit. In fact, the combination of sucralfate with agents that increase gastric pH is particularly unsound, in that sucralfate requires a pH of less than 4.5 for effective activity. Thus no specific recommendations for the choice of a prophylactic agent can be made at this time.

Chapter 100

1. **A.** Only about 10 percent of patients with acute upper gastrointestinal bleeding will be found to have gastroesophageal varices as the etiology. However, the mortality rate of 30 to 50 percent associated with gastroesophageal variceal bleeding is much higher than that found with acid-peptic causes of upper gastrointestinal hemorrhage.

2. **B.** Vasopressin is normally produced by the posterior pituitary in the regulation of the body's water balance (antidiuretic hormone). It also acts as a potent vasoconstrictor and can reduce portal venous blood flow. It may be useful in the management of acute gastroesophageal variceal bleeding due to portal hypertension, although there is a significant controversy over the absolute utility of this approach. Because the vasoconstriction that vasopressin produces is nonselective, it can constrict the vessels and impair tissue perfusion to other vital organs besides the gastrointestinal tract, such as the heart and brain. Therefore, its use is contraindicated in patients with preexisting conditions that impair circulatory oxygen delivery, such as severe peripheral vascular disease and coronary artery disease.

3. **C.** Most patients with variceal bleeding stop bleeding spontaneously, with only supportive care necessary. In cases of severe or persistent bleeding, endoscopic visualization is usually necessary to determine the etiology of the gastrointestinal hemorrhage, as not all patients with varices who have acute upper gastrointestinal bleeding are actually bleeding from their varices. If variceal bleeding is then found, sclerotherapy is most effective for the majority of patients. Placement of a Sengstaken-Blakemore (or Minnesota) tube for gastroesophageal variceal tamponade, or a Linton-Nachlas tube for gastric varices

alone, may be useful when endoscopic sclerotherapy has failed, although the complication rates are higher. Distal splenorenal shunts and the Sugiura procedure are surgical operations that are reserved for those patients in whom other nonoperative methods have failed to control the hemorrhage.

Chapter 101

1. **C.** Patients with hollow visceral disease can develop intestinal pseudo-obstruction, but they will also have problems with the motility of other hollow organs. The single most useful parameter to identify this pattern from the patient's history is the frequency of urination. Urination significantly more or less frequent than the normal five to six times per day (in the absence of acute cystitis) is a sign of abnormalities with smooth muscle motility. Occasionally, problems with ptosis or ophthalmoplegia can also provide clues to the presence of hollow visceral disease.

2. **D.** Surgical opening of the abdomen and handling of intestine appear to arrest intestinal contractile activity. However, most of this slowing appears to involve the colon and the stomach. The small intestine regains its function rapidly and may never really lose much activity secondary to uncomplicated surgery. Because of this, enteral feedings can be used at a very early period postoperatively, even in the recovery room. This is especially true for those enterally delivered nutrient systems that bypass the stomach (i.e., jejunal tubes) and contain little residue to be deposited into the atonic colon.

3. **B.** Intravenously delivered erythromycin appears to stimulate motor activity in the stomach and small intestine and may be beneficial in cases of paralytic ileus. A macrolide antibiotic, erythromycin acts as a motilin agonist in the intestinal tract. Naloxone, a narcotic antagonist, may be marginally beneficial in cases where excessive narcotic has led to intestinal slowing, although it would not be expected to work in other types of ileus. Simethicone can absorb excessive gas within the intestine and thus may provide some marginal benefit, although in serious cases of ileus it is not of significant help. Atropine would be contraindicated in cases of ileus because it would aggravate the intestinal atony.

Chapter 102

1. **E.** Colonic perforation is the greatest risk factor for death in cases of toxic megacolon. The mortality rate is 50 percent for those patients who develop perforation before surgical intervention is undertaken. Other factors associated with increased mortality include increased patient age (i.e., > 40 years) and a delay in surgical intervention. Early recognition and management of toxic megacolon have reduced the overall mortality of the condition to less than 15 percent.

2. **A.** Corticosteroids are frequently used in cases of toxic megacolon, although the issue of their use is subject to some controversy. In many cases of toxic megacolon, it is prudent to employ augmented doses of steroids for those patients who were taking steroids prior to the onset of the toxic condition. Furthermore, it does appear in clinical studies that the use of corticosteroids in patients with toxic megacolon increases the remission rate to as much as 70 percent, thus reducing the need for surgical intervention. Importantly, it has

been shown in clinical studies that patients managed without steroids had a higher mortality rate, regardless of the need for surgical intervention. However, prospective randomized trials of the issue are lacking, so the controversy over the appropriateness of steroid use in toxic megacolon is far from settled.

3. **D.** Perforation is an absolute indication for surgical intervention in patients with toxic megacolon. However, because the mortality rate is so high once perforation occurs, efforts at preventing this complication should be undertaken. The sign of impending perforation is an enlarged colon diameter (i.e., > 12 cm), which is an indication for emergent surgery to prevent the disastrous consequences of perforation, such as peritonitis, extreme fluid and electrolyte imbalance, and hemodynamic instability. Septic shock should also be an indication to desist with nonoperative therapy in an effort to eradicate the source of the septic complication. Some authors believe that conditions such as severe malnutrition or pregnancy should also mandate emergent surgery in patients with toxic megacolon.

Chapter 103

1. **B.** FHF is a severe complication of liver disease with devastating consequences. The single most important predictor of clinical outcome is the degree of encephalopathy. Higher survival rates are reported when the FHF is secondary to hepatitis A, hepatitis B, and acetaminophen toxicity, but not those failures due to idiosyncratic drug reactions, acute Wilson's disease, halothane hepatitis, and non-A, non-B hepatitis. In addition to helping to assess the overall prognosis, etiologic identification is very important for effective clinical management. Those cases due to toxicity may benefit from potential antidotes, while those due to infectious agents may require that adequate public health measures are taken. Liver transplantation is an important therapeutic tool, producing survival rates in excess of 50 percent in most series, but less than 20 percent without transplantation. Mortality following liver transplantation for FHF is usually due to sepsis and neurologic complications.

2. **E.** In patients with FHF, the most sensitive method for detecting the presence and degree of intracranial pressure elevations is through the use of intracranial pressure monitoring. The grade of encephalopathy can sometimes be a guide to the need for intracranial pressure monitoring, although it is neither sensitive nor specific. In general, patients with grade 3 or 4 encephalopathy should be monitored with an intracranial pressure monitor. Typical clinical manifestations of increased intracranial pressure, such as papilledema, bradycardia, vomiting, and headache, are frequently not evident in FHF. Computed tomography of the brain in FHF does not appear to correlate well with the presence of increased intracranial pressure.

3. **A.** Acute renal failure in a patient with FHF is an ominous sign. It occurs in up to 75 percent of patients with FHF due to acetaminophen toxicity, but in only about 30 percent of patients with FHF secondary to other causes. The most common causes for renal failure are intravascular volume depletion, acute tubular necrosis, and the hepatorenal syndrome, with many cases having a multifactorial etiology. The technique of continuous hemodiafiltration may offer advantages to patients with FHF who develop renal failure and require dialytic support.

Chapter 104

1. **B.** Diarrhea is the most common nonhemorrhagic gastrointestinal complication observed in critically ill patients. It occurs in 40 to 50 percent of patients in the intensive care unit, although it is often overlooked as a problem by clinicians. Furthermore, definitions of what actually constitutes diarrhea seem to vary, thus confusing the establishment of this clinical entity as a problem requiring clinical attention. Yet, failure to properly identify and manage diarrhea in the critically ill patient will usually lead to severe fluid, electrolyte, and nutritional abnormalities that will further complicate the patient's course.

2. **E.** Antibiotic-associated, or pseudomembranous, colitis is most notoriously linked to the use of clindamycin with the subsequent emergence of *Clostridium difficile*. However, it actually appears to develop following the use of other antibiotics such as ampicillin. Interestingly, it even occurs following the use of agents that are commonly used to treat antibiotic-associated colitis, vancomycin and metronidazole. Broad-spectrum cephalosporins have also been implicated in its development. It is also important to realize that pseudomembranous colitis can occur up to 6 weeks after discontinuation of the responsible antibiotic.

3. **E.** While the management of critically ill patients with diarrhea can be a very complex process, the most important early management issues concern effective management of fluid and electrolyte disturbances. Replacement of water, sodium, potassium, phosphorus, magnesium, and bicarbonate may all be necessary to varying degrees. In states of severe volume depletion, invasive hemodynamic monitoring may be necessary to more accurately guide resuscitative measures. Diagnostic procedures such as sigmoidoscopy may be necessary to establish the etiology for the diarrhea, but this is never the initial procedure. Agents such as vancomycin and metronidazole can be effective at controlling pseudomembranous colitis due to the emergence of *C. difficile*. However, such regimens should not be employed empirically but rather should be administered after the diagnosis of pseudomembranous colitis is established. Indeed, these agents have been implicated in the causation of some cases of pseudomembranous colitis themselves. While enteral feeding intolerance is frequently implicated in cases of diarrhea, enteral feedings should not be arbitrarily stopped until a clear relationship is established between the rate of infusion and the onset of diarrhea. Not infrequently, patients receiving enteral feedings often have their nutritional regimen discontinued as the initial response to the onset of diarrhea, yet there are a host of other potential etiologies that should be considered. Arbitrary discontinuation of enteral nutrition could impair the nutritional status and recovery of the patient without necessarily approaching or controlling the etiology of the diarrhea satisfactorily.

Chapter 105

1. **C.** Ultrasonography of the abdomen can be very helpful in evaluating the critically ill patient in whom it is suspected that a biliary problem exists. It is very sensitive and specific for determining the presence of dilated bile ducts as well as gallstones. Similarly, hepatobiliary scanning is very useful for demonstrating patency of the cystic duct as well as the presence of normal physi-

ologic function of the biliary tract. Both tests are noninvasive and can be done at the bedside in a critically ill patient, thus providing a significant advantage in this patient population. While computed tomography is also noninvasive and can show very specific findings, it is not a portable technique. Thus, ample justification should exist for seeking it over portable studies in a critically ill patient who may deteriorate during transport. One reason would be to provide a better view of the head of the pancreas than can be seen in many cases of ultrasonography. Both endoscopic retrograde cholangiopancreatography and percutaneous transhepatic cholangiography are invasive tests requiring fluoroscopy. As such, they are usually not employed as the initial diagnostic maneuver in critically ill patients with suspected biliary tract disease.

2. **B.** This patient is presenting with the classic signs of acute cholangitis (fever, right upper quadrant abdominal pain, and jaundice), also known as Charcot's triad. Under such circumstances, initial stabilization efforts should concentrate on maintaining an effective circulating volume status with intravenous fluids. Also, the systemic septic picture should be approached initially with broad-spectrum intravenous antibiotics after blood cultures are obtained. In many cases, a response will be seen, and the antibiotic regimen can be tailored pending further identification of the offending organism.

3. **D.** When the initial approach of fluid and antibiotic administration fails to achieve a significant beneficial response, or in patients who clearly have a complete obstruction of an infected biliary tree, emergent decompression of the biliary tract should be performed. This can be accomplished by a variety of different approaches, either endoscopic, percutaneous, or surgical, depending on the patient's condition and the available local resources and expertise. Removal of the gallbladder is not necessary at the initial setting. Rather, efforts to decompress the biliary tract must be the focus of the intervention. The gallbladder may be removed at a later date if the patient survives.

Chapter 106

1. **B.** One of the greatest risks of performing procedures in critically ill patients is that of producing hypoxemia. Patients with chronic obstructive lung disease and elderly patients are more likely to develop respiratory depression during endoscopy. Premedication is responsible for the greatest number of hypoxic events, although other factors can sometimes play a role, such as the presence of the endoscope in the hypopharynx or the use of topical anesthesia. Although it was initially thought to be more causative of respiratory depression, midazolam was shown in a large clinical study to be no more likely responsible for cardiopulmonary complications than diazepam. Allergy to sedation or narcotic premedication is extremely rare. However, allergy to intravenous contrast agents is not unusual. Nevertheless, anaphylaxis during endoscopic retrograde cholangiopancreatography has not been reported.

2. **D.** Flumazenil is a benzodiazepine-receptor antagonist that can block the action of benzodiazepines at receptor sites. This makes it useful for complete or partial reversal of oversedation due to benzodiazepines. However, it may be ineffective at reversing any hypoventilation and accompanying hypoxemia due to benzodiazepines. Furthermore, patients who have taken benzodiazepines chronically may experience seizures when given flumazenil. Naloxone is a narcotic antagonist and would not be expected to reverse the action of ben-

zodiazepines, although it could be useful if excessive narcotics were used in addition to the benzodiazepines.

3. E. The finding of free intraperitoneal air following a colonoscopic polypectomy indicates the presence of an intestinal perforation. Such a condition warrants surgical management to minimize the potential for overwhelming iatrogenic peritonitis. The other symptoms listed may be suggestive of the presence of a serious complication following colonoscopic polypectomy but may not mandate surgical exploration. These may be related to what has been termed the postpolypectomy coagulation syndrome, which can present within a few hours of colonoscopy. Treatment with antibiotics, bowel rest, and close observation for 48 to 72 hours is usually sufficient.

Chapter 107

1. C. The diagnosis of ischemic hepatitis can often be made on clinical grounds, making a liver biopsy unnecessary in many cases. The syndrome occurs in response to a period of reduced liver perfusion. The most striking finding is the pronounced rise in serum aminotransferases, AST and ALT. These can rise to levels 40 or more times the normal level. In contrast, the serum bilirubin and alkaline phosphatase levels are normal or modestly elevated. The elevated transaminases are brief and self-limited, usually only lasting 1 to 2 weeks at most.

2. D. TPN can produce abnormalities in liver function tests in 68 to 93 percent of patients who receive it for more than 2 weeks. Typically, elevations of ALT and, to a lesser extent, AST develop, with variable changes in serum bilirubin and alkaline phosphatase. No specific effect of TPN on coagulation parameters has been determined. With prolonged administration, cholelithiasis or alcalculous cholecystitis can develop, presumably related to gallbladder disuse and the development of biliary sludge. The pathophysiologic mechanisms underlying the effects of TPN on liver function are not known, although a number of issues are speculated to be involved. Enteral nutrition may help to prevent many of the abnormalities in liver function seen with TPN, although this is not always possible.

3. A. Although the complete pathophysiologic picture is not entirely known, it is thought by many that either an absolute or relative perfusion deficit develops. This may impair the liver's circulation itself and reduce the effectiveness of Kupffer cell and hepatocyte function. Furthermore, this altered perfusion may promote the absorption of endotoxin and other bacterial products from the intestinal tract, potentially overwhelming the liver's ability to detoxify these agents. While blood units contain bilirubin, which must be processed by the liver, it is not clear that the administration of blood products plays a significant role in further damaging liver function. Similarly, TPN does produce some clinically detectable abnormalities in liver function studies, but it has not been shown that this contributes to the liver function that is seen during sepsis and multiple organ failure, especially as the latter can develop in patients who are not receiving TPN.

VIII. Endocrine Problems in the Intensive Care Unit

108. Approach to the Acutely Ill Patient on Chronic Steroid Therapy

1. True or False. Patients receiving pharmacologic doses of glucocorticoids for only 10 days may have an abnormal cortisol response to adrenocorticotropic hormone (ACTH) infusion.

2. True or False. Hypotension during surgical stress is uncommon in adrenal-suppressed patients who fail to receive supraphysiologic glucocorticoid supplementation.

3. True or False. A glucocorticoid dose-equivalent to methylprednisolone, 60 mg IV every 8 hours, is necessary for adequate "stress" coverage.

4. True or False. Alternate-day therapy with glucocorticoids reduces the possibility of adrenal suppression.

109. Management of Diabetes in the Critically Ill Patient

1. Compensatory mechanisms to maintain normal blood concentrations of glucose during fasting and starvation include all of the following except

   A. Mobilization of hepatic glycogen.
   B. Release of amino acid precursors for gluconeogenesis.
   C. Inhibition of lipolysis.
   D. Central nervous system utilization of ketone bodies.

2. An 88-year-old man with a history of asthma and noninsulin-dependent diabetes mellitus underwent laparotomy for a perforated colonic diverticulum, resulting in a partial colectomy and descending colostomy. Two days postoperatively, he developed worsening bronchospasm despite frequent nebulized albuterol, and methylprednisolone was begun. Three days postoperatively, en-

teral feeding was initiated. The following day, his morning blood sugar was noted to be 410 mg per deciliter. The most appropriate management is

A. To discontinue methylprednisolone.
B. Continuous intravenous insulin infusion.
C. To discontinue enteral feeding.
D. Intermittent subcutaneous insulin.

110. The Diabetic Comas

1. Alcoholic ketoacidosis is characterized by all of the following except

A. Dehydration.
B. Hyperglycemia.
C. Lactic acidosis.
D. Increased free fatty acids.

2. Insulin deficiency results in

A. Decreased lipolysis.
B. Accelerated gluconeogenesis.
C. Reduced glucagon secretion.
D. Metabolic alkalosis.

3. A 29-year-old man presented to the emergency room with complaints of weakness, nausea, anorexia, thirst, and weight loss that has been progressive over the last 2 weeks. He denied prior significant medical problems and takes no medication. On examination, he appeared to be in moderate respiratory distress. His blood pressure was 96/64 mm Hg, supine. His pulse was 150 per minute and regular, respirations were 38 per minute, and his temperature was 36.6°C. The lungs were clear, the heart showed only the regular tachycardia, and the abdomen was mildly tender diffusely. Initial laboratory studies showed serum sodium, 142 mEq per liter; potassium, 6.2 mEq per liter; carbon dioxide, 5 mmol per liter; chloride, 105 mEq per liter; blood urea nitrogen, 62 mg per deciliter; creatinine, 2.1 mg per deciliter; and glucose, 820 mg per deciliter. Arterial blood gases revealed PO_2, 106 mm Hg; PCO_2, 21 mm Hg; and pH, 7.02. Urine was positive for sugar and ketones. The most appropriate immediate management is

A. Intravenous calcium for severe hyperkalemia.
B. Intravenous bicarbonate for severe acidosis.
C. Intravenous isotonic saline for dehydration.
D. Intravenous insulin for severe hyperglycemia.

111. Thyroid Storm

1. A 67-year-old woman with a history of insulin-dependent diabetes mellitus presented with a 2-week history of polydipsia and polyuria and a 1-week history of palpitations, fever, nervousness, and insomnia. Her temperature was 37.8°C. Pulse rate was 140 per minute, and the rhythm was irregular. Her electrocardiogram showed atrial fibrillation. A serum thyroxine level was markedly elevated. A true statement concerning this patient's condition is

A. Worsening diabetic control may occur in hyperthyroidism.
B. Tachycardia out of proportion to fever makes thyroid storm unlikely.
C. Atrial tachyarrhythmias during thyroid storm usually require less propranolol than given to the typical patient.
D. The fever of thyroid storm should not be treated.

2. True statements concerning treatment for thyroid storm include all of the following except

A. Salicylates should not be used to treat the fever.
B. Beta-blockade should not be used in the setting of congestive heart failure.
C. Iodide is useful to decrease thyroid hormone release.
D. Plasmapheresis and/or dialysis will remove thyroid hormone from the circulation.

112. Myxedema Coma

1. A patient with a history of bipolar disorder treated with lithium carbonate presented to the emergency room with a 7-day history of lethargy progressive to obtundation. A history of fatigue and weight gain over the previous 6 months was elicited from a family member. On examination, the patient was difficult to arouse. Blood pressure was 88/50 mm Hg, pulse rate 55 per minute, respirations 14 per minute, and temperature 35.8°C. Laboratory values included a blood sugar of 50 mg per deciliter, mildly elevated lithium level, markedly elevated thyroid-stimulating hormone, and a low serum free thyroxine index (FTI). True statements about this condition include all of the following except

A. Lithium may be responsible.
B. FTI is a calculation derived from the serum thyroxine level and the available thyroxine binding sites of thyroxine binding globulin.
C. Severe infections may precipitate this state.
D. Administration of concentrated dextrose solutions is contraindicated.

113. Hypoadrenal Crisis

1. A principle in the treatment of adrenal insufficiency is

A. You must confirm the diagnosis before initiating treatment.
B. 300 to 400 mg of methylprednisolone per day is equivalent to maximum adrenal glucocorticoid release.
C. A random serum cortisol less than 20 μg per deciliter in a critically ill patient is suggestive of adrenal insufficiency.
D. Secondary adrenal insufficiency from pituitary dysfunction often requires additional mineralocorticoid replacement.

114. Disorders of Mineral Metabolism

1. Select the correct answer. Elevated serum calcium in malignancy

   A. May be secondary to both humoral and localized destructive mechanisms.
   B. Was once thought to be caused by a circulating parathormone-like substance, but this has been disproved by a radioimmunoassay.
   C. Secondary to osteolytic processes is uncommon in metastatic breast cancer.
   D. Is treated the same regardless of the underlying disease or mechanism.

115. Lactic Acidosis

1. Select the correct answer. Bicarbonate therapy for severe lactic acidosis

   A. Improves cardiovascular hemodynamics.
   B. May worsen metabolic acidosis.
   C. Improves tissue hypoxia.
   D. May cause hyponatremia.

117. Sick Euthyroid Syndrome in the Intensive Care Unit

1. Changes in thyroid function tests observed in critically ill patients can include all of the following except

   A. Decreased serum triiodothyronine (T_3) level.
   B. Decreased serum thyroxine (T_4) level.
   C. Increased thyrotropin (TSH) level.
   D. Increased serum (T_4) level.

Answers

Chapter 108

1. **True.** Patients receiving therapeutic glucocorticoids for as little as 5 days have shown abnormal cortisol responses to ACTH infusion. As a rule, however, those who have taken glucocorticoids for at least 4 weeks are at greater risk.

2. **True.** It is rare for patients receiving only replacement doses of steroids to experience hypotension during surgical stresses, but supraphysiologic perioperative dosing is still recommended.

3. **False.** The maximal adrenal stress equivalent is 300 to 400 mg of hydrocortisone equivalent per day (60 to 80 mg of methylprednisolone).

4. **True.** Doses in glucocorticoids generally decrease adrenal and immune suppression.

Chapter 109

1. **C.** Lipolysis is accelerated, not inhibited, and peripheral tissues use free fatty acids for fuel. Glycogenolysis proceeds until hepatic glycogen stores are exhausted, and subsequently gluconeogenesis supplies glucose for obligate glycolytic tissues such as the central nervous system. If starvation is severe, lasting for more than 72 hours, the brain utilizes ketone bodies as alternative fuel.

2. **B.** The patient needs corticosteroids for asthma control and needs continued enteral feeding for gut mucosal integrity and nutrition. He requires insulin to decrease the blood sugar to the 150 to 250 mg per deciliter range to avoid metabolic, electrolyte, and possible infectious complication. Continuous intravenous insulin infusion is the preferred route to avoid large swings in glycemic control. Fingerstick blood glucose concentration should be monitored every 1 to 2 hours to ensure safety and efficacy.

Chapter 110

1. **B.** Patients with alcoholic ketoacidosis are often hypoglycemic. Fasting subjects with exhausted glycogen stores depend on the generation of glucose by gluconeogenesis, which is impaired in alcoholic ketoacidosis due to unavailability of NAD^+. NAD^+ is reduced during the metabolism of ethanol. Insulin levels are low, and free fatty acid levels are high. Lactic acidosis contributes to the metabolic acidosis perhaps related to poor tissue oxygenation from dehydration and/or impaired hepatic and renal lactate clearance.

2. **B.** Insulin deficiency is the cause of diabetic ketoacidosis. Lack of insulin results in no glucose entering cells. Glucagon secretion is increased, and gluconeogenesis is accelerated. Blood sugar rises and causes an osmotic diuresis, with water and electrolyte loss. To conserve muscle mass, free fatty acids are released and become the primary fuel source. Free fatty acids are metabolized in the liver to ketoacids, thus producing a metabolic acidosis.

3. **C.** This patient is in diabetic ketoacidosis and is severely dehydrated. Volume resuscitation with isotonic saline is the most important initial therapy. Hyperkalemia probably reflects the systemic acidemia, but total body potassium is severely depleted. The serum potassium value will fall rapidly with volume resuscitation, glucose control, and improving acidemia. Bicarbonate is not indicated for this level of acidemia. The metabolic acidosis will improve with volume and glycemic control. Insulin is essential in this patient's management, but volume resuscitation takes precedence in the initial emergency management.

Chapter 111

1. **A.** Diabetes mellitus and hyperthyroidism may occur in the same patient perhaps due to a common autoimmune etiology. Glycemic control will be more difficult if the patient is hyperthyroid. Tachycardia out of proportion to fever is characteristic of thyroid storm. Significant fever should be aggressively treated to control that component driving oxygen utilization. Atrial

tachyarrhythmias during thyroid storm may require higher doses and higher plasma levels of propranolol for rate control compared to the euthyroid patient.

2. **B.** Beta-blockade stops the peripheral effects of excess thyroid hormone, the cause of the congestive heart failure. Beta-blockers, sometimes combined with digoxin and diuretics, can be used. Large doses of salicylates displace thyroid hormones from serum binding proteins, and an alternative antipyretic should be used. Iodide is important in the early treatment of severe hyperthyroidism and acts by blocking hormone release from the gland. Plasmapheresis and dialysis may be useful in rare patients who do not respond to conventional treatment.

Chapter 112

1. **D.** This patient is in myxedema coma, and hypoglycemia is not uncommon. Supplemental concentrated dextrose or glucose should be administered if the serum value is low. Hypothyroidism is induced in 5 to 30 percent of patients on chronic lithium therapy. Trauma, infection, and cold exposure may precipitate myxedema coma in a hypothyroid patient. The FTI is a calculated value as indicated in B.

Chapter 113

1. **C.** Most seriously ill patients will have a serum cortisol well above 20 μg per deciliter if adrenal function is normal and they are not taking pharmacologic corticosteroids. Adrenal insufficiency is suspected on clinical grounds, and treatment including saline infusion, glucose supplementation, and glucocorticoid placement should be given quickly to seriously ill patients. Diagnostic tests, which involve checking the 1-hour cortisol response to synthetic adrenocorticotropic hormone (ACTH) infusion, can be initiated, but treatment should proceed on clinical grounds before definitive results are available. The most appropriate replacement steroid is hydrocortisone, 300 to 400 mg per day IV in divided doses. This also supplies mineralocorticoid replacement if it is needed. The maximal dose of methylprednisolone needed for glucocorticoid replacement would be 60 to 80 mg per day. Pituitary dysfunction resulting in adrenal failure rarely involves mineralocorticoid deficits, since ACTH is not critical to mineralocorticoid control.

Chapter 114

1. **A.** Hypercalcemia of malignancy can be caused by multiple mechanisms in the same patient. A circulating parathormone-like substance in many patients has been confirmed. Osteolytic bone disease can also cause hypercalcemia, especially in metastatic breast cancer. Treatment of hypercalcemia involves minimizing central nervous system, renal, and cardiovascular affects. This includes increasing renal clearance by saline hydration and addition of loop diuretics when intravascular volume has been expanded. Calcitonin, diphosphonates, and mithramycin inhibit osteoclast activity. Aggressive palliative treatment of the primary or metastatic tumor is essential if any long-lasting control is possible.

Chapter 115

1. **B.** Bicarbonate therapy for lactic acidosis is probably ineffective and may be harmful. A randomized trial failed to show improved hemodynamics in patients with lactic acidosis treated with bicarbonate. Bicarbonate may paradoxically worsen metabolic acidosis by increasing carbon dioxide at the tissue level, which crosses the cellular membrane. In addition, bicarbonate may transiently shift the oxyhemoglobin curve to the left, resulting in less tissue oxygen availability. Administration of sodium bicarbonate can cause hypernatremia.

Chapter 117

1. **C.** TSH levels are usually normal in early acute illness but often fall as the illness progresses. Dopamine and glucocorticoids have a direct inhibitory effect on TSH secretion. Thyrotropin-releasing hormone levels may also be depressed. Acute illness results in impairment of T_4 to T_3 conversion due to inhibition of the enzyme 5′-deiodinase. Therefore, T_3 levels fall shortly after onset of severe illness. Reverse T_3 (rT_3) levels will increase due to unaffected conversion from T_4 and slow degradation. T_4 levels may be elevated in early acute illness due to increased thyronine-binding globulin levels or the inhibition of 5′-deiodinase. Late in severe illness, however, T_4 level declines due to decreased binding to carrier proteins, decreased TSH level, and increased non-deiodinase metabolic pathways.

IX. Hematologic Problems in the Intensive Care Unit

118. Acquired Bleeding Disorders

True or False. Regarding the hemostatic and fibrinolytic processes:

1. Thromboxane A_2 mobilizes other platelets.

2. Platelet pseudopod extension and internal contraction are energy-dependent phenomena.

3. Fibrinogen is the bridge mediating platelet aggregation.

4. All of the clotting factors are serine proteases.

5. Factor XIII is a transglutaminase that introduces covalent bonds between lysine and glutamine residues.

6. Activated procoagulants do not inhibit their own further generation.

7. Antithrombin III appears to inhibit other clotting factors and not just inhibit activated thrombin.

8. Protein C requires activation by thrombin in conjunction with thrombomodulin for its effect on factors V and VIII.

9. Compartmentalization of reactions helps to limit the degree of coagulation.

10. Plasminogen formation of plasmin is an abnormal process that predisposes to clinical bleeding.

11. Which of the following statements regarding acquired bleeding disorders is true?

A. The most common cause of qualitative platelet disorders is autoimmune disease.
B. Desmopressin (DDAVP) offers no benefit to patients with functional platelet disorders.
C. Vitamin K deficiency can be commonly observed in critically ill patients.
D. The diagnosis of disseminated intravascular coagulation is easily made from the clinical appearance of the patient.
E. Aprotinin is of little value in the control of postbypass bleeding.

119. The Congenital Coagulopathies

1. Select the correct answer. Hemophilia A

A. Is an X-linked recessive disorder caused by decreased levels of properly functioning factor IX.
B. Is an X-linked recessive disorder caused by decreased levels of properly functioning factor VIII.
C. Is a Y-linked recessive disorder caused by decreased levels of properly functioning factor VIII.
D. Is a Y-linked dominant disorder caused by decreased levels of properly functioning factor VIII.
E. Is an X-linked dominant disorder caused by decreased levels of properly functioning factor VIII.

True or False. Regarding hemophilia:

2. Female carriers of hemophilia can manifest some bleeding tendencies.

3. Spontaneous hemorrhage does not usually occur unless the factor levels are less than 1 percent of normal.

4. Patients with factor levels 5 percent of normal activity or more will often not bleed unless stressed by surgery or trauma.

5. Intracranial bleeding is the single major cause of death.

6. For the treatment of life-threatening bleeding in the intensive care unit, a factor VIII level of at least 80 percent should be achieved.

7. Which of the following statements is true?

A. Hemophilia A is the most common congenital coagulopathy.
B. Factor VIII inhibitor antibody tends to develop in patients over 50 years of age who have received fewer than five treatments of factor concentrate.
C. Currently, roughly 20 percent of all U.S. hemophiliacs are seropositive for the human immunodeficiency virus (HIV).
D. Patients with type I von Willebrand disease do not respond to DDAVP.
E. Patients with type III von Willebrand disease do not respond to DDAVP.

120. Thrombocytopenia

1. Select the correct answer. Thrombocytopenia

A. Is defined as a platelet count below 250×10^9 per liter.
B. Is only seen when excessive platelet destruction occurs in the circulatory periphery.
C. Should be initially evaluated with a bone marrow biopsy.
D. Is rarely caused by increased platelet destruction in intensive care unit patients.
E. Is differentiated from pseudothrombocytopenia by reviewing the blood film.

True or False. Regarding the management of thrombocytopenia:

2. Prophylactic platelet transfusions are contraindicated in patients with heparin-induced thrombocytopenia.
3. Desmopressin (DDAVP) can lower the bleeding time in patients with uremia.
4. In many patients, the management is largely supportive while treatment of the underlying etiology is undertaken.
5. Vancomycin-induced thrombocytopenia does not require discontinuation of vancomycin for its treatment.
6. Corticosteroids have been shown to be highly effective in the management of most cases of thrombocytopenia seen in the intensive care unit.

7. Select the correct answer. Thrombocytopenia

   A. Is most likely cured by splenectomy when idiopathic thrombocytopenic purpura is the underlying condition.
   B. Is usually mild and brief in cases of post-transfusion purpura.
   C. Due to thrombotic thrombocytopenic purpura typically occurs in male children.
   D. Due to massive transfusion can be effectively prevented by the prophylactic administration of platelets in patients who receive large intravenous infusion volumes.
   E. Due to hypersplenism can cause severe bleeding and should be aggressively treated with splenectomy.

121. Antithrombotic Therapy

For questions 1 to 5, match each antithrombotic agent with its primary target(s). Each item in the second column should be used only once.

1. Heparin	A. Cyclooxygenase
2. Warfarin	B. Factors II_a, IX_a, X_a, XI_a, and XII_a
3. Dextran	C. Factors II, VII, IX, and X
4. Aspirin	D. Plasminogen
5. Streptokinase	E. Platelet adhesion and aggregation

6. Select the best answer. Heparin therapy

   A. Is best given by intermittent intravenous boluses.
   B. Is usually started with an initial dose of 2500 units per hour and titrated up or down as necessary.
   C. Is most commonly monitored by the activated partial thromboplastin time.
   D. Is achieved when the heparin concentration is 4 units per milliliter.
   E. Should be given for at least 4 weeks to be effective.

True or False. Regarding thrombolytic therapy:

7. Streptokinase is approved for fewer clinical indications than are other thrombolytic agents.

8. Thrombolytic agents have been shown to reduce the mortality from acute pulmonary embolism.
9. Large loading doses of streptokinase are necessary to overcome antistreptococcal antibodies.
10. Thrombolytic therapy does not usually require close monitoring of coagulation parameters.
11. In contrast to the anticoagulant agents, hemorrhage is not the major complication of thrombolytic therapy.

122. Hypercoagulability and the Pathophysiology of Thrombosis in the Critically Ill Patient

True or False. Regarding coagulation and fibrinolysis:

1. Flow promotes dilution and reduces the predisposition toward thrombosis.
2. The activity of antithrombin III is inhibited by heparin.
3. Activated protein C neutralizes activated factors V and VIII.
4. Protein S inhibits the activity of protein C.
5. Natural inhibitors exist for both plasmin and its activators.

For questions 6 to 10, match the acquired thrombophilic disorder with its characteristic. Each item in the second column should be used only once.

6. Antiphospholipid syndrome	A. Budd-Chiari syndrome
7. Polycythemia vera	B. Megakaryocyte hyperproliferation
8. Paroxysmal nocturnal hemoglobinuria	C. Treated by phlebotomy
9. Trousseau's syndrome	D. Presence of lupus anticoagulant
10. Essential thrombocythemia	E. Adenocarcinoma

11. Select the best answer. Prophylaxis against venous thromboembolism
    A. Is contraindicated in patients undergoing neurosurgical procedures.
    B. Requires the same dosage of anticoagulation that is required for the treatment of thromboembolic disease.
    C. Is of no benefit for patients recovering from a myocardial infarction.
    D. Has been shown to be beneficial for patients over 40 years of age undergoing abdominal surgery.
    E. Is not warranted for patients with stroke-in-evolution.

123. The Hemolytic Anemias

True or False. Regarding hemolytic anemia:

1. Intravascular hemolysis is characterized by increased plasma hemoglobin.

2. Extravascular hemolysis is characterized by elevated bilirubin.
3. In most cases of hemolysis, a bone marrow examination is mandatory.
4. The direct Coombs test detects the presence of antibodies in the patient's serum.
5. The indirect Coombs test detects the presence of antibodies in the patient's serum.

6. Select the correct answer. Autoimmune hemolytic anemia (AIHA)

   A. Is commonly associated with a negative direct Coombs test.
   B. Can be classified into six major categories.
   C. Is characterized by the presence of IgA antibodies in the case of the cold-reactive form.
   D. Is characterized by the presence of IgM antibodies in the case of the warm-reactive form.
   E. Can be improved by steroid therapy in most cases of warm-reactive AIHA, whereas steroids are ineffective in most cases of cold-reactive AIHA.

For questions 7 to 11, match each type of hemolytic anemia with its offending etiology or associated clinical finding. Each item in the second column should be used only once.

7. Paroxysmal nocturnal hemoglobinuria	A. Hemoglobin S
8. March hemoglobinuria	B. Sticky platelets
9. Osmotic erythrocyte injury	C. Rh incompatibility
10. Erythroblastosis fetalis	D. Physical injury to erythrocytes
11. Sickle cell anemia	E. Hypotonic intravenous infusions

124. Transfusion Therapy: Blood Components and Transfusion Complications

1. The hemoglobin level at which transfusion is warranted in red cell transfusion therapy is

   A. 12 gm per deciliter.
   B. 10 gm per deciliter.
   C. 8 gm per deciliter.
   D. 6 gm per deciliter.
   E. Dependent on the patient's clinical situation.

125. Granulocytopenia

1. Which of the following statements regarding cytokines is false?

   A. Granulocyte-macrophage colony stimulating factor primarily affects the granulocyte pool.

B. Granulocyte-macrophage colony stimulating factor primarily affects the macrophage pool
C. Granulocyte colony stimulating factor primarily affects the granulocyte pool.
D. Macrophage colony stimulating factor primarily affects the macrophage pool.
E. The various colony-stimulating factors prevent apoptotic cell death.

True or False. Regarding drug-induced granulocytopenia:

2. With most chemotherapeutic agents, the nadir of peripheral neutrophil counts occurs about 2 weeks following the onset of therapy.

3. Neutrophil counts usually take longer to recover following treatment with *cis*-chloronitrosourea (CCNU) than with other chemotherapeutic agents.

4. Chloramphenicol only causes an aplastic anemia affecting all cell lines.

5. Penicillin in high doses can cause neutropenia.

6. H_2-blockers have not been implicated in cases of neutropenia.

7. An oliguric patient who developed acute renal failure underwent dialysis, in which 2.5 liters of fluid was removed. During dialysis, the patient became acutely short of breath. Arterial blood gases revealed a PaO_2 of 54 mm Hg on 60% oxygen by face mask, with a $PaCO_2$ of 32 mm Hg. Vital signs revealed a tachycardia of 110 per minute, blood pressure of 124/82 mm Hg, and a respiratory rate of 28 per minute. The patient had an indwelling pulmonary artery catheter, showing a pulmonary capillary wedge pressure of 7 mm Hg, a cardiac index of 4.9 L/min/m^2, and a mixed venous oxygen saturation of 74 percent. Which of the following tests is most likely to reveal the etiology of the hypoxemia?

A. Serum calcium level.
B. Hematocrit determination.
C. White blood cell count determination.
D. Colloid oncotic pressure measurement.
E. Serum albumin determination.

126. The Acute Leukemias

1. Select the correct answer. Acute lymphoblastic leukemia (ALL)

A. Primarily affects the elderly.
B. Has three distinct immunologic subtypes.
C. Is incurable for the majority of patients it affects.
D. Has a good prognosis when associated with a chromosomal marker of the Philadelphia type.
E. Is of the T cell type in the majority of cases.

2. Select the correct answer. Acute myelogenous leukemia (AML)

A. Primarily affects children.
B. Is often associated with disseminated intravascular coagulation (DIC) in its promyelocytic form.
C. Has three subtypes in the French-American-British (FAB) classification system.

D. Cannot be treated with bone marrow transplantation.
E. Has an excellent response rate in the elderly.

True or False. Regarding the medical complications of acute leukemia:

3. Patients presenting with hyperleukocytosis have a poorer prognosis.

4. Respiratory failure rarely develops as a result of leukemic infiltration and/or infection.

5. Patients can develop lethargy and obtundation secondary to leukostasis within the cerebral circulation.

6. Patients can develop DIC as a result of the release of a procoagulant from the primary azurophilic granules of leukemic promyeloblasts.

7. Patients should not be started on antibiotics until inflammation is identified at the site of infection.

For questions 8 to 12, match the chemotherapeutic agent with its characteristic feature. Each item in the second column should be used only once.

8. Cytosine arabinoside	A. Toxicity treated with leucovorin
9. Daunorubicin	B. Toxic to bladder mucosa
10. Vincristine	C. Peripheral neuropathy
11. Methotrexate	D. Cardiotoxicity
12. Cyclophosphamide	E. Cerebellar toxicity

127. Oncologic Emergencies

1. Which of the following statements regarding the superior vena cava (SVC) syndrome is false?

A. Currently, most cases of SVC syndrome result from malignancies.
B. Swan-Ganz catheters can cause SVC syndrome.
C. The presence of azygous occlusion increases the likelihood of problems.
D. Thoracotomy is necessary to establish the etiology.
E. The mainstay of therapy is radiation.

2. Select the correct answer. Epidural metastatic tumor compression of the spinal cord

A. Is usually caused by metastatic prostatic cancer.
B. Typically presents initially with autonomic dysfunction.
C. Is rarely detected on plain radiography of the spine.
D. Mandates prompt lumbar puncture and myelography with neurosurgical backup.
E. Should be initially approached with radiation therapy in most cases.

3. Which of the following statements regarding the hypercalcemia of malignancy is false?

A. Hypercalcemia usually occurs late in the course of the disease in most cases.

B. Only about 15 percent of cancer patients with hypercalcemia do not have bone metastases.
C. Hypercalcemia appears to be precipitated by hormonal therapy in about 25 percent of breast cancer patients who develop elevated calcium levels.
D. Volume infusions and diuretic agents can help reduce the calcium level.
E. Approximately 80 percent of the total serum calcium is bound to protein.

Answers

Chapter 118

1. **True.**

2. **True.**

3. **True.**

4. **False.**

5. **True.**

6. **False.**

7. **True.**

8. **True.**

9. **True.**

10. **False.**

The process of blood coagulation is a highly complex system of cellular and molecular interactions. One of the key initiating events is platelet adhesion and activation. With activation, platelets release thromboxane A_2 as a result of initiation of the prostaglandin synthetic pathway. Thromboxane A_2, in turn, activates other platelets to amplify the initial response. With activation, platelets undergo a shape change, extruding pseudopods while internally contracting, a process requiring energy and the interaction of actin and myosin filaments. As a part of the shape changes on platelet membranes, the glycoprotein II_b-III_a complex is exposed, enabling fibrinogen binding to the platelet surface. Fibrinogen serves as the bridge linking platelets together during the phase of platelet adhesion and aggregation. Many of the clotting factors (specifically XII, XI, X, IX, VII, II, and prekallikrein) are called serine proteases because of the mechanism of their enzymatic reaction. On the other hand, factor XIII is not a serine protease but is a transglutaminase, stabilizing polymerized fibrin by introducing covalent bonds between lysine and glutamine residues.

Several mechanisms exist to control the process of fibrin formation so the circulation does not come to a frozen standstill of total body clotting. While some of the initial clotting processes serve to amplify their own formation (such as the activation of factor XII), many of the activated factors serve to inhibit their own further generation (for example, excess factor X_a inhibits factor VII activity). Antithrombin III is a major modulator of the coagulation cascade, affecting factors X_a, IX_a, XI_a, XII_a, and kallikrein, in addition to thrombin (factor II_a) itself. Protein C inhibits activated factors V and VIII after being activated by thrombin in conjunction with the endothelial cell membrane-based molecule thrombomodulin. Compartmentalization is a mechanism that helps to limit the spread of fibrin formation, in large part controlled by the requirement for phospholipid surface (membrane) binding for reactions to occur. Plasmin activation from plasminogen is a normal part of the clotting process, serving to keep fibrin formation from extending beyond areas where it is not being actively stimulated.

11. **C.** The most common cause of qualitative platelet disorders is drugs, with aspirin and other nonsteroidal anti-inflammatory medications being the main offenders. Desmopressin (DDAVP) is useful in some patients with functional platelet disorders such as uremia. Vitamin K deficiency can be commonly observed in critically ill patients because of the mechanisms that can produce this phenomenon, such as biliary disease, malnutrition, and antibiotic use. The diagnosis of disseminated intravascular coagulation is difficult and complicated by the fact that the clinical manifestations range from none at all to a severe hemorrhagic disorder; the definitive diagnosis is established in the laboratory. Aprotinin, a serine protease inhibitor that seriously affects plasmin, has recently been shown to decrease blood loss in patients following cardiopulmonary bypass.

Chapter 119

1. **B.** Hemophilia A is the name given to a congenital coagulation defect that results in inadequate levels of properly functioning procoagulant factor VIII. The disease is X-linked and recessive; thus it is a disease of males carried primarily by females. It accounts for roughly 80 percent of the true hemophilias. Hemophilia B is another X-linked bleeding disorder that results in decreased levels of functional procoagulant factor IX (Christmas factor).

2. **True.** Female carriers of hemophilia are not entirely immune from the condition, as they may show bleeding tendencies following surgery or trauma if their normal X chromosomes are more randomly expressed than normal. They may have factor levels less than 10 percent, similar to mild hemophiliacs.

3. **True.** In true hemophiliacs, spontaneous hemorrhage does not usually occur unless the factor levels are less than 1 percent of normal.

4. **True.** Those with factor levels of 5 percent or more will often not bleed unless stressed by surgery or trauma.

5. **False.** Intracranial bleeding had been the single major cause of death until the acquired immunodeficiency syndrome (AIDS) epidemic emerged.

6. **True.** While most major joint or muscle bleeding requires a factor VIII level of 50 percent, the treatment of life-threatening bleeding in the intensive care unit requires a level of at least 80 percent.

7. **E.** It is surprising for many to learn that the most common congenital coagulopathy is actually von Willebrand's disease and not hemophilia. Von Willebrand's disease occurs in approximately 1 in 200 of the general population, whereas hemophilia A occurs 10 to 15 times in every 100,000 males. In the

management of hemophilia A, repeated treatments can result in the development of an inhibitor antibody to factor VIII. Typically, this results after 5 to 30 treatments with factor concentrates in patients below the age of 5 years. A more severe problem in the treatment of hemophilia is AIDS, with about 70 percent of all U.S. hemophiliacs now seropositive for HIV. In the management of von Willebrand's disease, patients with the type I version respond very well to DDAVP, whereas those with type III do not respond to DDAVP.

Chapter 120

1. **E.** Thrombocytopenia can be defined in many ways. However, normal platelet counts range from 150×10^9 to 400×10^9 per liter. Most clinicians agree on platelet counts of less than 150×10^9 per liter as being indicative of thrombocytopenia, as this level is 2 standard deviations below the mean platelet count for a normal, healthy population. Thrombocytopenia can develop from one of four mechanisms: inadequate platelet production, hemodilution, platelet sequestration, and increased platelet destruction. Most cases of thrombocytopenia can be diagnosed from the history, physical examination, a complete blood count, and the peripheral blood film. Bone marrow biopsy is only warranted when the mechanism for thrombocytopenia remains obscure or in patients in whom decreased platelet production is suspected. It is rarely necessary in intensive care unit patients because they most commonly suffer from increased platelet destruction. Thrombocytopenia is differentiated from pseudothrombocytopenia by reviewing the blood film.

2. **True.**

3. **True.**

4. **True.**

5. **False.**

6. **False.**

The management of thrombocytopenia varies, depending on the particular etiology of the low platelet number. In many patients, the management is largely supportive while treatment of the underlying etiology is undertaken. While platelelet transfusions may be necessary in many cases of thrombocytopenia, they are actually contraindicated in patients with platelet-mediated thrombosis (i.e., heparin-induced thrombocytopenia, thrombotic thrombocytopenic purpura, hemolytic-uremic syndrome). Desmopressin (DDAVP) may be useful in some cases of functional platelet disorders (e.g., uremia, cirrhosis) where it can lower the bleeding time as long as the platelet count is not severely depressed (i.e., $> 20 \times 10^9$/L). Vancomycin-induced thrombocytopenia appears to affect IgG Fab binding to specific glycoprotein complexes (i.e., GPIIb/IIIa or GPIb/IX); treatment includes discontinuation of vancomycin and replacement (if necessary) with a non–cross-reactive agent. While corticosteroids may benefit some types of thrombocytopenia where excessive platelet destruction is involved, such as idiopathic thrombocytopenic purpura, they are not consistently beneficial for all types of thrombocytopenia.

7. A. Idiopathic thrombocytopenic purpura is a relatively common autoimmune condition characterized by premature destruction of platelets. While treatment is usually initiated with corticosteroids, splenectomy offers the best chance for a lasting cure. Post-transfusion purpura produces a severe, life-threatening thrombocytopenia that can last for days to weeks. Thrombotic thrombocytopenic purpura is a thrombotic microangiopathic disorder that occurs in middle-aged adults with a slight female predominance. Thrombocytopenia due to dilution is treated when platelet counts become severely diminished in patients with active bleeding, but prophylaxis is not warranted. Hypersplenism increases the circulating platelet pool through sequestration. The platelet count is usually not severely depressed, and thus splenectomy is not often useful unless it somehow contributes to the management of other pathophysiologies (i.e., portal hypertension).

Chapter 121

1. B.

2. C.

3. E.

4. A.

5. D.

Several pharmacologic agents are used clinically in modulating the hemostatic process for therapeutic or prophylactic reasons. Each agent has a particular area of primary activity that impacts the rationale for its use in a particular situation. Heparin is administered intravenously and serves as the specific cofactor for antithrombin III in its activity against activated free forms of the serine proteases, specifically factors II_a, IX_a, X_a, XI_a, and XII_a. Thus, heparin is useful in controlling uncontrolled activation of the clotting cascade and is only useful when adequate amounts of antithrombin III are present. Warfarin is the most commonly used oral anticoagulant. It interferes with the production of the vitamin K–dependent clotting factors (inactivated factors II, VII, IX, and X) by the liver. Thus, it is useful when oral administration is desired for the production of a chronic hypocoagulable state. Dextran is an intravenously administered polysaccharide that has mild effects on both platelet function and coagulation. With regard to its effects on platelets, dextran appears to inhibit platelet adhesion and adenosine diphosphate–induced aggregation. Thus, it is used following acute vascular surgery, where an acute, short-term, and mild impairment of hemostasis is consistent with safe post-operative patient management and the inhibition of platelet adhesion as a primary effect is important. Aspirin irreversibly acetylates cyclooxygenase, the key enzyme in the initial stages of the prostaglandin synthesis pathway. Because this renders the platelet essentially nonfunctional for its lifetime (about 10 days), aspirin is more useful when a more chronic impairment of platelet adhesion and aggregation is desired. Streptokinase binds to plasminogen, promoting the formation of plasmin, the circulation's primary fibrinolytic agent. Thus, streptokinase and other plasminogen activators (urokinase and tissue plasminogen activator) find their best use in the acute thromboembolic setting, where clot lodgement threatens tissue or whole body viability.

6. **C.** Heparin used to be given by intermittent intravenous boluses, until several clinical studies indicated that safer and more consistent management could be achieved with continuous intravenous infusion. Typically, a patient is loaded with a bolused dose of heparin ranging from 50 to 125 units per kilogram and then is maintained with an infusion of 1000 to 1200 units per hour. The dose is adjusted as necessary, usually monitoring against the patient's activated partial thromboplastin time, trying to keep it 1.5 to 2.5 times control values. Therapeutic heparin concentrations usually range from 0.2 to 0.6 units per milliliter. Usually, heparin is given for a period of 5 to 14 days, ensuring that the period during which the clot is nonadherent is fully covered by adequate anticoagulation.

7. **False.** The various thrombolytic agents are in various stages of evaluation and approval by the Food and Drug Administration for clinical indications. Streptokinase is approved for more indications than the other agents, primarily because of the longer history of experience with the drug.

8. **False.** Urokinase, tissue plasminogen activator, and streptokinase have been studied in the treatment of pulmonary embolism. While they have shown some benefits, there are no data to indicate any improvement in mortality, primarily because of limited study sample sizes.

9. **True.** Large loading doses of streptokinase must be given to overcome antistreptococcal antibodies; additionally, hydrocortisone should be given with streptokinase therapy to prevent side effects of the drug.

10. **True.** Typically, thrombolytic therapy does not require close monitoring of coagulation parameters because a fixed dose is usually given. For long-duration therapy, monitoring either the thrombin time or fibrinogen level may be beneficial in ensuring that a lytic effect has been achieved.

11. **False.** As with the anticoagulant agents, the most common complication of fibrinolytic therapy is bleeding.

Chapter 122

1. **True.**

2. **False.**

3. **True.**

4. **False.**

5. **True.**

   Coagulation and fibrinolysis represent a complex system of interrelated activities among a number of different protein species. The formation of a clot is naturally inhibited by properties that make up a normal circulation. Virchow's triad describes abnormalities that accelerate or promote in vivo clot formation, namely abnormalities of flow, abnormalities of the vessel wall, and abnormalities of the blood itself. The presence of flow tends to inhibit coagulation through the local dilution of clotting factors. Injury to the vessel wall can promote thrombosis by exposing the blood components to collagen and other negative charges, activating several members of the coagulation and inflammatory cascades.

Blood itself contains a number of products that promote, inhibit, and otherwise modulate clot formation. The several factors involved in the clotting cascade exist normally as procoagulants, awaiting activation by other activated components in the cascade. Most of the clotting factors are inhibited in their activity by antithrombin III. Antithrombin III is enhanced 1000- to 10,000-fold by the presence of heparin; indeed, heparin will not work without the presence of adequate amounts of antithrombin III. Activated protein C neutralizes activated factors V and VIII; protein S is a cofactor for protein C. Plasminogen activation is inhibited by plasminogen activator inhibitor-1, while plasmin itself is inhibited by α_2 antiplasmin.

6. **D.**

7. **C.**

8. **A.**

9. **E.**

10. **B.**

A number of acquired thrombophilic disorders have been described, with each having certain characteristics. The antiphospholipid syndrome defines a broad spectrum of abnormalities involving the presence of the lupus anticoagulant, thrombocytopenia, hemolytic anemia, leg ulcers, and a tendency for arterial and venous thrombosis. Polycythemia vera belongs to a group of myeloproliferative syndromes associated with recurrent thromboses; it is often treated with aggessive phlebotomy. Another myeloproliferative disorder, essential thrombocythemia, represents a hyperproliferation of megakaryocytes, with a resultant thrombocytosis. Paroxysmal nocturnal hemoglobinuria tends to promote thrombosis of splanchnic vessels, particularly the hepatic veins, producing the Budd-Chiari syndrome. Trousseau's syndrome represents the hypercoagulability associated with adenocarcinoma.

11. **D.** Because of the significant morbidity and mortality that accompany venous thromboembolism, the potential to prevent these consequences has attracted a great deal of scientific interest. In general, it can be summarized that there is a group of patients who are at risk for venous thromboembolic disease and who can have their risk significantly reduced through appropriate prophylactic measures. In general, this consists of the use of anticoagulant agents, although in some cases, such as in neurosurgical patients where the risk of bleeding mitigates against anticoagulant use, effective prophylaxis can often be achieved with intermittent pneumatic compression devices. It has been shown that the doses of anticoagulation necessary for prophylaxis are much lower than those usually required for the treatment of thrombotic disease. The patients who have been most thoroughly evaluated are those undergoing elective abdominal surgery, in whom prophylactic anticoagulation has been shown to be beneficial in patients over 40 years of age. Patients with recent myocardial infarction and those with stroke-in-evolution also appear to be aided by the use of prophylactic anticoagulation.

Chapter 123

1. **True.**

2. **True.**

3. **False.**

4. **False.**

5. **True.**

Hemolytic anemias can be characterized by whether the hemolysis occurs within or outside of blood vessels. Intravascular hemolysis is typically characterized by an acute anemia associated with increased plasma hemoglobin, hemoglobinuria, and reduced plasma haptoglobin. Extravascular hemolysis develops more slowly and is characterized by an elevated serum bilirubin with a minimal increase, if any, in plasma hemoglobin. In determining if the anemia is due to increased destruction or decreased production, the reticulocyte count is usually a good index of bone marrow activity, thereby negating the need for a bone marrow examination. The direct Coombs test is performed on the patient's red cells, whereas the indirect Coombs test detects the presence of antibodies in the patient's serum.

6. **E.** AIHA can be broken down into two major categories: cold-reactive and warm-reactive. This classification terminology is based on the best temperature range at which the offending antibodies react and agglutinate. In most cases of AIHA, a positive direct Coombs test identifies the presence of antibodies to the patient's own red cells. Cold-reactive AIHA is characterized by the presence of IgM antibodies that react best at low temperatures, whereas warm-reactive AIHA is usually associated with the presence of IgG antibodies that react best at body temperature. Corticosteroids are usually of no benefit in the case of cold-reactive AIHA, whereas they can help roughly 80 percent of patients with the idiopathic form of warm-reactive AIHA.

7. **B.**

8. **D.**

9. **E.**

10. **C.**

11. **A.**

Hemolysis of red cells can occur through a variety of mechanisms, both congenital and acquired. Paroxysmal nocturnal hemoglobinuria is an acquired stem cell disorder manifested by severe intravascular hemolysis, thrombocytopenia, and thrombotic events. A peculiar characteristic, that of abnormally sticky platelets, may be responsible for many of the thrombotic consequences of this disease. March hemoglobinuria appears to occur as a result of physical injury to red blood cells in the capillaries of the feet during excessive physical exertion. Osmotic erythrocyte injury is a transient episode of intravascular hemolysis that occurs following the intravenous infusion of hypotonic solutions. Erythroblastosis fetalis, or hemolytic disease of the newborn, occurs when an Rh-negative mother is sensitized to the presence of the Rh antigen in an Rh-positive fetus, affecting subsequent pregnancies. Sickle cell anemia is due to the homozygous presence of the abnormal hemoglobin, hemoglobin S.

Chapter 124

1. **E.** A National Institutes of Health Consensus Development Conference reviewed the available information regarding perioperative red cell transfusion and came to the conclusion that the arbitrary hemoglobin level of 10 gm per deciliter that clinicians have traditionally used was insupportable. The fundamental function of red blood cells is the transport of oxygen by hemoglobin to oxygen-dependent tissue beds, and transfusion should only be performed when oxygen delivery is seriously inadequate. Many otherwise normal patients can often tolerate hemoglobin levels of 7 to 8 gm per deciliter without adverse sequelae, and thus transfusing such patients would be wasteful. On the other hand, critically ill patients with circulatory insufficiency or impending organ failure may not have the reserve capable to tolerate even moderate degrees of anemia, and transfusion may be beneficial even if the hemoglobin already exceeds 10 gm per deciliter. A rational approach to red cell transfusion therapy ignores an arbitrary hemoglobin level and concentrates instead on signs of inadequate oxygen delivery.

Chapter 125

1. **B.** It has been possible in recent years to isolate and purify several growth hormones that control white blood cell development. Several are now in clinical use, primarily for the management of severely neutropenic patients. Granulocyte-macrophage colony stimulating factor and granulocyte colony stimulating factor primarily affect the granulocyte pool, while macrophage colony stimulating factor appears to act primarily on the macrophage population. These factors prevent apoptotic cell death in their respective cell lines.

2. **True.**

3. **True.**

4. **False.**

5. **True.**

6. **False.**

The list of potential drug causes of granulocytopenia is exhaustive. Granulocytopenia resulting from drug administration can be produced through decreased production or increased destruction. Chemotherapeutic agents used in the treatment of cancers are notorious for their ability to produce granulocytopenia, affecting as they do the more rapidly dividing cells. With most of these agents, the nadir of the white cell count occurs some 10 to 14 days following the beginning of chemotherapy administration, roughly paralleling the life span of neutrophils. A notable exception to this time course occurs with those chemotherapeutic agents that affect stem cells, such as CCNU, BCNU, melphalan, and busulfan, where the duration of granulocytopenia is significantly longer, lasting up to 6 weeks, with the nadir occurring roughly 1 month following the onset of treatment. Antibiotics of many types can cause granulocytopenia. Even penicillin in high doses has been found to produce neutropenia through a drug-hapten mechanism. Chloramphenicol classically produces aplastic anemia, although cases of isolated neutropenia have been described. H_2-blockers such as cimetidine and ranitidine appear to produce neutropenia through receptor blockade.

7. **C.** On occasion, patients undergoing hemodialysis can develop an acute neutropenia associated with pulmonary sequestration of neutrophils. This appears to develop from complement activation through exposure of complement to the cellophane dialysis membranes. Hypoxemia and pulmonary infiltrates can be observed. The pulmonary edema that develops transiently is due to alterations in permeability of the pulmonary capillary membrane and is not likely to result from excessive hydrostatic forces. With the patient's pulmonary capillary wedge pressure of 7 mm Hg, it is exceedingly unlikely for a low colloid oncotic pressure or a low albumin to contribute to the pulmonary edema and hypoxemia.

Chapter 126

1. **B.** ALL is primarily a disease of children, although it can affect adults on occasion. Roughly 60 to 70 percent of children can now be cured of their disease. It can be characterized on the basis of immunologic characteristics into three different subtypes. The most common type, accounting for about 70 percent of cases, is due to pre-B cells carrying the CD10 antigen on their surface. The next most common type is T cell ALL, making up approximately 25 percent of cases. The remainder are B cell type ALL, which is likely a variant of Burkitt's lymphoma. The presence of a type of Philadelphia chromosome (t(9;22)) in the pre-B cell variety of ALL portends an especially poor prognosis.

2. **B.** AML primarily affects adults, although it occasionally occurs in children. The disease appears to be more resistant to chemotherapy in older patients. The FAB classification system identifies seven AML subtypes, distinguished primarily by the different manifestations of the disease. The acute promyelocytic leukemia subtype is often associated with DIC. In some cases of AML, bone marrow transplantation has been employed, using bone marrow from a human leukocyte antigen (HLA)–matched sibling or unrelated donor or the patient's own remission bone marrow treated in vitro by chemotherapy or autologous monoclonal antibodies.

3. **True.**

4. **False.**

5. **True.**

6. **True.**

7. **False.**

A number of medical complications can develop as a result of acute leukemia. In many of these cases, the complications result from the leukemic infiltration of white cells into tissues, occluding the circulation of various body organs. In general, patients with hyperleukocytosis have a worse prognosis than those without it. Leukemic infiltration in the pulmonary and cerebral circulations can produce symptoms referable to those organs, such as dyspnea and obtundation, respectively. The promyelocytic form of acute leukemia is associated with a high frequency of DIC because of the release of a procoagulant from the primary azurophilic granules of promyeloblasts. Because a leukemic patient is often unable to produce the normal inflammatory response to infection, patients who, on the basis of fever, are suspected of being infected should not have antibiotic therapy withheld merely because no inflammatory focus can be identified.

8. E.

9. D.

10. C.

11. A.

12. B.

The chemotherapeutic agents employed in the management of acute leukemia can all produce toxicities related to their general mechanism of effectiveness. Cytosine arabinoside (Ara-C, Cytarabine) can cause severe intestinal mucositis, especially when used in a high-dose bolus regimen. In the worst cases, this can produce severe ileus and gram-negative sepsis. Cytosine arabinoside can also produce cerebellar toxicity. Daunorubicin and other anthracyclines and anthraquinones are prone to producing cardiotoxicity, especially as the cumulative dose increases. Vincristine, a vinca alkaloid, inhibits microtubular formation and can produce a peripheral neuropathy. Methotrexate inhibits dihydrofolate reductase. Toxicity can include mucositis, hepatitis, and pulmonary fibrosis. Methotrexate-induced toxicity can be treated with leucovorin (folinic acid) to overcome the metabolic block produced by the chemotherapeutic agent. Cyclophosphamide can be toxic to bladder mucosa.

Chapter 127

1. D. The SVC syndrome is usually an oncologic emergency because the most common etiology is malignant tumors of the upper thorax. In recent reports, indwelling central catheters, such as Swan-Ganz catheters, have been implicated as causes of the SVC syndrome. If patent, the azygous vein allows a collateral pathway for blood return, thereby minimizing symptomatology. Thoracotomy is rarely necessary to establish the diagnosis of the etiology for the SVC syndrome; usually, the histologic diagnosis should be made by the simplest, least invasive method available. The mainstay of treatment for SVC syndrome has been radiation, the dose and rate being determined by the histology.

2. D. Epidural compression of the spinal cord from metastatic tumors most commonly results from lymphoma, multiple myeloma, and, in children, sarcoma and neuroblastoma. Pain is the initial symptom in the majority (>80%) of patients, with weakness as a physical finding on presentation in most of these cases. Sensory deficits are rarely the presenting symptom, and autonomic dysfunction is a late and poor prognostic sign. Plain radiographs are beneficial in the evaluation of extradural compression, providing useful data in 80 percent of patients. Other diagnostic techniques that are useful for this condition are bone scanning, computed tomography, magnetic resonance imaging, myelography, and cerebrospinal fluid analysis. Lumbar puncture should be combined with myelography because the removed spinal fluid may not reaccumulate if there is a complete blockage above. Additionally, because up to 8 percent of patients develop paralysis within 48 hours of lumbar puncture, neurosurgical backup for the lumbar puncture activity should be available. Although surgical decompression was initially the mainstay of therapy, radiation therapy is now considered the treatment of choice in most cases of epidural tumor compression of the spinal cord.

3. E. Hypercalcemia is not an infrequent finding in patients with cancer, particularly those with bony metastases. The results of one study indicate that only 15 percent of cancer patients with hypercalcemia did not have evidence of bone metastasis. Typically, elevated calcium levels occur late in the course of the malignancy, with about 98 percent of the patients already having had their cancer detected. Interpretation of the total calcium level requires some judgment, in that about 40 percent of the total calcium pool is bound to protein, mostly albumin; thus, any reduction in albumin concentration will reduce the total calcium level, although the metabolically active ionized calcium may be normal or even elevated. Measurement of ionized calcium is physiologically more precise. In up to 25 percent of breast cancer patients who develop hypercalcemia, it appears to be precipitated by a course of hormonal therapy, such as androgens, estrogens, antiestrogens, progestins, or ablative surgery. One of the primary treatments of severe hypercalcemia is the combination of volume infusions and diuretic agents.

X. *Overdoses and Poisonings*

128. General Considerations in the Evaluation and Treatment of Poisoning

1. The most effective gastrointestinal decontamination procedure for oral poisonings or overdosage is

A. Activated charcoal.
B. Saline gastric lavage.
C. Syrup of ipecac.
D. Lactulose.

130. Acetaminophen Poisoning

1. Select the correct answer. Acetaminophen hepatotoxicity

A. Correlates poorly with measured serum concentrations.
B. Is associated with high hepatic levels of reduced glutathione.
C. Uncommonly progresses to severe liver failure and death.
D. Is characterized by an almost immediate increase in hepatic transaminases.

2. Select the correct answer. *N*-Acetylcysteine (NAC) therapy for acute acetaminophen toxicity

A. Is associated with frequent anaphylactic or anaphylactoid reactions.
B. Is more effective when administered intravenously.
C. Should be administered even if more than 8 hours has elapsed since ingestion.
D. Is unnecessary if initial liver enzymes are normal and the patient is asymptomatic.

131. Antiarrhythmic Poisoning

1. Polymorphic ventricular tachycardia (torsades de pointes) is associated with antiarrhythmic drug use and

A. Is most common with drugs that prolong repolarization.

B. Is usually associated with toxic antiarrhythmic drug levels.
C. Is invariably associated with baseline interval prolongation.
D. Rarely occurs in the first 4 weeks of antiarrhythmic therapy.

2. Lidocaine half-life is prolonged, and the risk of toxicity is increased in the setting of each of the conditions below except

A. Cirrhosis.
B. Congestive heart failure.
C. Old age.
D. Renal failure.

132. Alcohols and Glycols

1. An intoxicated patient with positive serum and urine ketones but no metabolic acidosis has most likely ingested

A. Isopropanol.
B. Methanol.
C. Ethylene glycol.
D. Ethanol.

2. Urgent hemodialysis is indicated for each clinical scenario below except

A. Methanol ingestion with a severe metabolic acidosis.
B. Ethylene glycol ingestion of approximately 175 mg per kilogram.
C. Visual acuity complaints in a patient with suspected methanol ingestion.
D. Ethanol ingestion with metabolic acidosis.

133. Anticholinergic Poisoning

1. The actions of physostigmine include which of the following?

A. It reversibly blocks the action of acetylcholine at the motor end plate.
B. It decreases receptor sensitivity to acetylcholine.
C. It inhibits acetylcholine release from the presynaptic neuron.
D. It prevents enzymatic degradation of acetylcholine.

134. Anticonvulsant Toxicity

1. Shortly into an intravenous loading dose of phenytoin, a patient develops bradycardia and hypotension. The most likely etiology is

A. Propylene glycol.
B. Metabolic acidosis.
C. Phenytoin metabolites.
D. Phenytoin anaphylaxis.

2. A 32-year-old woman with a history of seizures presented to the emergency room with a history of intentional carbamazepine overdose. She was comatose but hemodynamically stable. The carbamazepine level was 26 μg per milliliter. The patient's mental status gradually improved over the next 12 hours, but she subsequently worsened, with increasing somnolence and hypotension. In addition to hemodynamic and airway support, the next most appropriate procedure is

   A. Sodium bicarbonate intravenously.
   B. More activated charcoal by nasogastric tube.
   C. Physostigmine intravenously.
   D. Flumazenil intravenously.

135. Beta-Blocker Poisoning

1. A 62-year-old man was brought to the emergency room after an intentional overdose of propranolol. On examination he was confused and had a blood pressure of 81/40 mm Hg and a pulse rate of 32 per minute. His electrocardiogram showed sinus bradycardia with a P–R interval of 0.28 second and an intraventricular conduction delay. Intravenous fluids were started, and atropine, 1.0 mg, was given intravenously with minimal results. The most appropriate drug to try in order to stabilize this patient is

   A. Isoproterenol.
   B. Dopamine.
   C. Glucagon.
   D. Dobutamine.

136. Calcium Channel Blocker Poisoning

1. Acute cardiovascular toxicity from diltiazem may cause hypotension, bradycardia, and atrioventricular block. The most effective treatment for these complications is

   A. Glucagon.
   B. Calcium.
   C. Amrinone.
   D. Atropine.

137. Cholinergic Agents

1. A 65-year-old farmer was brought to the emergency room by his family 24 hours after spraying organophosphate pesticides on several acres of crops. Three hours after he had finished work, he noted nausea, vomiting, and diarrhea. Since then he has complained of blurred vision, shortness of breath, and mild weakness in his arms and legs. Following the pesticide spraying, he had removed his work clothes and bathed. On examination, he was diaphoretic and

confused. His heart rate was 52 per minute, blood pressure 100/60 mm Hg, and respiratory rate 30 per minute. Pupils were miotic, and there was excess tearing. Scattered expiratory wheezes were present. Abdominal examination showed mild diffuse tenderness and hyperactive bowel sounds. There was slight diffuse symmetric extremity weakness. Routine blood studies were unremarkable, and a chest x-ray was normal. Serum and red blood cell cholinesterase levels were requested. The electrocardiogram showed sinus bradycardia. Initial prescribed treatment should include

A. Pyridostigmine.
B. A transvenous pacemaker.
C. Succinylcholine and endotracheal intubation.
D. Atropine.

138. Cocaine Poisoning

1. Select the best answer. Chest pain following cocaine ingestion

A. Is unlikely to represent myocardial ischemia in patients without a prior history of coronary artery disease.
B. Should be treated presumptively with beta-adrenergic blocking drugs.
C. Often presents days after the acute ingestion.
D. May represent coronary artery spasm.

139. Corrosive Poisoning

1. A 24-year-old woman attempted suicide by ingesting acidic toilet bowl cleaner. Initial endoscopy showed diffuse severe esophagitis and marked inflammation in the gastric antrum. She was treated with water dilution of her gastrointestinal tract, and she was started on total parenteral nutrition. On the sixth postingestion day, she became more febrile and complained of shortness of breath and substernal pain. Crepitance was noted on both sides of the neck. Chest radiograph showed pneumomediastinum and a left pleural effusion. Contrast swallowing study showed a lower midesophageal perforation. The most appropriate management is

A. Intravenous corticosteroids.
B. Intravenous antibiotics and tube thoracostomy.
C. Thoracotomy with drainage and attempted esophageal repair.
D. Upper gastrointestinal endoscopy with stent placement.

140. Cyclic Antidepressant Poisoning

1. A 42-year-old man presented to the emergency room after ingesting "a bottle" of imipramine tablets. He was somnolent but arousable. His blood pressure was 90/60 mm Hg, pulse was 130 per minute, and respiratory rate was 18 per minute. Physical examination was unremarkable except for tachycardia. The electrocardiogram showed sinus tachycardia with a QRS interval of 0.12 second. Arterial blood gases on a 40% face mask showed pH 7.32, PCO_2 42 mm Hg, and PO_2 126 mm Hg. Intravenous access was established, and normal saline was started. A nasogastric tube was placed and activated charcoal administered. A serum drug screen was sent. The most appropriate next procedure is

A. Intravenous physostigmine.
B. Intravenous sodium bicarbonate.
C. Intravenous phenytoin.
D. To continue supportive therapy pending drug level.

141. Digitalis Poisoning

1. Cardiac glycoside–induced ventricular arrhythmias are most appropriately treated with

A. Phenytoin.
B. Procainamide.
C. Quinidine.
D. Bretylium.

2. A 62-year-old man was hospitalized with an exacerbation of his congestive failure. He was noted to have mild renal insufficiency with a serum creatinine of 2.3 mg per deciliter. Several days later he complained of nausea, weakness, and dizziness on standing. His pulse rate was 42 per minute, his blood pressure was 80/45 mm Hg, and his electrocardiogram showed 2:1 atrioventricular block. The digoxin level returned 6.4 mg per milliliter. The serum potassium was 4.2 mEq per milliliter. Digoxin-specific Fab fragments were administered, and atropine, 1.0 mg, was given intravenously. Intravenous fluids were started, and the patient was moved to the intensive care unit. Within a few minutes, the patient was in sinus tachycardia with a normal P–R and QRS interval and clinically stable. A repeat digoxin level, however, was 14.8 mg per milliliter. The most appropriate treatment now is

A. Repeat digoxin-specific Fab fragment administration.
B. To continue current support.
C. Dilantin administration.
D. Hemodialysis.

142. Envenomations

1. A 27-year-old woman suffered a snakebite on the calf while hiking in the mountains near Denver, Colorado. She recognized the snake as a rattlesnake, and she felt the bite was deep. Her hiking companions should

A. Capture the snake for identification, even if this takes some time.
B. Place a tourniquet around the leg and use snow to immediately cool the limb.
C. Immobilize and splint the extremity and make immediate arrangements for hospital transfer.
D. Avoid incising and mechanically suctioning the bite, even if there is an anticipated delay in hospital transfer.

2. The patient in question 1 arrived in her companion's truck at an emergency room approximately 90 minutes after the snakebite. She was diaphoretic and confused. Her blood pressure was 82/52 mm Hg and her pulse was 180 per minute. A bloody discharge was coming from the bite wound. Large-bore intravenous lines were placed. A urinary catheter drained dark red urine. Blood studies showed a hematocrit of 22 percent, prothrombin time 2.8 times control, and a partial thromboplastin time of 88 seconds. Proper management includes

A. To correct coagulopathy first.
B. Intravenous volume expansion and administration of antivenin.
C. Immediate skin testing to antivenin to assess potential hypersensitivity.
D. Local administration of antivenin into the wound.

147. Lithium Poisoning

1. A 28-year-old woman with a history of manic-depressive illness presented to the emergency room 12 hours after intentional overdose of an unknown number of lithium tablets. She was confused and had slurred speech. Her vital signs were stable except for a pulse rate of 56 per minute and a blood pressure of 100/60 mm Hg. Physical examination was unremarkable except for diffuse hyperreflexia. Laboratory studies showed serum sodium of 152 mEq per liter, potassium of 3.8 mEq per liter, and creatinine of 1.2 mg per deciliter. The electrocardiogram showed sinus bradycardia with an intraventricular conduction delay and a Q–T interval of 0.58 second. She was given intravenous fluids, nasogastric lavage, and activated charcoal down a nasogastric tube in the emergency room, and she was admitted to the intensive care unit. Serum lithium level returned at 3.9 mEq per liter. The most appropriate management is

A. Emergent hemodialysis.
B. Transvenous temporary pacemaker.
C. Subcutaneous vasopressin.
D. More activated charcoal.

148. Methylxanthines

1. A 72-year-old man with chronic obstruction pulmonary disease (COPD) presented to the emergency room complaining of shortness of breath, nausea, and tremors. He reported taking "extra" theophylline tablets for the previous 4 days because of worsening shortness of breath. On examination he was tachycardic and tremulous, but awake and alert. His blood pressure was normal. The chest showed decreased breath sounds but was otherwise clear. There was mild diffuse abdominal tenderness. The electrocardiogram showed sinus tachycardia at 124 per minute with occasional unifocal premature ventricular contractions. The chest radiograph showed changes typical of COPD and no infiltrates or edema. The theophylline level was 34.8 μg per milliliter. Serum potassium was 3.6 mEq per milliliter. The most appropriate treatment is

A. Propranolol.
B. Urgent hemodialysis.

C. Oral activated charcoal.
D. Charcoal hemoperfusion.

2. Select the correct answer. Theophylline-induced seizures

A. Respond rapidly to intravenous diazepam.
B. Only occur with theophylline levels greater than 35 μg per milliliter.
C. Are an indication for charcoal hemoperfusion.
D. May respond to vecuronium.

149. Monoamine Oxidase Inhibitor Toxicity

1. Which of the following sympathomimetic drugs should be used with caution in patients taking a monoamine oxidase inhibitor (MAOI) for depression?

A. Epinephrine.
B. Dopamine.
C. Norepinephrine.
D. Isoproterenol.

2. A severe drug reaction between meperidine and MAOIs that may lead to cardiovascular and neurologic crises has been described. Other agents that have been implicated in similar reactions include all of the following except

A. Metoclopramide.
B. Sumatriptan.
C. Fluoxetine (Prozac).
D. Dextromethorphan.

151. Opiate Overdose

1. Seizures associated with meperidine abuse or overdose are likely to be secondary to

A. Idiosyncratic drug reaction.
B. Toxic metabolite accumulation.
C. Occult central nervous system lesion.
D. Drug adulterants.

154. Salicylate and Other Nonsteroidal Antiinflammatory Drug Poisoning

1. Select the best answer. Metabolic acidosis secondary to severe salicylate intoxication

A. Is not anion gap in character.
B. Occurs early after toxicity when salicylate levels are high.

C. Is often associated with hypoglycemia.
D. May be associated with increased ketoacids.

155. Sedative-Hypnotic Poisoning

1. Flumazenil properties include all of the following except

A. Reversal of benzodiazepine-associated hypotension.
B. Reversal of benzodiazepine-associated sedation.
C. Potential for seizures in benzodiazepine-dependent patients.
D. Persistence of benzodiazepine-associated amnesia.

157. Systemic Asphyxiants

1. A chemist ingested 1 gm of potassium cyanide in a suicide attempt. An ambulance was called by a co-worker, and the patient arrived in the emergency room approximately 1 hour after ingestion. He was anxious, tachycardic, and vomiting. A true statement about his poisoning is

A. One gram is not a fatal dose.
B. Cyanosis should be present.
C. Hypoxemia should be present.
D. Metabolic acidosis should be present.

158. Withdrawal Syndromes

1. Delirium tremens secondary to alcohol withdrawal is commonly characterized by all of the following except

A. Hallucinations.
B. Seizures.
C. Autonomic instability.
D. Fever.

2. The most appropriate agent for controlling the addiction associated with alcohol withdrawal and preventing progression to delirium tremens is

A. Chlorpromazine.
B. Haloperidol.
C. Lorazepam.
D. Ethanol.

Answers

Chapter 128

1. **A.** Activated charcoal is probably the most effective single procedure for gut decontamination and prevention of chemical absorption. Gastric lavage may

result in aspiration, especially in patients who are not awake and alert. There is no substantial evidence that gastric lavage improves outcome when compared to administration of activated charcoal alone. Syrup of ipecac is likewise associated with increased numbers of side effects and complications, but it continues to be useful for home management of some accidental ingestions. Cathartics may be helpful in enhancing bowel motility of ingested toxins that have significant anticholinergic activity, but they do not affect gut chemical absorption significantly.

Chapter 130

1. C. Although severe hepatitis is possible in acetaminophen toxicity, death is unusual. Reports of mortality in untreated patients have varied from 5.3 to 24 percent. Patients treated with *N*-acetylcysteine within 8 hours of drug ingestion have a mortality of less than 1 percent. The risk of liver injury correlates well with the measured blood levels of acetaminophen when the interval from ingestion is known. Reduced glutathione detoxifies reactive toxic acetaminophen metabolites oxidized by the P-450 mixed-function oxidase system. Depletion of reduced glutathione is responsible for increased toxicity. Initial transaminase values are often normal after toxic acetaminophen overdose and may not increase until 24 to 36 hours after ingestion.

2. C. Even if there is substantial delay from acetaminophen ingestion to initiation of NAC, antidote therapy decreases mortality and morbidity presumably from effects other than those on acetaminophen metabolites and reduced glutathione stores. Serious side effects from NAC are rare. Although nausea and vomiting are common, the efficacy of oral NAC is the same as intravenous drug, and the intravenous form is not available in the United States. Initial liver enzymes may be normal even in the case of severe poisoning, and the necessity of therapy should be based on measured levels and nomogram interpretation.

Chapter 131

1. A. Polymorphic ventricular tachycardia occurs most commonly in association with class IA and class III antiarrhythmic drugs that prolong repolarization and increase the Q–T interval. The arrhythmia most often occurs with normal or therapeutic drug levels. One study found that less than half of patients with polymorphic ventricular tachycardia had baseline significant prolongation of the Q–T interval. Most episodes occur within the first 4 days of drug treatment, and the vast majority occur within the first month.

2. D. Lidocaine is metabolized in the liver, and liver disease and congestive heart failure (decreased hepatic blood flow) prolong the drug half-life and lead to drug accumulation. The elderly also often metabolize the drug more slowly. Renal failure does not affect levels or the elimination of the active drug.

Chapter 132

1. A. Isopropanol has twice the central nervous system depressant potency of ethanol. Acetone is the primary metabolite, and acetone cannot be further oxidized to an acid. Therefore, ketones (acetone) are positive, but metabolic acidosis does not occur. Toxicity with methanol and ethylene glycol is associated with metabolic acidosis. These intoxicants are metabolized to acids, and methanol also interferes with the mitochondrial electron transport chain, producing a lactic acidosis in addition. Alcoholic ketoacidosis occurs usually when ethanol levels are low to absent and is attributable to liver glycogen depletion, impaired gluconeogenesis, free fatty acid mobilization, and subsequent ketoacid formation.

2. **D.** Ethanol is primarily metabolized and cleared by the liver. Therapy of alcohol ketoacidosis is supportive, with intravascular volume and electrolyte replacement, glucose, and thiamine. Methanol and ethylene glycol are metabolized to acids that have the potential to produce severe end-organ damage and marked metabolic acidemia. Clearance is accelerated by hemodialysis, and this should be performed early at any indication of significant ingestion.

Chapter 133

1. **D.** Physostigmine binds reversibly to acetylcholinesterase and prevents this enzymatic degradation of acetylcholine, resulting in persistent action. Physostigmine is used in selected cases of anticholinergic poisoning. The drug penetrates the blood-brain barrier more effectively than neostigmine or pyridostigmine.

Chapter 134

1. **A.** Phenytoin is a weak acid and soluble only in alkaline media. The parenteral is therefore delivered in propylene glycol. If the intravenous infusion is too rapid (> 50 mg/min), hemodynamic and cardiac toxicity may occur secondary to the propylene glycol. The treatment is discontinuation of the infusion, at least temporarily, and routine hemodynamic support if necessary.

2. **B.** Carbamazepine may form concretions in the gastrointestinal tract that result in drug depots capable of persistent or intermittent release and absorption of drug over hours or days. A single dose of activated charcoal is inadequate to neutralize large amounts of ingested drug, and multiple doses are necessary. Because of the anticholinergic properties of carbamazepine, however, gastrointestinal decontamination procedures must be done cautiously. Alkalinization does not affect carbamazepine clearance. Flumazenil and physostigmine are not recommended in carbamazepine toxicity.

Chapter 135

1. **C.** Glucagon exerts positive inotropic and chronotropic effects through activation of adenyl cyclase independent of beta-adrenergic receptors. Therefore, glucagon will increase cardiac contractility and heart rate even with complete beta-adrenergic blockade. Other beta-agonists may be helpful if given in large doses, but the effect is inconsistent.

Chapter 136

1. **B.** Supplemental intravenous calcium improves the negative inotropy and atrioventricular conduction disturbances in calcium channel blocker toxicity.

The effect on heart rate is less predictable, and additional beta-sympathomimetic treatment may be needed. Glucagon and amrinone may improve the hemodynamic complications of calcium channel blocker toxicity, but clinical experience with these agents is minimal. Atropine is less effective than beta-agonists in treating the bradycardia.

Chapter 137

1. **D.** Atropine is the primary treatment for cholinergic poisoning. Large doses are sometimes necessary, often in combination with pralidoxime, which reactivates acetylcholinesterase. Pyridostigmine, an anticholinesterase agent, is obviously contraindicated. Transvenous cardiac pacing may eventually be needed if the patient is refractory to atropine and pralidoxime or develops more hemodynamic instability. Intubation and mechanical ventilation may also be necessary for patients with severe bronchospasm or respiratory muscle weakness, but there is no definite indication for this patient. Succinylcholine must be avoided because its effect may be very long lasting in the presence of cholinesterase inhibitors.

Chapter 138

1. **D.** Chest pain following cocaine use may represent myocardial ischemia regardless of the patient's age or cardiac history. The mechanisms of ischemia may be multifactorial including coronary artery spasm, direct toxicity, or induced ischemia in patients with prior disease due to increased myocardial oxygen consumption. Patients will most often complain of pain within 3 hours of ingestion, but rarely chest pain will present days later. Use of beta-blockers is controversial in cocaine toxicity, and some have raised concerns about increased complications from unopposed alpha-adrenergic effects if beta-blockade is imposed.

Chapter 139

1. **C.** This patient has developed esophageal perforation after caustic ingestion, a life-threatening complication. Immediate thoracotomy is indicated to attempt repair of the defect, isolation of the midesophagus, or possible colonic interposition. Intravenous corticosteroids in corrosive esophageal/gastric injuries are controversial but may decrease stricture formation when started prophylactically. They have no place in this patient's management at this time. Upper gastrointestinal endoscopy is unnecessary and may make the esophageal defect worse. The patient will need antibiotics and chest tube drainage, but thoracotomy and attempt at repair are critical.

Chapter 140

1. **C.** Cardiac arrhythmias and conduction abnormalities in tricyclic antidepressant overdoses can be suppressed by increasing the arterial pH to alkalemic ranges. Increasing the pH also increases plasma protein binding of the drug and decreases the available free drug. Increasing the extracellular sodium concentration has similar effects. Physostigmine will antagonize the sinus tachy-

cardia and altered mental status, but the potential for cholinergic toxicity makes this agent rarely indicated. Phenytoin use is controversial and may actually increase the incidence of ventricular tachycardia. This patient has obvious severe toxicity based on his central nervous system and cardiovascular manifestations, and basing treatment decisions on a drug level is inappropriate at this time.

Chapter 141

1. **A.** Phenytoin increases the ventricular fibrillation threshold and speeds conduction through the atrioventricular node. Procainamide and quinidine decrease atrioventricular nodal conduction and are contraindicated. Lidocaine has also been used successfully for digoxin-induced ventricular arrhythmias and can be used safely in the presence of atrioventricular block. Bretylium may also be successful in some cases, but animal models of digoxin toxicity have shown some proarrhythmogenic effects from bretylium.

2. **B.** Digoxin-specific Fab fragments rapidly bind free serum digoxin, and a concentration gradient results that moves tissue-based digoxin into the blood, where it is bound. The total bound and unbound digoxin is measured in the blood assay, and the level will be markedly increased after Fab treatment. Further therapy should be based on the patient's clinical and electrocardiographic status, not the measured drug level. The Fab-digoxin complex is excreted by the kidneys, and the level may be elevated for days. In severe renal failure, dissociation of the complex may occur over time, and increasing free digoxin levels could lead to further toxicity. The digoxin-Fab complex is not cleared by dialysis.

Chapter 142

1. **C.** Initial first aid for venomous snakebites should include placement of a wide constricting band on the extremity proximal to the bite with enough tension to occlude only superficial veins and lymphatics. An arterial tourniquet should be avoided. An involved extremity should be immobilized and splinted at heart level, and immediate transportation to an emergency room should be arranged. Cooling affected limbs is inappropriate, and some believe that cooling may actually drive venom deeper into tissues. Incision of the bite parallel to the axis of the extremity and mechanical suctioning for 30 to 60 minutes may be of benefit if there is an anticipated delay in hospital transfer. Almost all venomous snakebites in the United States are inflicted by pit vipers, and there should never be a delay in stabilization of the patient or hospital transfer while attempting to capture the snake.

2. **B.** Systemic manifestations of envenomation include shock, hemolysis, consumptive coagulopathy, hemorrhage, and acute renal failure. Proper management includes volume expansion and administration of intravenous antivenin. Testing for potential hypersensitivity to antivenin is inappropriate in this clinical situation, since the patient requires the therapy. The patient will be monitored closely, and any reaction should be treated with epinephrine and slowing of the infusion rate. Administration of blood products in an envenomated patient with consumptive coagulopathy should follow treatment with anti-

venin. Local administration of antivenin is not helpful since binding of toxins occurs rapidly and cannot be reversed.

Chapter 147

1. **A.** Hemodialysis effectively removes lithium, and the patient is suffering severe toxicity. Despite a lithium level below 4.0 mEq per liter, the neurologic and cardiovascular abnormalities present may progress without prompt treatment. Lithium absorption may be delayed for up to 72 hours after ingestion, and the acutely determined level may not represent the peak potential for toxicity. Repeated dialysis sessions may be necessary, as lithium slowly leaves that tissue compartment for the circulation. A pacemaker may be necessary, but dialysis should be initiated first, since reduction of lithium levels may stabilize the cardiovascular toxicity. This patient may have drug-induced nephrogenic diabetes insipidus reflected by the elevated serum sodium concentration, but this will not respond to vasopressin. Continued crystalloid volume replacement is the most effective therapy. Lithium is not bound effectively by activated charcoal, and additional treatment is necessary unless there is suspicion of ingestion of additional drugs.

Chapter 148

1. **C.** Serial oral activated charcoal will enhance elimination of theophylline by decreasing absorption and promoting the diffusion of theophylline out of the splanchnic circulation into the gut lumen. Theophylline clearance can be increased twofold by this treatment. Charcoal hemoperfusion is even more effective at drug removal, but the time and delay involved in initiating this procedure and this patient's clinical manifestations make hemoperfusion unnecessary. Hemodialysis also accelerates clearance, but it is comparable to serial oral charcoal. Propranolol may be useful in controlling toxic manifestations of theophylline, but it is not clearly indicated in this patient at this time.

2. **C.** Theophylline-induced seizures are a life-threatening complication, and hemoperfusion should be employed to rapidly decrease the theophylline level. Even with this intervention, however, seizures may be persistent and refractory. Failure to respond to usual doses of diazepam or phenytoin is typical. High-dose barbiturates may be the best anticonvulsant regimen. Theophylline-induced seizures have been described in patients with "high normal" drug levels. Vecuronium is a nondepolarizing neuromuscular blocker, not an anticonvulsant. It may be useful temporarily to control refractory tonic-clonic activity, but it will not affect electrical status epilepticus.

Chapter 149

1. **B.** Treatment with an MAOI results in decreased intraneuronal degradation of catecholamines. The administration of indirectly acting adrenergic agents such as dopamine results in release of stored catecholamines, which may precipitate a crisis. The other sympathomimetic drugs listed act directly on postsynaptic receptors.

2. **A.** All of the drugs listed except for metoclopramide have been associated with severe drug-MAOI reactions, although the data concerning morphine are inconsistent. The drug effect is felt to be an exacerbation of MAOI-induced increases in central nervous system serotonin. In one experimental report, metoclopramide decreased the symptoms of meperidine-MAOI interaction in an animal model.

Chapter 151

1. **B.** Meperidine is metabolized to normeperidine, which has reduced analgesic and euphoric potency but twice the convulsant potential of the parent drug. Normeperidine also has a prolonged elimination half-life, leading to metabolite accumulation after repeated doses or a single large dose. The seizures are usually short-lived, but repeated events may necessitate anticonvulsant therapy. Naloxone is not effective as an antagonist for normeperidine-induced seizures.

Chapter 154

1. **D.** Anion gap metabolic acidosis characteristically occurs greater than 24 hours after acute massive ingestion of salicylates. The mechanism is unclear but probably represents an effect of salicylates on normal oxidative phosphorylation processes and a stimulation of gluconeogenesis, glycolysis, and lipolysis. This leads to accumulation of acids, including ketoacids and lactic acid. Hypoglycemia may be present.

Chapter 155

1. **A.** Acute benzodiazepine overdose, especially parenteral overdose may produce hypotension. This does not usually respond to flumazenil. Flumazenil is a competitive inhibitor at the benzodiazepine receptor and effectively reverses sedation. Amnesia, however, is often retained. Benzodiazepine-dependent patients are at risk for withdrawal seizures with flumazenil administration, and the drug should be avoided if dependence is suspected.

Chapter 157

1. **D.** Cyanide binds to the ferric ion of mitochondrial cytochrome oxidase, blocking the terminal reaction of oxidative phosphorylation. Production of adenosine triphosphate is stopped, and anaerobic metabolism begins, leading to lactic acid production and metabolic acidosis in significant poisoning. Tissue and mixed venous oxygen tensions may be slightly increased. The problem is not hypoxemia, which occurs in late poisoning complicated by respiratory arrest. Ingestion of as little as 200 mg of cyanide can be fatal in an adult.

Chapter 158

1. **B.** Delirium tremens usually begins 48 to 72 hours after the cessation or reduction in alcohol consumption. Seizures rarely occur during the delirium tremens phase. If they should appear, it should prompt concern for an etiology other than the alcohol withdrawal. The most common time for alcohol withdrawal seizures is 8 to 48 hours after abstaining from drinking. The other signs and symptoms listed are characteristic findings.

2. **C.** Benzodiazepines are most effective at controlling agitation and potential self-harm, and they demonstrate cross-tolerance to ethanol, possibly preventing progression to delirium tremens. Phenothiazines and butyrophenones may lower the seizure threshold and do not prevent severe ethanol withdrawal, and they should be avoided. Alcohol will suppress withdrawal reaction, but the duration of action is short and central nervous system side effects are common. In addition, this practice fails in addressing the underlying abusive behavior.

XI. Surgical Problems in the Intensive Care Unit

159. Diagnosis and Management of Intraabdominal Sepsis

1. Which of the following statements regarding peritonitis is false?

A. In cases of perforated diverticulitis, the complication rate from primary anastomosis is significantly higher than when resection with end colostomy is performed.
B. Increased intraabdominal pressure can result in compression of mesenteric and renal veins.
C. Planned relaparotomy has been shown to reduce the mortality rate for diffuse peritonitis.
D. It is important to evacuate all purulent collections in patients with diffuse peritonitis.
E. Anastomotic leakage can increase mortality.

2. Which of the following statements regarding percutaneous drainage of intraabdominal abscesses is true?

A. Percutaneous drainage techniques are capable of removing infected necrotic tissue from the abdomen.
B. Follow-up imaging is rarely necessary for percutaneous drainage of abdominal abscesses.
C. It is not acceptable to cross the peritoneal space to drain an extraperitoneal abscess.
D. Percutaneous drainage can be used to temporize prior to an operation that may be necessary to adequately evacuate infected tissue or treat the underlying cause of the peritonitis.
E. It is not possible to drain lesser sac collections percutaneously.

3. Which of the following statements regarding the antibiotic management of intraabdominal infections is false?

A. The most common organisms isolated from intraabdominal infections are the Enterobacteriaceae and *Bacteroides fragilis*.
B. Aminoglycosides no longer represent the "gold standard" for therapy of intraabdominal infections.
C. Ceftazidime is recommended for general empiric therapy because of its broad spectrum of antimicrobial coverage.

D. Dosage regimens for cell-wall–active agents in critically ill patients should use sufficiently short dosage intervals to ensure that serum levels remain above the minimum inhibitory concentration.
E. Most authorities believe that anti-enterococcal therapy should be given for intraabdominal infection only when enterococci are the only organism isolated or when they are isolated from the blood.

160. Acute Pancreatitis

1. Which of the following drugs is **not** currently thought to be capable of causing acute pancreatitis?

   A. Dideoxyinosine.
   B. Pentamidine.
   C. Azathioprine.
   D. Furosemide.
   E. H_2-blockers.

2. Which of the following techniques usually provides the best imaging of acute pancreatitis?

   A. Plain abdominal radiographs.
   B. Abdominal ultrasound.
   C. Computed tomography (CT).
   D. Percutaneous transhepatic cholangiography.
   E. Endoscopic retrograde cholangiopancreatography (ERCP).

3. Which of the following is **not** considered a grave prognostic sign in acute pancreatitis?

   A. Age over 55 years.
   B. Serum calcium level below 8 mg per deciliter.
   C. PaO_2 below 60 mm Hg.
   D. White blood cell count over 15,000 per cubic millimeter.
   E. Serum amylase level over 1000 IU per deciliter.

161. Necrotizing Fasciitis and Other Soft Tissue Infections

True or False. Regarding skin and soft tissue infections:

1. The presence of gas in a soft tissue infection is diagnostic of clostridial myonecrosis.
2. All clostridial infections occur in muscle.
3. A combination of streptococci and staphylococci can cause a necrotizing fasciitis that is clinically identical to that produced by oral or enteric bacteria.
4. Cellulitis after animal bites is usually due to *Pasteurella multocida.*
5. The mortality rate for nonclostridial myonecrosis appears higher than that of clostridial myonecrosis.

6. The most effective means of establishing the diagnosis of necrotizing fasciitis is

A. Physical examination and needle aspiration.
B. Surgical exploration.
C. Plain radiographs of the area demonstrating gas.
D. Wound sonography.
E. Computed tomography.

162. Management of the Postoperative Cardiac Surgical Patient

1. Which of the following does not reduce the endocardial viability ratio (EVR)?

A. A decrease in aortic diastolic pressure.
B. An increase in heart rate.
C. An increase in aortic systolic pressure.
D. An increase in left ventricular diastolic pressure.
E. A decrease in heart rate.

2. Prophylactic treatment of all post–heart surgery patients with which of the following agents reduces the incidence of atrial fibrillation?

A. Lidocaine.
B. Procainamide.
C. Propranolol.
D. Digoxin.
E. Bretyllium.

3. Which of the following statements regarding postoperative bleeding in the cardiac surgical patient is false?

A. Heparin rebound is the most common cause for a prolonged partial thromboplastin time (PTT) and thrombin time (TT).
B. Platelets should be transfused when platelet dysfunction is suspected as an etiology for a bleeding diathesis.
C. Cardiac surgery patients with emergency exploration for bleeding performed in the intensive care unit have a poor survival rate, and this procedure should not be attempted.
D. A normal reptilase time confirms the diagnosis of heparin rebound.
E. Autotransfused blood has been extensively defibrinated.

166. Pressure Sores

1. Which of the following statements regarding the pathophysiology of pressure sores is true?

A. Skin is less able to resist pressure injury than are fat and resting muscle.
B. Elderly patients are not at increased risk for the development of pressure sores.
C. Tissue pressure decreases from the skin inward.

D. Shea's clinical grading system for pressure sores appears to correlate well with their pathophysiology, emphasizing the progressive inward tissue destruction.
E. A harder resting surface has no impact on the effective tissue pressure.

2. Which of the following statements is true?

A. Pressure sores are unlikely to produce fatalities.
B. Anaerobes such as *Bacteroides fragilis* are rarely involved in pressure sore infections because the open nature of such wounds inhibits anaerobic growth.
C. The definitive diagnostic maneuver for pressure sore infection is tissue and bone biopsies for quantitative bacterial analysis.
D. Radionuclide scanning is frequently helpful in confirming the diagnosis of infection in a pressure sore.
E. Infection in pressure sores can often be suspected by the presence of fever and an elevated white blood cell count.

3. Which of the following statements regarding the management of pressure sores is false?

A. Occlusive dressings can hide and promote wound infections.
B. Occlusive dressings can reduce pain.
C. Split-thickness skin grafts are useful in providing permanent coverage after a pressure sore has been thoroughly debrided.
D. Bone that has been infected or necrotic should be thoroughly debrided.
E. Myocutaneous flaps fill large irregular defects, bring in new blood supply, and provide padding.

168. Epistaxis

1. Most posterior nosebleeds are due to rupture of the

A. Anterior ethmoidal artery.
B. Posterior ethmoidal artery.
C. Lateral branch of the sphenopalatine artery.
D. Septal branch of the sphenopalatine artery.
E. Greater palatine artery.

2. Kisselbach's plexus is

A. A cluster of nerve fibers near the carotid body.
B. Considered an abnormality whenever it is encountered.
C. The area responsible for 90 percent of all nosebleeds.
D. Located on the superior-posterior portion of the nasal septum.
E. A site where ectopic pheochromocytomas are known to occur.

3. Select the correct answer. Posterior epistaxis

A. Commonly results from branches of the superior labial artery.
B. Is usually controlled with balloon catheters.
C. Is best controlled with direct visualization and control of the bleeding vessel.
D. Is more easily controlled than is anterior epistaxis.

E. Is usually controlled with cotton strips soaked in cocaine or tetracaine/phenylephrine.

169. Esophageal Perforation and Mediastinitis

1. Which of the following factors does not predict a poor prognosis following esophageal perforation?

A. Nonoperative management.
B. Poor general medical condition.
C. Spontaneous perforation (in contrast to instrumental or traumatic esophageal perforation).
D. Intrathoracic or intraabdominal perforation (in contrast to cervical perforation).
E. More than 24 hours of delay prior to the institution of therapy.

2. The most frequent isolates responsible for mediastinitis following cardiac surgery are

A. *Klebsiella* species.
B. *Candida* species.
C. Anaerobes.
D. *Staphylococcus* species.
E. *Enterococcus* species.

3. Which of the following signs is **not** suggestive of esophageal perforation?

A. Chest pain and dyspnea following esophageal instrumentation.
B. Intraabdominal free air on plain roentgenograms.
C. Thoracentesis fluid with a pH greater than 6.
D. Mediastinal free air on plain roentgenograms.
E. Thoracentesis fluid with an elevated amylase level.

170. Obstetric Problems in the Intensive Care Unit

1. Select the correct answer. During pregnancy

A. The heart rate increases during the first and second trimesters.
B. The systemic vascular resistance decreases during the first and second trimesters.
C. The cardiac output increases during the first and second trimesters.
D. The stroke volume increases during the first and second trimesters.
E. All of the above are true.

2. Select the correct answer. Fetal blood oxygen content

A. Is highly dependent on the vascular tone of the maternal uterine vessels.
B. Is lower than that of maternal blood because of the lower PO_2.

C. Is not dependent on maternal blood pressure.
D. Is very close to that of maternal blood because of the greater oxygen affinity of fetal hemoglobin.
E. Is lower than that of maternal blood despite a similar PO_2.

3. Which of the following drugs is **not** considered safe to administer to a pregnant patient?

A. Diazepam.
B. Warfarin.
C. Penicillin.
D. Nitroglycerin.
E. Clindamycin.

Answers

Chapter 159

1. C. Perforated diverticulitis usually produces a severe contamination to the peritoneal cavity. In such cases, it is important to resect the involved area and provide a diverting end colostomy to gain control over the septic state. All purulent collections should be evacuated to prevent persistent or recurrent infection. Attempts at primary anastomosis increase the complication rates, with significant mortality attributed to anastomotic leakage. Because of the bowel and abdominal wall edema that occurs with diffuse peritonitis, many of these patients may be difficult to close without exerting a severe amount of pressure intraabdominally. Such intraabdominal pressure elevations can compress mesenteric and renal veins, potentially producing bowel ischemia or renal failure. Because of this concern and because of the severe contamination that would be enclosed with a primary fascial repair, many centers have attempted a technique of temporary fascial prosthetic closure with substances such as Marlex, Silastic, or polytetrafluoroethylene. Planned relaparotomies can then be easily performed to reduce the level of peritoneal contamination through irrigation and debridement, with removal of the prosthesis and definitive abdominal closure when the abdomen is less heavily contaminated and a closure is mechanically feasible. Clinical studies have yet to demonstrate that this technique provides superior outcomes over more traditional methods of management, however.

2. D. Percutaneous drainage of abdominal abscesses represents a major therapeutic improvement in the management of peritonitis. In some patients, the technique may allow for the complete avoidance of a laparotomy that would have been required for drainage. In others, the presence of infected tissue prevents the percutaneous technique from completely evacuating the infectious process. Yet, such patients can often be temporized by using the percutaneous method to relieve the pressure within the collection and reduce the infectious load, thereby potentially improving the patient's clinical condition prior to the required surgical operation. While it is generally not considered prudent to cross the pleural space with a percutaneous approach for fear of producing an empyema, it is acceptable to cross the peritoneal space to drain an extraperitoneal collection. Furthermore, lesser sac collections can often be approached, using either a transgastric approach or a transhepatic route.

3. C. Intraabdominal infections represent serious clinical problems and often involve difficult decisions for the clinician, who is faced with a wide variety of antibiotic choices. The most common organisms isolated from these infections are the Enterobacteriaceae and *Bacteroides fragilis*, and antimicrobial therapy should be targeted against these bacteria. Although aminoglycosides were the "gold standard" for management of gram-negative infections for 30 years, they no longer are the only or even the preferred therapy, as many other agents have been developed that effectively cover the spectrum with less toxicity. Third-generation cephalosporins such as ceftazidime offer a broad range of coverage; however, wide use of this agent is associated with diminishing susceptibility of *Pseudomonas aeruginosa* and emergence of enterococcal superinfections. Therefore, ceftazidime is not recommended for initial empiric therapy. Beta-lactam agents should be given in adequate dosages and with sufficiently short dosing intervals to ensure that their tissue levels remain consistently above the minimum inhibitory concentrations for the organisms being attacked. Although frequently involved in intraabdominal infections, most authorities believe that enterococci should only be covered when they are the predominant organism on culture or they are isolated from the bloodstream.

Chapter 160

1. E. Several drugs appear to be capable of causing acute pancreatitis. Previously, diuretic agents such as furosemide and others were considered the most likely drugs to produce acute pancreatitis. However, recently, other drugs such as dideoxyinosine, pentamidine, and azathioprine have more commonly been observed to produce acute pancreatitis, although this may represent a shift in drug usage patterns as the treatment of acquired immunodeficiency syndrome and transplant patients has become more commonplace. Once considered likely to cause pancreatitis, H_2-blockers are no longer believed to be capable of producing acute pancreatitis.

2. C. CT is the most useful imaging modality in early acute pancreatitis. CT can image the pancreas without being obscured by overlying bowel gas, as is ultrasound examination of the acute abdomen. Plain abdominal radiographs of acute pancreatitis are not very helpful, merely providing suggestions of the etiology, such as a "sentinel loop" overlying the pancreas or retroperitoneal air if a gas-forming organism is involved. Percutaneous transhepatic cholangiography is unlikely to image the pancreas or the pancreatic ducts. ERCP is more likely to image the ducts, although this may not reveal the etiology in cases of acute pancreatitis; furthermore, ERCP could exacerbate the inflammatory process in the pancreas.

3. E. The clinical presentation of acute pancreatitis can vary widely. A worse outcome is often predictable based on indicators of a more severe disease state. Several grave prognostic indicators have been identified by Ranson and by Imrie. These include such findings as age over 55 years, a white blood cell count of over 15,000 per cubic millimeter, a low arterial partial pressure of oxygen, a low serum calcium level, and indicators of hypovolemia or fluid sequestration. Interestingly, the level of serum amylase does not appear to figure as a predictive parameter, although it is commonly used to detect the presence and follow the course of acute pancreatitis.

Chapter 161

1. **False.** While the term "gas gangrene" is an old and popular term for clostridial myonecrosis, clostridial soft tissue infection can occur without the presence of obvious gas formation. Clostridial abscesses can occur without myonecrosis, and nonclostridial myonecrosis can also produce gas in the wound.

2. **False.** Not all clostridial infections occur in muscle, as they can also occur in injured or ischemic subcutaneous tissue. In general, clostridia tend to thrive in poorly perfused tissue, as they are obligate anaerobes.

3. **True.** The combination of streptococci and staphylococci can cause a necrotizing fasciitis that is clinically identical to that produced by other organisms; from animal model work, this appears as though it could be due to the synergistic effects of staphylococcal alpha-lysin and *Streptococcus pyogenes.*

4. **True.** Cellulitis resulting from animal bites is usually due to infection with *P. multocida*, which is commonly susceptible to penicillin.

5. **True.** Nonclostridial myonecrosis can appear in patients with impaired host defenses, such as those with advanced age, diabetes, renal failure, obesity, or atherosclerosis, and is commonly due to a combination of mixed enteric bacteria. Probably because of the poor general health of the patients who develop the condition, nonclostridial myonecrosis appears to carry a higher mortality rate than clostridial myonecrosis, with most of the survivors having extremity infections that lend themselves to amputative control.

6. **B.** The physical examination of a patient with necrotizing fasciitis may be conclusive, especially if extensive superficial necrosis is evident, as can be seen in the scrotal skin infarction of the Fournier syndrome. Needle aspiration of the inflamed area may recover fluid, but a negative aspiration may have missed a deep area of necrosis. Gas and fluid may or may not be visible on plain radiographs, wound sonography, or computed tomography, but none of these conclusively eliminates the possibility of an infectious necrotic process. The most secure means of establishing or eliminating the diagnosis of necrotizing fasciitis in patients who are at risk for the process is through surgical exploration.

Chapter 162

1. **E.** The EVR is defined as the ratio of the diastolic pressure-time index to the systolic pressure-time index. The pressure-time index, in turn, is defined as the time-based integral of the area between the aortic pressure tracing and the left ventricular pressure tracing in either systole or diastole. The EVR represents the effect of hemodynamics on the myocardial oxygen supply and demand. Myocardial perfusion depends on the integrated pressure difference between aortic diastolic pressure and the left ventricular diastolic pressure. A longer diastole with a larger diastolic pressure gradient between the aorta and the left ventricle promotes improved myocardial blood flow and increases the EVR by increasing the numerator in the ratio. Conditions that reduce the EVR include a decrease in aortic diastolic pressure, an increase in left ventricular diastolic pressure, an increase in heart rate, an increase in aortic systolic pres-

sure, or a decrease in left ventricular systolic pressure. A decrease in heart rate would increase the EVR by providing a longer diastole for myocardial perfusion.

2. **C.** Atrial fibrillation and other supraventricular tachycardias are frequently observed in the initial days following cardiac surgery. Propranolol has been shown to reduce the incidence of atrial fibrillation in patients who have recently undergone heart surgery. This is an important consideration for patients taking beta-blockers prior to surgery. Procainamide may be useful after the atrial fibrillation has occurred. Digoxin can slow atrioventricular conduction of a rapid atrial fibrillation but is not very effective as a preventive measure. Lidocaine and bretylium primarily treat ventricular arrhythmias.

3. **D.** Postoperative bleeding in the cardiac surgery patient is a serious condition that can result from multiple potential etiologies. Heparin rebound can occur postoperatively, where a full reversal of heparin after the operation is overcome by release of heparin from body fat stores into the blood. This is the most common cause of a prolonged PTT and TT. A normal reptilase time will confirm that the prolonged TT is due to excessive heparin and not fibrinolysis or consumption. Platelet dysfunction can occur frequently because of preoperative aspirin use or prolonged cardiopulmonary bypass effects. When this condition is suspected as a cause for excessive bleeding, platelets should be transfused. Autotransfusion is being used increasingly to transfuse shed autologous blood and reduce homologous blood use. Autotransfused blood appears to be extensively defribrinated, but it does not appear to contribute to a coagulopathy when it is transfused. Rapid surgical bleeding that makes cardiac arrest imminent is best approached by an immediate reopening of the sternotomy incision in the intensive care unit, with finger control of the bleeding site and vigorous volume resuscitation, to be followed by definitive control in the operating room. This practice appears to produce a survival rate of 60 percent.

Chapter 166

1. **D.** Pressure sores are an all too common and serious problem in chronically ill, paralyzed, or debilitated patients. The pathophysiology of pressure sores relates to the application of an external pressure on an area of tissue that impedes adequate tissue perfusion. In general, it appears that the ischemic and necrotic process extends as a deep area of cavitation outward. Bony prominences are important anatomic foci for the development of pressure sores, as it appears that tissue pressure increases with proximity to bony prominences. Furthermore, subcutaneous fat and resting muscle are less resistant to pressure injury than is the skin, contributing to the cavitation process. Thus, the clinical grading system proposed by Shea does not appear to correlate well with the pathophysiologic process, in that the grading system suggests a progressive inward evolution from a grade I to grade IV status, starting with skin breakdown and ending with bony involvement.

   Elderly patients can be at a significantly increased risk for the development of pressure sores. Their skin is much thinner and much less elastic with poorer peripheral perfusion, all contributing to heightened tissue fragility. When this is combined with mental and physical debilitation as well as incontinence, the chances for decubitus ulceration can become near certain.

   A harder surface provides a smaller area for weight distribution. Pressure is defined as force per unit area. Thus, when gravitational force is applied to a smaller area, pressure increases. The effective pressure in an unpadded wooden chair can increase to 300 mm Hg, compared to 75 mm Hg for a padded chair.

2. **C.** Infection in pressure sores is not uncommon and can produce very serious sequelae. Systemic sepsis produced by pressure sores carries a 50 percent mortality rate despite surgical debridement and systemic antibiotics. The most common organisms encountered are *Staphylococcus aureus* and gram-negative bacilli, including anaerobes such as *Bacteroides fragilis*, attesting to the ischemic and anaerobic nature of these wounds despite the fact that the skin is open over them. The diagnosis of infection in pressure sores can be difficult, as colonization of such wounds is the rule and the debilitated patients in whom these ulcers develop may not demonstrate the typical responses to infection, such as a fever or an elevated white blood cell count. A high level of clinical suspicion for the presence of a pressure sore infection is necessary for effective management. Radionuclide scanning is of little value, although adjuncts such as standard radiographs, contrast-enhanced sinographs, and computed tomography may be helpful. The definitive diagnostic manuever is to biopsy the suspected tissue and bone to perform quantitative bacteriologic analysis, serving to differentiate infection from colonization and to help direct surgical and antibiotic therapy.

3. **C.** At first glance, occlusive dressings appear to provide many advantages in the management of pressure sores. They appear to promote tissue healing, require little attention, decrease pain, and can be left in place for days. Yet, they interfere with the detection of necrosis and infection in the wound. Furthermore, they provide a moist, warm, closed environment that is advantageous for bacterial proliferation. Thus occlusive dressings should be used only on thoroughly viable wounds with minimal bacterial colonization density, a condition that does not often exist in pressure sores.

   In the course of caring for pressure sores, all infected or necrotic bone should be thoroughly debrided to eliminate its potential as a smoldering source for persistent infection. Skin grafts are poor choices for coverage of tissue defects where a pressure sore has been debrided because they are totally dependent on the nutrient blood supply of the residual tissue bed, which may still be compromised. Myocutaneous flaps have revolutionized the management of pressure sores because of their ability to fill large and irregular tissue defects with well-perfused tissue and to provide padding that serves to distribute the patient's weight over a broader surface, thereby reducing the tissue pressure.

Chapter 168

1. **D.** Five arteries supply the internal nose: the anterior ethmoidal and posterior ethmoidal arteries (both branches of the ophthalmic artery, which in turn is a branch of the internal carotid artery), the sphenopalatine and greater palatine arteries (both branches of the internal maxillary artery, which in turn is a branch of the external carotid artery), and the septal branch of the superior labial artery (coming from the facial artery, which is also a branch of the external carotid artery). The septal branch of the sphenopalatine artery supplies most of the middle and posterior parts of the septum and thus is most commonly responsible for posterior nosebleeds.

2. C. Ninety percent of all nosebleeds occur in an area known as Kisselbach's plexus, or Little's area. It is located on the anterior-inferior portion of the nasal septum. It represents a plexus of the end branches of several different source vessels supplying the septum, such as the sphenopalatine, the anterior ethmoidal, the greater palatine, and the superior labial arteries.

3. B. Posterior epistaxis is commonly responsible for bleeding that is more difficult to control than is anterior epistaxis. It usually results from a rupture of the septal branch of the sphenopalatine artery. Although the same techniques used for anterior epistaxis should be initially attempted for posterior bleeding, they are often ineffective, and some form of posterior packing is usually employed. Traditionally, the technique of posterior packing employed gauze packs that were pulled into the posterior pharynx and secured. However, these have now been largely replaced by balloon catheters that can occlude both the posterior and anterior nasal passages.

Chapter 169

1. E. Several published series have identified clinical factors that paint a poor prognosis for patients who have experienced esophageal perforation. A poor general medical condition is one such factor, especially if the perforation occurs in the setting of an associated esophageal cancer. Similarly, any spontaneous perforation carries a worse prognosis than perforations that result from instrumentation or trauma, presumably because it speaks to a worse general overall condition. Intraabdominal and intrathoracic perforations have worse prognoses than perforations that occur in the neck, most likely because of the reduced dissemination of contamination that occurs with the latter location. A delay of more than 24 hours prior to establishing the diagnosis of perforation and instituting treatment is also predictably associated with a poorer outcome. Interestingly, nonoperative management does not appear to carry a worse mortality rate than surgery, although case selection no doubt has a significant amount of influence on which patients are not approached operatively.

2. D. Because of the increase in cardiac surgery approached through a median sternotomy incision, sternal wound infections and mediastinitis have become increasingly common entities in modern intensive care. A variety of organisms have been found to be responsible, although staphylococcal species and other gram-positive organisms are more frequently isolated. Patient mortality can approach 20 percent and is largely related to concomitant medical problems, which in turn could also have contributed significantly to the risk for mediastinitis in the first place.

3. C. Esophageal perforation is a not uncommon consequence of esophageal instrumentation, such as upper gastrointestinal endoscopy and esophageal dilation. The potential for the existence of esophageal perforation should be considered in all such patients who present suddenly with chest pain and dyspnea, although intraabdominal perforations can present with signs of peritonitis and epigastric pain. Plain roentgenograms may show the presence of free air in the neck, mediastinum, pleural space, or intraabdominally. The presence of pleural fluid can often provide a clue if thoracentesis is performed, as the presence of food particles, an elevated amylase level, or a pH of less than 6 is virtually pathognomonic for esophageal perforation.

Chapter 170

1. **E.** Because of the increased demands for oxygen delivery that the placenta and developing fetus place on the maternal circulation, a number of hemodynamic changes are commonly found in the uncomplicated pregnant patient. There is an increase in both the stroke volume and heart rate during the first and second trimester. These combine to produce an increase in the cardiac output that peaks during the second trimester to nearly 50 percent above normal values. Associated with these changes, the calculated systemic vascular resistance decreases to a similar degree. In later stages of pregnancy, the cardiac output can be compromised whenever the patient assumes a supine position because of compression of the inferior vena cava produced by the gravid uterus.

2. **D.** Fetal oxygen delivery is dependent on arterial oxygen content, the uterine arterial blood flow, the placental transfer of oxygen, and the affinity of fetal hemoglobin for oxygen. Because uterine blood vessels are normally maximally dilated, uterine blood flow is directly related to maternal blood pressure. The greater oxygen affinity of fetal hemoglobin overcomes the relatively inefficient placental oxygen transfer and provides the fetus with a blood oxygen content that is very close to that of maternal blood. This occurs despite the fact that the PO_2 in fetal blood is substantially lower than that in the mother.

3. **B.** Concerns are commonly expressed over drugs administered to pregnant women because of the potential for adverse effects on the developing fetus. In general, drug administration should be avoided in all patients unless the potential benefits outweigh the potential risks. In pregnant patients, however, the risks are often greater than in normal individuals because of the presence of the fetus. Yet, several drugs have a long and established track record of safety during pregnancy that makes their use acceptable. Among these are diazepam, the penicillins and cephalosporins, clindamycin, and nitroglycerin, to name a few. Warfarin is associated with a syndrome of developmental defects and should therefore be avoided in early pregnancy.

XII. Shock and Trauma

171. Shock: An Overview

1. Which of the following statements regarding circulatory shock is correct?

A. It has been proved that all patients in shock require higher cardiac outputs than normal.
B. The pulmonary capillary wedge pressure should always be raised to 18 cm H_2O or higher in shock patients.
C. It is important to keep the patient's oxygen delivery at supply-dependent levels.
D. A drop in blood pressure always means that decreased perfusion to tissues is occurring.
E. When oxygen consumption is supply dependent, anaerobic metabolism and lactate production increase, and metabolic acidosis ensues.

2. Which of the following conditions would **not** be considered likely to produce a hypovolemic form of shock?

A. Acute pancreatitis.
B. Bilateral femur fractures.
C. Intestinal obstruction.
D. Tension pneumothorax.
E. Second-degree burns covering 40 percent of body surface area.

3. Which of the following statements concerning the compensatory stage of hypovolemic shock is false?

A. Compensatory mechanisms act to preserve coronary and cerebral perfusion at the expense of perfusion to skin, skeletal muscle, kidneys, and splanchnic viscera.
B. Resuscitation efforts cannot usually be started until this stage is completed because it cannot be detected.
C. Vasoconstriction and transcapillary refill can partially restore the effective intravascular volume.
D. Damage to vital tissues is generally not produced.
E. Myocardial contractility and heart rate usually increase as efforts toward maintaining the cardiac output.

172. Hemorrhage and Resuscitation

1. Which of the following statements regarding fluid resuscitation is true?

A. Resuscitation of hemorrhagic shock patients with isotonic crystalloid solutions increases the amount of pulmonary edema that develops over that seen in patients resuscitated with colloid solutions.
B. Hypertonic saline solutions may be able to provide effective resuscitations with relatively small fluid volumes.
C. An improved mortality rate is observed when trauma patients are resuscitated with colloid solutions.
D. The higher cost of colloid solutions is justified by the more rapid resuscitations that are achieved through their use.
E. The colloid oncotic pressure is more important than the capillary hydrostatic pressure in determining the amount of transvascular fluid movement in the pulmonary circulation.

2. Which of the following conditions would be the **weakest** indication for the transfusion of red blood cells?

A. A serum hemoglobin concentration of 8 gm per deciliter.
B. A mixed venous oxygen saturation of 45 percent.
C. An oxygen extraction ratio of 52 percent.
D. A mixed venous PO_2 of 25 mm Hg.
E. A serum hemoglobin concentration of 3 gm per deciliter.

3. Prophylactic administration of blood components is warranted in which of the following circumstances?

A. Platelet transfusion with every 6 units of red blood cell transfusion during an episode of massive transfusion.
B. Fresh-frozen plasma transfusion with every 6 units of red blood cell transfusion during an episode of massive transfusion.
C. Fresh frozen plasma transfusion with every 2 units of red blood cell transfusion during an episode of massive transfusion.
D. Cryoprecipitate transfusion with every 6 units of fresh frozen plasma transfusion during an episode of massive transfusion.
E. Platelet transfusion for anyone with a platelet count below 10,000 per cubic millimeter.

173. Septic Shock

1. Which of the following conditions would not be considered essential in the definition of the systemic inflammatory response syndrome (SIRS)?

A. Fever or hypothermia.
B. Tachycardia.
C. Tachypnea.
D. Alteration of the white blood cell count.
E. Hypotension.

2. Which of the following statements is true?

A. Lipopolysaccharide (LPS) appears to mediate septic shock, as anti-LPS antibody therapy in humans prevents it.
B. Gram-negative bacteria appear to be the only microbial agents responsible for septic shock.
C. The O-specific side chain of gram-negative bacteria is highly variable.
D. Tumor necrosis factor alpha (TNF-α) has no effect on nitric oxide synthesis.
E. Humans rendered tolerant to LPS resist signs of illness when infected with viable gram-negative bacteria.

3. Which of the following substances is **not** thought to mediate the hypotension of septic shock?

A. Naloxone.
B. Nitric oxide.
C. Tumor necrosis factor alpha.
D. Interleukin-1.
E. Calcitonin gene–related peptide.

174. Trauma: An Overview

1. The primary reason for early death or central nervous system dysfunction in trauma patients is

A. Shock.
B. Bleeding.
C. The presence of a severe closed head injury.
D. Hypoxia.
E. Arrhythmias.

175. Head Trauma

1. In a patient with a closed head injury who manifests systemic circulatory hypertension, attempts to lower the blood pressure with vasodilators

A. May improve cerebral blood flow.
B. May decrease the cerebral perfusion pressure (CPP).
C. May decrease brain edema.
D. May prevent intracranial hemorrhage.
E. Is considered standard therapy.

2. Which of the following statements regarding blood coagulation in patients with head trauma is true?

A. Laboratory evidence of disseminated intravascular coagulation is reported in nearly 25 percent of head-injured patients.
B. Levels of fibrin degradation products correlate with the extent of brain tissue damage.

C. Patients with higher concentrations of fibrin degradation products have poorer functional outcomes.
D. Abnormal prothrombin times (PT), partial thromboplastin times (PTT), or platelet counts are seen in 55 percent of patients who develop delayed intracranial hematomas.
E. All of the above.

3. What percentage of patients develop an increased cerebral A-$\dot{V}DO_2$ during hyperventilation therapy?

A. 0 percent.
B. 20 percent.
C. 40 percent.
D. 60 percent.
E. 80 percent.

4. What proportion of head-injured patients with an altered level of consciousness have an elevated ICP?

A. 0 percent.
B. 20 percent.
C. 40 percent.
D. 60 percent.
E. 80 percent.

5. Which of the following statements is true?

A. Fluid restriction of the head-injured patient consistently reduces ICP.
B. Corticosteroids used in the head-injured patient consistently reduce ICP.
C. Empiric hyperventilation of the head-injured patient improves clinical outcomes.
D. Mannitol reduces brain water primarily in normal (uninjured) brain.
E. Barbiturates used in the head-injured patient consistently reduce ICP.

176. Spinal Cord Trauma

1. The skeletal and ligamentous elements that compose the middle column, providing spinal stability, are the posterior longitudinal ligament, the posterior annulus fibrosis, and the

A. Anterior wall of the vertebral column.
B. Posterior wall of the vertebral column.
C. Anterior longitudinal ligament.
D. Ligamentum flavum.
E. Apophyseal joint capsules.

2. The finding of sacral sparing in a patient with spinal cord injury indicates

A. A higher lesion in the cord than is indicated by the patient's dermatome level.
B. A lower lesion in the cord than is indicated by the patient's dermatome level.
C. The absence of a central cord syndrome.

D. A more favorable prognosis than exists when sacral sparing is not present.
E. The presence of spinal shock.

3. Which of the following statements concerning corticosteroid use in spinal cord trauma is **not** true?

A. Steroids must be administered within 8 hours of injury to provide a beneficial effect.
B. The steroid protocol for reduction of spinal cord morbidity requires a period of administration that encompasses 24 hours.
C. The steroid protocol for reduction of spinal cord morbidity requires a period of administration that encompasses 8 hours.
D. High-dose corticosteroids have been shown to improve motor and sensory function following spinal cord injury.
E. A short course of high-dose corticosteroids administered for spinal cord injury has not been shown to increase the morbidity or mortality rate.

177. Thoracic Trauma

1. A 28-year-old man who was involved in a motor vehicle crash 4 hours prior to arrival in the emergency department is found to have a right hemopneumothorax on a chest radiograph. A straight 36 Fr. chest tube is inserted in the right fourth intercostal space, and 750 ml of blood is evacuated. A follow-up chest radiograph demonstrates that the lung is still incompletely expanded, with some residual clot present. What steps should be taken to inflate the right lung?

A. The patient should be endotracheally intubated with application of positive end-expiratory pressure (PEEP) to help inflate the collapsed lung.
B. Suction on the chest tube drainage chamber should be increased to 80 cm H_2O.
C. Urokinase should be injected into the chest tube to lyse the clot that is present.
D. A chest tube should be inserted through a more cephalad intercostal space.
E. Vigorous pulmonary toilet with therapeutic bronchoscopy, another chest tube on the right side, or operative removal of the pleural clot may be required.

2. A 38-year-old man is thrown from his motorcycle at high speed onto a car in a parallel lane. At the scene of the collision, his initial vital signs show a blood pressure of 90/70 mm Hg, a heart rate of 112 per minute, and a respiratory rate of 42 per minute. He is noted to have a large open pneumothorax involving the left chest. The paramedics apply an occlusive dressing over the wound, taping it tightly on only three of the four sides of the dressing. They also insert two 14-gauge intravenous catheters and infuse Ringer's lactate rapidly. During transport, after the infusion of 1500 ml of IV solution, they note that his blood pressure increases to 132/82 mm Hg, his heart rate slows to 78 per minute, and his breathing appears much easier at a rate of 16 per minute. His IV rate is accordingly decreased. However, on his arrival in the emergency department, he is noted to be acutely diaphoretic, cyanotic, and in respiratory distress, with a blood pressure of 70/40 mm Hg, a heart rate of 140 per minute, and a respiratory rate of 44 per minute. At the sternal notch, his trachea appears to be deviated to the right. What should be the initial response?

A. Emergency tracheostomy.
B. Increase the IV infusions once more, and type and cross for blood.
C. Administer intravenous epinephrine.
D. Remove the dressing over the open pneumothorax.
E. Perform an emergency left thoracotomy.

3. Which of the following radiologic signs is **not** strongly associated with a mediastinal hematoma or a traumatic tear of the thoracic aorta?

A. Fracture of the first rib.
B. Mediastinal widening greater than 8 cm.
C. Depression of the left mainstem bronchus.
D. Deviation of the trachea to the right.
E. Presence of an apical cap.

178. Abdominal Trauma

1. Which of the following statements is true?

A. Overwhelming postsplenectomy infection (OPSI) is more likely to occur in adults following splenectomy than in children.
B. *Mycoplasma pneumoniae* infections are among those that commonly occur in splenectomized patients.
C. Thrombocytosis following splenectomy should be treated with antiplatelet agents.
D. Administration of the Pneumovax vaccine is recommended for all patients who have undergone splenectomy.
E. Transient periods of hypotension in patients with known splenic trauma require no operative intervention as long as intravenous fluid and blood administration can reestablish normal vital signs.

2. A 34-year-old woman was injured in a motor vehicle crash. She was hemodynamically stable on arrival with normal vital signs and was neurologically intact. She was found to have a right clavicular fracture, fractured ribs 9 through 11 on the right posteriorly, and a fracture of the right transverse process of the L2 vertebra. An abdominal computed tomography (CT) scan showed no other abnormalities. She was admitted to the hospital for observation and recovery. Roughly 24 hours following her injury, she began to develop a fever to 103°F, associated with a pulse of 140 per minute, a blood pressure of 100/70 mm Hg, and a respiratory rate of 36 per minute. A chest radiograph revealed the presence of atelectasis at both bases. A flat plate of the abdomen revealed the presence of some retroperitoneal air outlining the right kidney, but no other abnormalities. What should be done at this point?

A. A laparotomy.
B. An abdominal CT scan.
C. Obtain blood cultures.
D. An intravenous pyelogram (IVP).
E. An endoscopic retrograde cholangiopancreatogram.

3. Which of the following treatments is **not** generally recommended for the management of patients with rectal wounds?

A. Diverting colostomy.
B. Performance of a low rectal anastomosis with the EEA stapler.
C. Distal rectal washout.
D. Presacral drainage.
E. Systemic antibiotics.

179. Burn Management

1. Today, the mean burn size associated with a 50 percent mortality in healthy young adults is

A. 30 percent.
B. 50 percent.
C. 70 percent.
D. 90 percent.
E. 100 percent.

2. The Parkland burn formula calls for resuscitation with

A. 2 ml of Ringer's lactate per kilogram of body weight per percent of body surface area burned to be given in the first 8 hours following the burn.
B. 4 ml of Ringer's lactate per kilogram of body weight per percent of body surface area burned to be given in the first 8 hours following the burn.
C. 2 ml of Ringer's lactate per kilogram of body weight per percent of body surface area burned to be given in the first 24 hours following the burn.
D. 4 ml of Ringer's lactate per kilogram of body weight per percent of body surface area burned to be given in the first 24 hours following the burn.
E. Both A and C are correct.

3. Which of the following statements regarding nutritional support of burn injury is **not** true?

A. Acutely burned patients need at least 50 percent to 60 percent of their calories to be in the form of carbohydrate.
B. Patients receiving calorie-to-nitrogen ratios of 100:1 have a better survival rate than patients receiving calorie-to-nitrogen ratios of 150:1.
C. Early wound closure immediately reverses the metabolic rate toward normal.
D. Large protein losses can occur through the burn wound.
E. Daily weights are often inaccurate in burn patients.

4. Select the incorrect answer. Pneumonia in burn patients

A. Is emerging as a more frequent infectious cause of death.
B. Can often be prevented through the use of prophylactic antibiotics.
C. Is usually due to penicillin-resistant *Staphylococcus* when it occurs in the first 3 days postburn.
D. Is usually due to gram-negative organisms when it occurs later in the postburn course.
E. May be preventable in some cases through the use of sucralfate instead of H_2-blockers for stress ulcer prophylaxis.

180. Compartment Syndromes

1. Which of the following is most representative of the capillary perfusion pressure in the systemic circulation?

A. 5 mm Hg.
B. 25 mm Hg.
C. 45 mm Hg.
D. 65 mm Hg.
E. 85 mm Hg.

2. A 21-year-old man was injured in a motorcycle accident in an isolated area of desolate country. At the scene of the accident, he was noted to be ventilating spontaneously and adequately, but he was hypotensive, with a blood pressure of 86/56 mm Hg and a heart rate of 140 per minute. He had an apparent closed pelvic fracture and closed fractures of his right tibia and fibula. Two large-bore intravenous catheters were placed by the paramedics, and large volumes of Ringer's lactate were infused. Also, military antishock trousers (MAST) were applied, and both the abdominal and extremity segments were inflated. The nearest hospital was over an hour away and the nearest trauma center even further. He received a total of 6500 ml of fluid during transport, arriving at the trauma center some 2½ hours after the paramedics had arrived at the scene. On arrival, his blood pressure was 92/62 mm Hg, but after receiving 4 units of packed red blood cells and application of a pelvic external fixator, his blood pressure increased to 112/72 mm Hg and remained stable, even after removal of the MAST device. Computed tomography (CT) scan of the head was unremarkable, and CT of the abdomen revealed only the pelvic fracture and a large surrounding pelvic hematoma. In addition to stabilizing his right tibia and fibula, which of the following should probably be performed?

A. A right leg fasciotomy.
B. Measurement of the patient's intraabdominal pressure.
C. Therapeutic embolization of the pelvic vessels.
D. Bilateral leg fasciotomies.
E. Measurement of bilateral lower extremity compartment pressures.

3. A stable normotensive patient who has sustained a tibial fracture has compartment pressures measured in the involved leg. The highest pressures recorded read 27 mm Hg. What should be done at this point?

A. Perform a fasciotomy in the involved leg.
B. Administer 25 gm of mannitol intravenously.
C. Continue to monitor the compartment pressures closely.
D. Administer 2 ampules of sodium bicarbonate intravenously.
E. Perform nerve conduction studies.

181. Derangements of Oxygen Transport in Shock States and Sepsis

1. Systemic oxygen delivery is defined as

A. The product of the arterial PO_2 times the mean arterial blood pressure.

B. The product of the arterial PO_2 times the cardiac output.
C. The product of the arterial oxygen content times the mean arterial blood pressure.
D. The product of the arterial oxygen content times the cardiac output.
E. The product of the arteriovenous oxygen content difference times the cardiac output.

2. Select the best answer. Pathologic supply dependency

A. Only exists in animal models of sepsis.
B. Describes a pattern in the oxygen consumption-delivery relationship in which the plateau is higher and the critical oxygen delivery is right-shifted.
C. Can only be found in patients with the adult respiratory distress syndrome (ARDS).
D. Indicates the need for dopexamine infusions.
E. Does not exist.

Answers

Chapter 171

1. E. Under normal conditions, oxygen consumption is independent of the amount of oxygen delivery available (Pfluger's law). However, with significant impairments in oxygen delivery below a critical level, oxygen consumption can decline because of insufficient substrate; thus, oxygen consumption can become supply dependent. Under these conditions, cells are dependent on anaerobic metabolism for energy production, with resultant accumulation of pyruvate because of inability to enter the Krebs cycle. Hydrolysis of adenosine triphosphate produces increasing acidosis, and lactate ions accumulate through the combined effect of increased pyruvate and proton accumulation. With prolonged anaerobiosis, the progressive lack of high-energy phosphate compounds will significantly impair cellular functions and even viability. Thus, supply dependency can produce an oxygen deficit that could ultimately lead to cell death and should therefore be avoided.

While some patients in shock may benefit from higher cardiac outputs than normal levels, it is not clear that all shock patients have these requirements. In general, many patients with septic shock appear as though they may fare better if their cardiac outputs achieve supranormal levels, while most patients with cardiogenic shock may only need normal cardiac outputs at best. The pulmonary capillary wedge pressure should be titrated to achieve the optimal cardiac output in shock patients. While this may occasionally warrant high levels, such is not always the case. Furthermore, the potential impact of pulmonary capillary wedge pressure elevation on pulmonary transvascular fluid extravasation should be carefully judged in each patient. Traditionally, a drop in blood pressure was equated with a drop in perfusion. However, it is becoming increasingly appreciated that there can be several instances where a low blood pressure may be associated with normal or even elevated levels of perfusion, as is often seen in septic shock.

2. D. Effectively identifying the pathophysiologic mechanisms responsible for producing the circulatory shock state in individual patients significantly benefits effective clinical management. The general shock categories of hypovolemic, cardiogenic, and other (i.e., septic) appear relatively consistent among the shock classifications that have been proposed.

Several potential causes can lead to the syndrome of hypovolemic shock.

Acute pancreatitis produces a massive sequestration of fluid in the peritoneal cavity and the retroperitoneum around the inflamed pancreas. This fluid is drawn from the circulating volume, often dropping circulatory performance to critical levels, producing a state of shock. Bilateral femur fractures can also be associated with circulating volume losses primarily due to the sequestration of blood and extracellular fluid from ruptured vessels around the fracture site. Intestinal obstruction also sequesters fluid internally in the intestinal lumen as well as intraperitoneally; vomiting can exacerbate these fluid losses. Severe burns can lose huge amounts of fluid through evaporative losses as well as some tissue sequestration, thus producing a hypovolemic state.

A tension pneumothorax is not specifically linked to any deficit in circulating volume. Rather, the condition prevents effective venous return, thereby limiting the resulting cardiac output. This then produces more of a cardiogenic type of shock (even though the heart is not primarily dysfunctional).

3. **B.** The first stage of circulatory shock is considered a compensatory and reversible stage in which mechanisms are invoked that work to maintain an adequate circulation without permanent tissue damage. As circulatory shock progresses to decompensation, permanent damage can develop, with increased morbidity and mortality. Because of the favorable prognosis, resuscitation efforts should begin as early as possible while compensatory mechanisms are still effective. Though subtle, the signs of compensation can be detected clinically. Tachycardia provides evidence of increased myocardial activity seeking to preserve the cardiac output in the face of a diminished circulatory volume. A narrowed pulse pressure can provide evidence of the vasoconstriction that helps to normalize the effective circulating volume and redistribute blood flow away from nonvital beds. The presence of cool, clammy skin is also evidence of this redistribution as flow to vital organs such as the brain and heart is preserved.

Chapter 172

1. **B.** There has been a long and complex controversy in clinical medicine regarding the optimal fluid for circulatory resuscitation. To date, comparison studies have failed to show any significant benefit in resuscitating hemorrhagic shock or trauma patients with colloid solutions that would justify their significantly higher cost. In fact, a meta-analysis of several clinical studies indicated that the mortality rate for trauma patients appears to be better when resuscitated with crystalloid solutions, although there seemed to be a slight advantage to resuscitating the nontrauma patient with colloid solutions. Even though colloid solutions may be able to resuscitate patients more rapidly because of the smaller volumes required, the outcomes are not obviously different, and thus the higher costs cannot be justified. Elevations in pulmonary microvascular pressure are the major determinants governing the transvascular movement of fluid into the pulmonary interstitium, and thus pulmonary capillary wedge pressure monitoring can be crucial in ensuring a safe and effective resuscitation. Preliminary studies with hypertonic saline solutions indicate that these solutions may effectively resuscitate hypovolemic shock patients with relatively small volumes.

2. **A.** Although a long-held tradition, the use of a particular hemoglobin level as a "transfusion trigger" no longer seems valid. Basic experimental studies indicate that an arbitrary hemoglobin level does not necessarily produce diminished oxygen transport until levels below 3.5 gm per deciliter are reached.

Rather, indicators of impaired oxygen delivery relative to oxygen consumption demands appear to more accurately indicate the absolute physiologic need for red blood cell transfusion. Thus, indicators such as a high oxygen extraction ratio or a low mixed venous saturation or PO_2 would be more appropriate indicators of a transfusion need. Furthermore, these parameters should also be coupled with the patient's overall condition to make an appropriate assessment. For example, a patient with severe coronary artery disease will likely be less able to compensate safely for the effects of anemia than a patient without such a condition and thus may benefit from a transfusion that would otherwise be unnecessary in a normal individual.

3. **E.** The concept of administering blood components prophylactically implies that the components are being given to prevent an undesired complication. To that end, physicians have traditionally administered platelets, fresh frozen plasma, or both during massive resuscitation efforts in the attempt to prevent serious coagulopathy from dilution. However, prospective studies have failed to show that such regimens are effective at preventing the coagulopathies that develop in association with massive transfusion episodes. Hence, the coagulation status should be closely monitored, and deficits should be replaced only if they actually develop rather than in anticipation of a potential problem. Patients with severe thrombocytopenia ($<10,000/mm^3$) may be at risk for spontaneous intracerebral hemorrhage from their prolonged bleeding time, and thus, most clinicians still consider prophylactic platelet administration warranted under such circumstances.

Chapter 173

1. **E.** The *systemic inflammatory response syndrome (SIRS)* is a new term used to designate a commonly appreciated clinical condition that can result from infectious or noninfectious etiologies. It is defined by the presence of two or more of the following signs or symptoms: (a) an abnormal body temperature, (b) tachycardia, (c) tachypnea, or (d) an alteration in the white blood cell count. Hypotension is not a designated component of SIRS but rather would tend to indicate the presence of septic shock (where severe SIRS is caused by infection).

2. **C.** Gram-negative bacteria contain a substance known as lipopolysaccharide (LPS) within their cell walls. LPS is a glycolipid composed of two components: an O-specific side chain and a core lipid region. The O-specific side chain is highly variable from species to species. It is a polymer of oligosaccharides that confers antigenic specificity to gram-negative bacteria. The lipid core consists of a unique sugar, 2-keto-3-deoxyoctonate (KDO), and a glycolipid called lipid A. It appears that lipid A confers toxic properties to the LPS molecule. While these toxic properties may account for a significant degree of the pathophysiology observed in human septic shock, it is apparent that LPS is not the only toxic substance at work. In clinical trials, anti-LPS antibodies have been administered to humans with infections, sepsis, and septic shock, with controversial findings at best and certainly without an obvious curative effect. However, to date, no study of the preventive use of these agents has been published. Furthermore, the hemodynamic and metabolic manifestations of septic shock can occur when patients are infected with organisms other than gram-negative bacteria. Also, human volunteers who are rendered tolerant to LPS still manifest signs of illness when infected with viable gram-negative bacteria. It may be that many endogenous mediators

such as TNF-α could also participate in some of the phenomena observed in septic shock patients. Among other things, TNF-α appears to induce nitric oxide synthase, especially in vascular smooth muscle, thus promoting at least some of the vasodilation observed in sepsis.

3. **A.** One of the common features of early septic shock is hypotension in the face of often elevated cardiac output, thus producing a dissociation between blood pressure and blood flow. Several agents have been implicated in this process of septic vasodilation. Tumor necrosis factor alpha and interleukin-1 are two cytokines that have received a great deal of recent attention because of the fact that they appear capable of producing many of the stigmata of septic shock. Among other effects, these cytokines appear to be able to induce nitric oxide synthase, the enzyme responsible for the production of nitric oxide, from smooth muscle cells. Nitric oxide, in turn, is a potent vasodilator that increasingly appears to be highly involved in the septic shock response. Other potential mediators of the hypotension of septic shock are the release of calcitonin gene–related peptide, opening of adenosine triphosphate–sensitive K^+ channels in vascular smooth muscle cells, and alterations in adrenergic signal transduction by vascular smooth muscle cells. Naloxone is an opioid antagonist that was initially thought to be of potential benefit in septic shock because of promising results from animal studies, but it has failed to show benefit in human clinical trails.

Chapter 174

1. **D.** While several conditions can produce adverse outcomes, hypoxia remains the primary reason for early death or central nervous system dysfunction in trauma patients. Because of this problem, effective airway management at the trauma scene is critical. If an airway and adequate ventilation are not provided, death or severe disability will result before transport to a trauma center can occur. Airway management takes primacy over all other concerns in the initial assessment and resuscitation of the injured patient.

Chapter 175

1. **B.** The development of intracranial hypertension often produces a syndrome of systemic hypertension and bradycardia, known as the Cushing response. Effective management of the Cushing response employs efforts to reduce the intracranial pressure (ICP), as that is the etiology of the syndrome. In this circumstance, the use of vasodilators to lower blood pressure is probably not beneficial. A reduction in blood pressure with no change in the ICP will produce a reduction of the CPP, represented by the difference between the mean systemic blood pressure and the ICP. If the CPP falls below a critical level, cerebral perfusion becomes impaired, thereby potentially producing cellular swelling through ischemic mechanisms. This in turn could lower the CPP still further because of the resulting increases in ICP.

2. **E.** Coagulation abnormalities are a frequent occurrence in head-injured patients. Presumably, this is because the brain is rich in thromboplastins, which may be released into the circulation on injury. (In fact, rabbit brain thromboplastin is often used by clinical laboratories as an activator for performance of the PT.) Nearly one-quarter of head-injured patients demonstrate at least laboratory evidence of disseminated intravascular coagulation. Furthermore,

55 percent of patients who develop delayed intracranial hematomas manifest abnormal clotting tests (e.g., PT, PTT, and platelet count). It appears that there is a correlation between the extent of brain tissue damage and the levels of fibrin degradation products that can be observed. In fact, elevated levels of fibrin degradation products may occasionally indicate brain damage that is below the limits of sensitivity for computed tomography scans. Poorer functional outcomes are generally realized with patients who have higher concentrations of fibrin degradation products; also, such patients are at greater risk to develop the adult respiratory distress syndrome.

3. B. Hyperventilation therapy is frequently used in the management of patients with elevated intracranial pressures. By reducing the $PaCO_2$, cerebral vasoconstriction is produced, thereby reducing the volume of intracerebral contents provided by cerebral blood flow. This reduction in intracerebral volume in turn reduces ICP. If the mean arterial pressure is unchanged, the CPP should be improved, as the CPP results from the difference in mean arterial pressure and ICP. This process occurs in most patients with intracranial hypertension. However, in some patients, so-called luxury perfusion may not exist, and the cerebral vasoconstriction produced by hyperventilation may reduce cerebral blood flow sufficiently to threaten the adequacy of cerebral perfusion for tissue health and viability. In nearly 20 percent of patients, a wide cerebral $A\text{-}V\dot{D}O_2$ results during hyperventilation therapy, indicating an increased extraction of oxygen off hemoglobin across the cerebral circulation as a result of the decreased perfusion. Because of this phenomenon, it is often useful to monitor cerebral oxygen extraction by using a jugular bulb venous saturation monitor or catheter during hyperventilation therapy. In some cases of increased oxygen extraction resulting from excessive cerebral vasoconstriction, actual increases in ICP may result. In such situations, mannitol may be a more effective intracranial volume reducing strategy.

4. C. The neurologic examination is a useful tool in roughly assessing the degree of derangement of intracranial pathophysiology. Still, it is not entirely reliable, and significant variation can occur. It is very rare that a patient who is alert and able to follow commands will have an elevated ICP. On the other hand, a patient with an altered level of consciousness is more likely to have an elevated ICP, although not consistently so. It appears that 40 to 50 percent of head-injured patients who have an altered level of consciousness will be found to have an elevated ICP. A raised ICP is more likely as the Glasgow Coma Scale score drops to levels below 8, although not consistently so. ICP elevations may be more consistently found when obtunded patients also demonstrate Cushing's triad of hypertension, bradycardia, and respiratory irregularity. Pupillary dilatation may indicate transtentorial herniation.

5. D. Among other techniques used to reduce ICP is the use of diuretics, such as mannitol. Osmotic diuresis with this agent can reduce brain tissue volume, primarily by reducing the amount of brain water in normal brain. Because the blood-brain barrier is often not intact in injured brain, mannitol may have little effect in the abnormal regions. Furthermore, because of its blood volume expanding capabilities, mannitol can increase regional cerebral blood flow without changing blood pressure or even ICP. Maximal reductions in ICP can be achieved with large rapid boluses of mannitol, especially if followed by furosemide. The empiric use of mannitol administered as a routine infusion does not alter the morbidity or mortality over mannitol infusions given only for control of ICP elevations.

Fluid restriction does not reduce brain tissue volume or ICP in experimental animals. Glucocorticoids have failed to show any significant benefit in head injury. Barbiturates do not appear to reduce the incidence of intracranial hypertension or improve clinical outcomes, although it may benefit some patients with refractory intracranial hypertension. The effects of barbiturates on ICP are not consistent, however. Empiric hyperventilation may actually worsen neurologic outcome and mortality rates when compared with patients managed with normocarbic ventilation.

Chapter 176

1. **B.** The determination of whether a spinal injury is clinically stable is important in the management of such patients. Patients with stable injuries can be more readily mobilized, thus helping to prevent pulmonary and other complications that appear to develop during prolonged immobilization, whereas those with unstable injuries must have their spine adequately stabilized by some type of intervention before safe mobilization can be undertaken. The three-column theory advanced by Denis helps in the understanding and application of the concept of clinical stability. The anterior column is considered to be made up of the anterior longitudinal ligament, the anterior annulus fibrosis, and the anterior part of the vertebral body. The middle column is formed by the posterior longitudinal ligament, the posterior annulus fibrosis, and the posterior wall of the vertebral column. Finally, the posterior column is made up of the posterior bony arch, the posterior ligamentous complex (i.e., the supraspinous and interspinous ligaments), the capsules of the apophyseal joints, and the ligament of flavum. Disruption of any two of the three columns produces clinical instability. Furthermore, isolated middle column damage can be potentially unstable through herniation of material into the spinal canal.

2. **D.** *Sacral sparing* is a term applied to the clinical finding of a preservation of perineal sensation in a patient with spinal cord injury. It implies an incomplete lesion of the spinal cord, with preservation of the cord's lateral aspects, namely the sensory fibers of the ascending spinothalamic tract. Usually, this finding is associated with a central cord lesion, with the potential for significant recovery. Spinal shock is defined as the absence of sensorimotor function and the presence of flaccidity below the injured segment. Deep tendon reflexes, the bulbocavernosus reflex, and the anal wink reflex are absent during spinal shock.

3. **C.** Recently, the national acute spinal cord injury study (NASCIS-2) demonstrated that a short (24-hour) course of high-dose methylprednisolone administered within 8 hours of spinal cord injury could improve the motor and sensory outcomes of patients who received the drug over those who received placebo. If the treatment were started more than 8 hours following injury, however, no benefit was seen. The mortality and major morbidity rates did not differ between the treatment and placebo groups.

Chapter 177

1. **E.** When the lung fails to expand completely after placement of a chest tube, several possibilities should be considered. The chest tube could be improperly positioned. Generally, a chest tube for a traumatic hemopneumothorax should

be placed between the fourth and fifth intercostal spaces in the anterior axillary line. More cephalad placement is rarely necessary, but more caudal placement runs the risk of being subdiaphragmatic. Chest tube suction could be inadequate, although it should rarely if ever exceed 60 cm H_2O. While an attractive possibility for clearing clot out of chest tubes, the use of urokinase in the acute trauma setting is unproved and has a significant possibility of producing a severe hemorrhagic condition. Intubation and use of PEEP should only be employed if oxygenation failure warrants mechanical ventilation and high inspired oxygen concentrations become necessary to oxygenate the bloodstream. The accepted and effective remedies for the condition presented in this scenario address the possibilities of airway occlusion by blood or secretions and occlusion of the chest tube by clotted blood. Vigorous pulmonary toilet, which may include therapeutic bronchoscopy, can clear secretions that may be interfering with effective lung inflation. Another chest tube could overcome the presence of clot in the chest tube already placed. In some cases, however, the clotted hemothorax is so difficult to evacuate that a thoracotomy may become necessary if lung inflation is to be achieved.

2. D. This patient has just developed a tension pneumothorax on the left side. The application of the semi-occlusive dressing over the open pneumothorax is an effective way to aid lung expansion by producing a flap-valve mechanism. Ideally, air can escape the pleural space but not be sucked back into it. However, it is possible for such a dressing to trap air and produce a tension pneumothorax if there is a leak of air into the chest (i.e., from injured lung tissue) that cannot escape as rapidly as it enters. The findings of an acutely hypotensive patient with the trachea deviated away from the injured side support the diagnosis of a left tension pneumothorax. Quick removal of the occlusive dressing off the left chest will relieve the tension, converting the left chest to a simple pneumothorax, which should have significantly less severe hemodynamic consequences.

3. A. The diagnosis of a torn thoracic aorta in an injured patient can be lifesaving if the aorta is repaired prior to its rupture. Although infrequently encountered, this condition provides a window of opportunity in some patients who survive the initial accident to make it to a hospital. Determining the likelihood of an aortic injury is based on the mechanism of injury (typically a deceleration force) and radiographic signs of a mediastinal hematoma. The signs include mediastinal widening greater than 8 cm, a ratio of mediastinal width to chest width greater than 0.25, abnormality of the aortic contour, opacification of the aortopulmonary window, depression of the left mainstem bronchus, deviation of the trachea to the right, deviation of a nasogastric tube to the right, the presence of an apical cap, widening of the right peritracheal stripe, and a left hemothorax. While the presence of upper rib fractures indicates that a severe blow to the thorax has been sustained, studies of large series of patients indicate that there is no increased association of aortic injury among such patients compared to those who do not have upper rib fractures.

Chapter 178

1. D. Patients who have had a splenectomy performed are at risk for developing OPSI. Children who are splenectomized appear to be at greater risk for this complication than are adults. Encapsulated organisms, particularly *Streptococcus pneumoniae*, *Haemophilus influenzae*, or *Neisseria meningitidis*, appear to be frequently involved in OPSI cases; *Mycoplasma pneumoniae* is not encapsulated. Because of this risk, the Pneumovax vaccine is generally recommended for all patients who have undergone splenectomy, since it provides immunity for many of the pneumococcal strains involved in OPSI. However, Pneumovax does not confer protection against all OPSI organisms, and long-term prophylactic antibiotics are often used, although the ultimate effectiveness of such an approach is not known.

Splenectomized patients frequently develop thrombocytosis postoperatively. While concerning, it does not appear that thrombotic risks are increased in such patients. Therefore, treatment with antiplatelet agents is not warranted unless other indications exist.

One should always attempt to preserve the spleen wherever possible, and nonoperative management of the patient with a known splenic injury is certainly one way to achieve that goal. However, a patient with recurrent bouts of hypotension that require repeated episodes of fluid and blood administration has a source of continued blood loss that should be controlled. If the spleen appears to be the source of bleeding, a laparotomy should be performed, and hemostatic operative techniques can often be used to salvage the spleen. In many cases, it may be necessary to sacrifice the spleen to obtain hemorrhagic control.

2. A. The presence of retroperitoneal air outlining the right kidney in this septic-appearing patient who has sustained blunt abdominal trauma indicates a ruptured duodenum. Although rare, it is a serious injury that can produce devastating infectious complications if untreated. The initial CT scan could easily miss such an injury in the early stages. A CT scan is not necessary at this point, as a hollow viscus rupture is demonstrated by the presence of retroperitoneal air without any other obvious explanations. The most expedient measure in this patient would be to perform an emergent laparotomy, with repair and drainage of the injury.

3. B. Rectal injuries represent a serious risk for infectious complications. Because of the huge bacterial concentrations resident in the rectal flora, pelvic infections are a likely consequence of rectal wounds unless the wounds are handled exceptionally well. Toward this end, several techniques are usually advocated as being beneficial in the management of patients with rectal wounds. These include (a) administration of large doses of broad-spectrum antibiotics, (b) placement of a proximal diverting colostomy, (c) thorough irrigation of the distal rectum, and (d) placement of perineal drains in the presacral space. Use of the EEA stapling device or any other technique for rectal anastomosis is generally not warranted, although most authorities recommend that the rectal wound be repaired, if possible.

Chapter 179

1. C. The outcome from burn injury has improved significantly over the past century. Fifty years ago, the mean burn size associated with a 50 percent mortality in healthy young adults was only about 30 percent, whereas today a burn size of approximately 70 percent is associated with a 50 percent mortality rate. There are several contributing reasons for this improvement. They include a better understanding of burn pathophysiology, which in turn has led to more effective management, improved methods of fluid administration and monitoring, improved antimicrobial agents, more effective nutritional maintenance, and an increased understanding of the need for early removal of necrotic burn tissue and skin grafting to minimize the degree and duration of physiologic stress.

2. **E.** Extracellular circulatory fluid losses through transudation, evaporation, and tissue edema are the natural consequences of burn injury. The amount of volume loss is directly related to the amount of burned skin surface area affected. If the circulatory fluid losses are not replaced, the consequences of hypovolemic underperfusion can result. There are several fluid management protocols that have been advocated for burn resuscitation. The Parkland formula is one of the more commonly used regimens. It calls for 4 ml of Ringer's lactate per kilogram of body weight per percent of body surface area burned to be given in the first 24 hours following the burn, with half of the total volume (i.e., 2 ml of Ringer's lactate per kilogram of body weight per percent of body surface area burned) to be given in the first 8 hours following the burn.

3. **C.** Acutely burned individuals are usually hypermetabolic and can become severely catabolic. Effective nutritional support of these patients is often key to their ultimate survival. Monitoring of the nutritional requirements of burn patients is problematic, however. Daily weights are often inaccurate because of the marked fluid shifts that can occur as well as the variable weight that can be provided by wound dressings. Nitrogen balance studies are also often inaccurate because of the large protein losses that can occur through the burn wound. The burn wound appears to be an obligate glucose consumer. Therefore, at least 50 to 60 percent of the calories should be administered in the form of carbohydrate. However, protein supplementation is also very important. It has been observed over the years that patients receiving lower calorie-to-nitrogen ratios (i.e., 100:1) experience an improved survival probability over those receiving more traditional ratios (150:1). While early burn wound excision and closure appear to improve clinical outcome and may contribute to an ultimate reduction in hypermetabolism, the reversal of the metabolic rate toward normal is not immediate following closure.

4. **B.** Because of the declining incidence of burn wound sepsis, pneumonia is now emerging as a more frequent infectious cause of death among burn patients. Unfortunately, the prophylactic use of antibiotics has failed to effectively prevent these pneumonias from occurring and will often predispose to the selection of antibiotic-resistant bacteria. Better preventive measures include effectively clearing pulmonary secretions, avoidance of microaspiration around the endotracheal tube, and early extubation. The use of sucralfate instead of H_2-blockers for the prevention of stress ulcers may reduce the incidence of pneumonia. When pneumonias occur early postburn (i.e., within the first 3 days), they are commonly due to penicillin-resistant staphylococcal organisms. However, when they occur later in the postburn course, the pneumonias are more likely due to gram-negative enteric bacilli or *Pseudomonas*.

Chapter 180

1. **B.** Normal precapillary and postcapillary hydrostatic pressures are roughly 25 and 16 mm Hg, respectively. This information becomes important in conditions where tissue pressures could exceed perfusion pressure, thereby limiting nutrient blood flow. An example of such a situation is that of compart-

ment syndrome, wherein intrafascial compartment pressures rise as a result of increased volume accumulation within a closed nonexpansive space. Unless the compartment pressure is promptly released, tissue ischemia will result, with eventual muscle necrosis. Other clinical situations in which the systemic capillary pressure becomes important include the management of intracranial hypertension, the assessment of elevated abdominal pressure as a potential etiology for oliguria, and the upper limit for endotracheal tube cuff pressure.

2. E. This patient is at great risk of developing compartment syndromes, not only in his injured right leg, but in both lower extremities as a result of the prolonged application of the MAST in the face of hypotension. Normally, systemic hydrostatic pressure is roughly 25 mm Hg. When tissue pressures exceed hydrostatic microvascular pressures (as occurs during MAST inflation), perfusion to the tissues may become impaired. Furthermore, the presence of hypovolemic shock, due primarily to the large fluid losses imposed by the pelvic fracture, could have reduced the systemic microvascular hydrostatic pressure even further. Thus, it is quite likely that perfusion pressures were exceeded for a significant duration, thereby rendering the leg muscles ischemic. With prolonged ischemia as well as venous and lymphatic compression, tissue edema could occur, aggravating the compartment syndrome. At the very least, an expedient measurement of the tissue pressures in all four compartments in both legs should be performed, as this patient will likely require bilateral fasciotomies to preserve muscle and nerve viability.

3. D. A patient with a tibial fracture is at risk to develop a compartment syndrome. This patient's compartment pressures are elevated, but not yet to severe levels. It appears that the threshold compartment pressure at which fasciotomy is warranted tends to vary from authority to authority. Most would not recommend a fasciotomy in a normotensive patient when the compartment pressures are less than 30 mm Hg, however. Therefore, continued close monitoring of this patient would be important to determine if the compartment pressures go to higher levels so that a prompt fasciotomy can be performed at that time. Nerve conduction studies may provide a functional test of the nerves that run through the involved compartments and can demonstrate the presence of muscle viability. However, at these levels of compartment pressure, it is likely that the muscle is viable. Furthermore, nerve conduction velocity measurements require specially trained personnel for their performance and can produce false-positive results from other reasons.

While such patients are at risk for myoglobinuria and acute renal failure as a result, no evidence has been provided that this patient has increased levels of myoglobin release. A test for myoglobin in the urine should probably be performed prior to the administration of agents such as mannitol or sodium bicarbonate.

Chapter 181

1. D. Systemic oxygen delivery is defined as the product of the arterial oxygen content times the cardiac output. The arterial oxygen content, in turn, is the sum of hemoglobin-bound oxygen and dissolved oxygen in the blood. Hemoglobin-bound oxygen can be determined by the product of the hemoglobin concentration, the arterial oxygen saturation, and the hemoglobin binding coefficient for oxygen (1.34). Dissolved oxygen is the product of the arterial PO_2

times the solubility coefficient for oxygen in blood (0.003). The product of the arteriovenous oxygen content difference times the cardiac output defines the oxygen consumption according to the Fick principle.

2. **B.** The relationship between systemic oxygen delivery and oxygen consumption appears to be biphasic in controlled situations where oxygen delivery can be progressively changed. An oxygen supply–dependent phase exists on the lower end of the spectrum, wherein the amount of oxygen consumed is directly dependent on the amount of oxygen delivery. On the higher end of the spectrum is an oxygen supply–independent phase wherein the amount of oxygen delivered has no impact on the amount of oxygen consumed. In clinical practice, it is more difficult to observe the biphasic relationship between oxygen consumption and oxygen delivery because there is less independent control over the variables in question. Indeed, it is quite likely that patients can change their oxygen consumption dependency state from moment to moment, thus distorting or skewing the observed pattern. In many cases, this can make it appear that critically ill patients are supply dependent across the entire spectrum of oxygen delivery. While such a relationship appears commonly in patients with ARDS, it is also occurs in patients who do not have ARDS. Many clinicians consider evidence of oxygen supply dependency as an indication for further circulatory support in the hope of achieving a supply-independent state. Inotropes such as dopamine, dobutamine, amrinone, milrinone, or dopexamine may be useful in this process. However, there is no clear consensus that this approach is completely beneficial or that the potential risks (i.e., arrhythmias) outweigh the potential benefits.

XIII. Neurologic Problems in the Intensive Care Unit

183. Evaluating the Patient with Altered Consciousness in the Intensive Care Unit

1. Select the best answer. The locked-in state

A. Describes a state of mild cerebral obtundation.
B. Is most commonly caused by a destructive process at the base of the pons.
C. Is characterized by having absolutely no muscle movement detectable.
D. Can only be diagnosed by the electroencephalogram.
E. Can only be diagnosed by computed tomography.

184. Metabolic Encephalopathy

1. Which of the following factors does **not** contribute to a poor outcome in Reye's syndrome?

A. Age less than 1 year.
B. Serum ammonia levels greater than five times normal at their peak.
C. The presence of seizures.
D. A prothrombin time greater than 20 seconds.
E. Very rapid progression of liver failure in the first 48 hours.

2. Which of the following statements regarding uremic encephalopathy is true?

A. The electroencephalogram (EEG) typically correlates with mental status changes.
B. The level of the blood urea nitrogen (BUN) is directly related to the cognitive state.
C. The creatinine level is directly related to the cognitive state.
D. The EEG is not changed at higher levels of BUN.
E. The pathophysiology of uremic encephalopathy is not known.

True or False. Regarding metabolic encephalopathies:

3. Rapid correction of hyperglycemic hyperosmolality with intravenous hydration and insulin results in cerebral water intoxication and signs of increased intracranial pressure.

4. Adrenocortical insufficiency, like many other metabolic encephalopathies, is associated with increased muscle tone and deep tendon reflexes.

5. In a patient with Wernicke's encephalopathy, prompt administration of 100 mg of thiamine will restore the impairment of ocular movements completely.

185. Generalized Anoxia/Ischemia of the Nervous System

1. Select the correct answer. In cases of out-of-hospital cardiac arrest

A. The prognosis for recovery is not related to cardiopulmonary resuscitation (CPR) time if the duration of untreated cardiac arrest is less than 6 minutes.
B. Over half of patients make a good recovery when CPR is done for over 30 minutes if the duration of untreated cardiac arrest is less than 6 minutes.
C. Only 3 percent of patients have a neurologic recovery if CPR time is over 30 minutes.
D. Only 3 percent of patients recover if the untreated cardiac arrest time is over 6 minutes, despite the fact that the actual CPR time is less than 5 minutes.
E. Recovery is quite likely even if attempts fail to resuscitate patients prior to their arrival in the emergency room.

2. Select the correct answer. In cases of nontraumatic coma

A. The absence of brainstem reflexes during the first 48 hours following an anoxic event has no impact on prognosis.
B. The most valuable prognostic information is obtained from the physical examination.
C. Only 30 percent of patients who do not regain at least two brainstem reflexes within 48 hours fail to recover.
D. The presence of decerebrate or decorticate posturing at 24 hours often portends a favorable outcome.
E. Children have the same recovery rates as adults.

3. Seizures occur in what percentage of patients in anoxic coma?

A. 5 percent.
B. 10 percent.
C. 25 percent.
D. 50 percent.
E. 90 percent.

186. Status Epilepticus

True or False. Regarding status epilepticus:

1. Myoclonic status epilepticus in adults is almost always associated with mental retardation syndromes.

2. The most common cause of status epilepticus in known epileptics is a change in antiepileptic drug serum levels.

3. Lesions of the occipital lobe are more likely to produce status epilepticus than lesions at other sites in the brain.

4. Initial treatment for status epilepticus should be intravenous lorazepam, simultaneous with a loading dose of phenytoin.

5. Roughly how much time is required on average for death to result from status epilepticus?

A. 5 minutes.
B. 30 minutes.
C. 4 hours.
D. 13 hours.
E. 3 days.

187. Cerebrovascular Disease

1. Which of the following statements concerning heparin use in ischemic cerebrovascular disease is **not** true?

A. Heparin therapy should be considered within 24 to 48 hours of the event for patients with cardioembolic stroke.
B. It has been definitively demonstrated that heparin therapy impedes the progression of stroke-in-evolution.
C. Patients with large cerebral infarcts should generally not receive heparin.
D. Heparin should be administered as a continuous infusion.
E. A randomized, double-blind trial of heparin versus placebo in the setting of acute partial stable stroke demonstrated no benefit.

2. Select the incorrect answer. Primary intracranial hemorrhage

A. In about 50 percent of cases results from long-standing hypertension.
B. Is defined as bleeding within the brain parenchyma without an underlying cause such as a neoplasm, vasculitis, bleeding disorder, prior embolic infarction, aneurysm, vascular malformation, or trauma.
C. Has increased in incidence over the last 30 years.
D. Was probably misdiagnosed as bland infarcts in previous years.
E. Carries lower apparent fatality rate than seen in previous years.

3. The most frequent site of occurrence for nontraumatic intracranial hemorrhage is

A. The pons.

B. The putamen.
C. The cerebellum.
D. The subcortical white matter.
E. The thalamus.

188. Neurooncologic Problems in the Intensive Care Unit

Match the term in the first column with the appropriate term in the second column:

1. Peritumoral edema	A. Intracellular edema
2. Vasogenic edema	B. Extracellular edema
3. Cytotoxic edema	
4. Responsive to steroid therapy	

5. The steroid most commonly used for the treatment of brain tumors is

A. Methylprednisolone.
B. Hydrocortisone.
C. Dexamethasone.
D. Aldosterone.
E. Prednisone.

189. The Guillain-Barré Syndrome

1. Select the correct answer. The Guillain-Barré syndrome (GBS)

A. Was first described by Dr. Strohl Guillain-Barré in 1902.
B. Has an annual incidence of 1 case per 1,000,000 population.
C. Is a congenital disorder of neurons.
D. Often occurs 2 to 4 weeks after a flulike illness.
E. Is a weakness that classically descends from the arms to the legs.

True or False. Regarding GBS:

2. Surgery can be an antecedent event that precedes the onset of GBS.

3. Most patients have recurrent bouts of GBS after the initial episode.

4. Over half of GBS patients will require mechanical ventilation at some point in their clinical course.

5. Disturbances of the autonomic nervous system are common and potentially lethal.

6. The cerebrospinal fluid (CSF) typically shows an elevated protein and minimal cellularity, with a normal glucose and opening pressure.

7. Plasmapheresis has been shown to offer no benefit to patients with GBS.

190. Myasthenia Gravis in the Intensive Care Unit

1. Select the correct answer. Myasthenia gravis

A. Is an autosomal dominant disorder.
B. Affects males four times more frequently than females.
C. Is an exceedingly rare disorder, occurring once in every 4,000,000 people.
D. Is produced when circulating antibodies react with parts of acetylcholine receptors in postsynaptic membranes, blocking receptor activation and accelerating receptor degradation.
E. Is usually a disease of children.

True or False. Regarding myasthenia gravis:

2. Respiratory muscles are the most frequently involved.

3. Edrophonium hydrochloride (Tensilon) is a fast, short-acting parenteral cholinesterase inhibitor that transiently accentuates the muscle weakness in myasthenics.

4. Antiacetylcholine receptor antibodies are often absent from patients with purely ocular myasthenia.

5. The antiacetylcholine receptor antibody titer correlates well with the severity of the disease.

6. The antiacetylcholine receptor antibody titer does not correlate well with the response to treatment.

7. Arterial blood gases are the best indicators of impending respiratory failure in the myasthenic patient.

8. Neuromuscular blocking agents should never be administered to myasthenics in the intensive care unit.

9. Corticosteroids are beneficial in the majority of myasthenics in whom they are attempted.

10. Thymectomy should be considered early in the course of myasthenia.

11. Select the best answer. Plasmapheresis for myasthenia gravis

A. Offers little benefit.
B. Is often followed by increased sensitivity to cholinesterase inhibitors.
C. Helps by removing abnormal neurotoxins that cannot be metabolized by myasthenic patients.
D. Requires several weeks of therapy to show a favorable response in most patients.

191. Miscellaneous Neurologic Problems in the Intensive Care Unit

True or False. Regarding suicidal hanging:

1. A patient who appears dead following hanging is not resuscitatable.

2. Hanging is the third most common means of committing suicide.

3. Hyperthermia can develop following hanging as a result of hypoxic damage to the hypothalamus.

4. A fracture of the odontoid requires immediate neurosurgical or orthopedic intervention to stabilize the cervical spine and protect the cord from injury.

5. Complete or partial recovery is rare in most patients who survive the initial event.

True or False. Regarding electrical injuries:

6. Electrical injuries account for about 100 deaths annually in the United States.

7. Direct current is more dangerous than alternating current.

8. Spinal cord injury is the most common of the neurologic sequelae that can result from an electrical injury.

9. Myoglobinuria and acute renal failure can result from muscle damage.

10. Seizures are common following electrical injury.

11. Select the correct answer. Carbon monoxide

A. Can be lethal at concentrations of 0.001%
B. Has a distinctive odor.
C. Can be emitted from charcoal-burning grills.
D. Is not elevated in the bloodstream of cigarette smokers.
E. Is not normally formed in vivo.

12. Which of the following statements regarding carbon monoxide poisoning is false?

A. Headaches can occur with concentrations of less than 10%.
B. The classic cherry-red color on the lips usually requires carboxyhemoglobin levels of 30% to 40% to be evident.
C. 100% oxygen should be immediately administered to any patient suspected of having carbon monoxide poisoning.
D. Steroids have been shown to be effective at controlling the intracranial hypertension resulting from carbon monoxide poisoning.
E. Roughly 75 percent of affected individuals recover within a year of the carbon monoxide poisoning insult.

13. Which of the following statements regarding decompression sickness is false?

A. The onset of symptoms occurs within 12 hours of the decompression event in 97 percent of patients.
B. Four-fifths of patients with decompression sickness have neurologic symptoms.
C. The patient should be placed in the head-up position lying on the right side to prevent systemic gas embolization.
D. Air embolism is a serious form of decompression injury, producing symptoms within 5 minutes of decompression.
E. Recompression is the primary definitive treatment.

ANSWERS

Chapter 183

1. **B.** The locked-in state is a state of paralysis without loss of consciousness. It is commonly caused by destruction of the base of the pons. Less frequent etiologies include acute polyneuritis (Guillain-Barré syndrome), acute poliomyelitis, toxins that block transmission at the neuromuscular junction, and myasthenia gravis. The patient is completely paralyzed except for vertical eye movements and blinking, which operate by muscles innervated by midbrain structures. Consciousness is preserved through the ascending reticular activating system, which is located in the tegmentum of the pons and is therefore dorsal to the damaged area. The diagnosis is commonly made through clinical neurologic examination.

Chapter 184

1. **C.** Reye's syndrome is a morbid form of acute hepatic encephalopathy in children, usually between the ages of 1 and 10, that follows a viral infection combined with aspirin therapy. Treatment for Reye's syndrome is directed at decreasing intracranial hypertension through aggressive reduction of cerebral edema, as well as controlling seizures and providing adequate nutritional and metabolic support during the period of liver failure. The prognosis for Reye's syndrome has improved significantly in recent years, with a mortality and morbidity rate of 10 to 20 percent at the current time (compared to 40–50% in previous decades).

   Factors that appear to contribute to a poor outcome are patient age of less than 1 year, a serum ammonia level that peaks higher than five times the normal level, a prothrombin time longer than 20 seconds, very rapid progression of liver failure within the first 48 hours, and the presence of renal failure.

2. **E.** Uremic encephalopathy is one of the many metabolic encephalopathies that can be seen in the intensive care unit population. It is often a complication of systemic diseases that independently affect the central nervous system, such as collagen vascular disease, malignant hypertension, drug overdoses, diabetes mellitus, or bacterial sepsis. The clinical presentation is quite variable, with no direct correlation seen between the cognitive state and the level of BUN or any other biochemical marker. Interestingly, the EEG is slower at higher levels of BUN, but it does not correlate with the mental status either. Fundamentally, the pathophysiology of uremic encephalopathy remains unknown.

3. **True.** The hyperosmolality that accompanies hyperglycemia causes a shift of water from the intracerebral tissue space to the intravascular space. This, in turn, produces brain tissue shrinkage that makes the brain susceptible to water intoxication and signs of increased intracranial pressure if rehydration is accomplished too rapidly.

4. **False.** Unlike other metabolic encephalopathies, adrenocortical insufficiency produces decreased muscle tone and deep tendon reflexes that do not clear until cortisone replacement is given along with treatment of any associated electrolyte imbalances.

5. **True.** Wernicke's encephalopathy develops acutely in alcoholics and malnourished individuals, producing a striking impairment of ocular movements. Ocular function can be completely restored with the prompt intravenous and oral administration of 100 mg of thiamine. Cerebral symptoms resolve more slowly on thiamine therapy.

Chapter 185

1. **C.** For the brain, it is vitally important that circulation be restored as promptly as possible. In cardiac arrests that occur outside the hospital, the prognosis is related to the duration of CPR efforts if the duration that the arrest goes untreated is less than 6 minutes. Thus, when CPR lasts less than 30 minutes before the circulation is restored, over half the patients make a good neurologic recovery. On the other hand, if CPR lasts longer than 30 minutes, only 3 percent of patients make a good neurologic recovery. If the duration of the untreated arrest is longer than 6 minutes, up to 50 percent of patients can still recover if the CPR time is less than 5 minutes. However, longer periods of CPR are associated with poorer outcomes. If resuscitative efforts fail prior to the patient's arrival in the emergency room, the prognosis is quite bleak.

2. **B.** Nontraumatic coma is often prognosticated best by the physical findings. The presence of brainstem reflexes (pupillary light, corneal, and vestibulo-ocular) within the first 48 hours following an anoxic event provides a more favorable prognosis than if they are absent. On the other hand, essentially no patients recover who do not regain at least two of these brainstem reflexes within 48 hours. The persistence of decerebrate or decorticate posturing at 24 hours after the event mitigates against a favorable outcome. In general, children appear to have better prospects for return of neurologic function than do adults.

3. **C.** Roughly 25 percent of patients in anoxic coma develop seizures. These can usually be managed like other seizures with loading and then maintenance doses of phenytoin. Alternatively, phenobarbital can be used if phenytoin administration is at all problematic, such as in patients with cardiac conduction abnormalities.

Chapter 186

1. **False.** Myoclonic status epilepticus is a rare form of convulsions. In children, it usually occurs in association with chronic epilepsy and mental retardation. However, in adults, myoclonic states are almost always secondary to toxic, metabolic, viral, or degenerative causes of acute or subacute encephalopathies.

2. **True.** The most common cause of status epilepticus among known epileptics appears to be a change in antiepileptic drug serum levels. Indeed, the incidence of status epilepticus has increased over the past century despite the introduction of antiepileptic drugs, implying a link between the use of these drugs and status epilepticus.

3. **False.** Status epilepticus is more likely to be produced by lesions of the frontal lobes than by lesions at other sites in the brain.

4. **True.** The initial management of status epilepticus is best approached with intravenous lorazepam for immediate, short-term arrest of any ongoing seizure activity. A loading dose of phenytoin should be administered simultaneously with the lorazepam to establish maintenance therapy. If these drugs fail to control the seizures, phenobarbital should be added, and if necessary, barbiturate coma should be induced.

5. **D.** The duration of status epilepticus profoundly affects patient outcome. The mean duration of status epilepticus for patients who died as a result of their status was 13 hours in one clinical study. Patients who had no neurologic sequelae from their status had an average status duration of 90 minutes, whereas those with neurologic sequelae had an average status duration of 10 hours.

Chapter 187

1. **B.** Although anticoagulants have been used for many years in ischemic cerebrovascular disease, definitive proof of their efficacy is lacking. Acute anticoagulation is generally considered for patients with cardioembolic strokes, where it is generally given within 24 to 48 hours of the event to prevent recurrence. Also, heparin therapy is often given to patients with stroke-in-evolution to prevent progression, although there is no definitive proof that it works. Heparin therapy is also often given to patients with multiple transient ischemic attacks to prevent stroke development, although again there is no proof of efficacy. A recent randomized, controlled, double-blind clinical trial in the setting of acute partial stable strokes demonstrated no benefit of heparin over placebo. When given, heparin should be administered as a constant infusion, generally aiming to maintain the partial thromboplastin time at 1.5 to 2 times control.

2. **C.** Primary or spontaneous intracranial hemorrhage and rupture of saccular aneurysms and arteriovenous malformations account for a majority of cases of nontraumatic intracranial hemorrhage. Primary intracranial hemorrhage is defined as bleeding within the brain parenchyma without an underlying cause such as a neoplasm, vasculitis, bleeding disorder, prior embolic infarction, aneurysm, vascular malformation, or trauma. However, it does appear that about half of the cases of primary intracranial hemorrhage actually result from long-standing and uncontrolled hypertension, thus suggesting it is actually a secondary process as well. Interestingly, the incidence of spontaneous intracranial hemorrhage has dropped over the past 30 years, due in large part no doubt to the aggressive modern approach to systemic hypertension. This reduction in incidence is despite the fact that computed tomography scans now more readily identify small hemorrhages that were once misdiagnosed as bland infarcts. Also, because of the inclusion of these small spontaneous hemorrhages, the apparent fatality rate for nontraumatic intracranial hemorrhage has declined.

3. **B.** The most frequent site of occurrence for nontraumatic intracranial hemorrhage is the putamen, where it occurs in 30 to 50 percent of cases. Here, the bleeding is from a lenticulostriate vessel, and the clinical syndrome typically produced is one of sudden flaccid hemiplegia, hemisensory disturbances, homonymous hemianopsia, and paralysis of conjugate gaze to the side opposite the lesion. The subcortical white matter is involved in 15 percent of cases, where

the condition is often called a lobar hemorrhage. These hemorrhages produce syndromes dependent on the location of the bleed and generally have the lowest mortality and the best prognosis. Thalamic intracranial hemorrhages account for 10 percent of cases and produce unilateral sensorimotor deficits in which the sensory findings predominate. Pontine intracranial hemorrhages carry the highest mortality and also account for 10 percent of intracranial hemorrhages. Cerebellar hemorrhages account for 10 percent of cases and have a mortality of up to 60 percent.

Chapter 188

1. **B.**

2. **B.**

3. **A.**

4. **B.**

   In addition to cellular growth, brain neoplasms tend to increase extracellular edema. Consequently, this form of edema is also termed peritumoral edema, and because of its association with altered capillary permeability, it is known as vasogenic edema. Vasogenic edema is typically very responsive to steroid therapy. In contrast, intracellular edema usually results from cellular membrane pump failure and thus is termed cytotoxic edema.

5. **C.** Dexamethasone remains the most commonly used steroid in the treatment of brain tumors. It is a very potent glucocorticoid and yet has minimal mineralocorticoid effects. Yet, it has a relatively long onset of action and is therefore not as useful for the acute reduction of elevated intracranial pressure as are other measures, such as hyperventilation or mannitol administration.

Chapter 189

1. **D.** GBS was first described by Guillain, Barré, and Strohl in 1916. It is the most common cause of rapidly progressive weakness, with an annual incidence of roughly 1 case per 100,000 population. It appears to have an immunologically mediated mechanism and classically occurs some 2 to 4 weeks after a flulike illness. The typical presentation is that of a progressive ascending weakness that moves from the legs to the arms, then the respiratory and bulbar muscles.

2. **True.** Several clinical conditions appear to precede the onset of GBS. These include flulike illnesses, viral infections (including human immunodeficiency virus), immunization, surgery, and renal transplantation.

3. **False.** The nadir of the clinical course is achieved in the large majority of patients within 1 month. Only 2 to 5 percent have recurrent GBS.

4. **False.** Between 10 and 25 percent of patients will require ventilator assistance within 18 days after the onset of the condition.

5. **True.** About 50 percent of patients can have disturbances of the autonomic nervous system that are potentially lethal, taking the form of cardiac arrhythmias, hypotension, and hypertension.

6. **True.** The CSF typically shows an albuminocytologic dissociation (an elevated protein with minimal pleocytosis). The CSF glucose and opening pressure are typically normal.

7. **False.** Plasmapheresis appears to improve the course of GBS, with patients who receive plasmapheresis walking sooner on average than those who do not.

Chapter 190

1. **D.** Myasthenia gravis is an autoimmune disease, resulting from the production of circulating antibodies that attack parts of acetylcholine receptors in the postsynaptic membranes of muscles. This blocks the acetylcholine receptors from full activation and may accelerate the actual degradation of receptors. It is a relatively common disorder, affecting roughly 1 in 20,000. The female-male ratio is 3:2. The incidence peaks in women in their third decade and in men in the fifth and sixth decades.

2. **False.**

3. **False.**

4. **True.**

5. **False.**

6. **True.**

7. **False.**

8. **True.**

9. **True.**

10. **True.**

The ocular muscles are the most frequently involved muscle group in myasthenia gravis, commonly producing ptosis. Respiratory muscle involvement is not rare, producing respiratory insufficiency with some frequency. The Tensilon test is evoked by edrophonium hydrochloride (Tensilon), a short, fast-acting parenteral cholinesterase inhibitor that transiently strengthens the affected muscles of a myasthenic patient. Because myasthenia gravis is an autoimmune disease, the presence of antiacetylcholine receptor antibodies is a strong indication of the disease's presence, although they are often absent in patients with purely ocular myasthenia. However, the antibody titer does not correlate with the severity of the disease or the response to treatment. The best parameters to monitor the myasthenic for potential respiratory failure are the forced vital capacity, maximum inspiratory pressure, and the maximum expiratory pressure. Neuromuscular blocking agents should never be administered to myasthenics in the intensive care unit because they will usually have prolonged and excessive effects. Because of the immunologic nature of myasthenia, immunotherapy has now become the mainstay for treating myasthenia. Corticosteroids are associated with a response rate of 80 percent. Because of the excellent response to thymectomy, it should be considered early in the course of myasthenia, except in those patients who are too unstable or frail to undergo operation.

11. **B.** Because of the immunologic nature of myasthenia gravis, plasmapheresis has been attempted with favorable results. Most patients respond within 48 hours of the initiation of plasmapheresis, although therapy must be continued on an intermittent basis. Many patients develop increased sensitivity to cholinesterase inhibitors after plasmapheresis, mandating a reduction in their maintenance dosage of these drugs.

Chapter 191

1. **False.** A patient who appears dead following hanging could still be resuscitatable, likely requiring endotracheal intubation, mechanical ventilation, restoration of a normal cardiac rhythm and circulation, and control of intracranial hypertension.

2. **True.** Hanging is the third most common means of committing suicide, occurring more commonly in males (3:1).

3. **True.** Hyperthermia can be observed following hanging as a result of hypoxic damage to the hypothalamus.

4. **True.** A fracture of the odontoid should mandate immediate neurosurgical or orthopedic consultation to protect the spinal cord from injury by stabilizing the cervical spine.

5. **False.** Despite the initially poor appearance, most patients who survive the initial event recover partially or completely.

6. **False.** Electrical injuries account for about 1000 deaths and 4000 injuries annually in the United States.

7. **False.** Because of the tetanic contractions that prevent voluntary release from the current source, alternating current is more dangerous than direct current. It is also more likely to produce cardiac arrhythmias and respiratory arrest.

8. **True.** Neurologic sequelae result in over 25 percent of patients with electrical injuries. Spinal cord injury is most commonly involved because of the common occurrence of extremity-to-extremity current flow, thereby going through at least some part of the cord.

9. **True.** Myoglobinuria and acute renal failure can result from the extensive muscle damage that can occur.

10. **False.** Seizures are uncommon following electrical injury.

11. **C.** Carbon monoxide is a colorless, tasteless, odorless gas that is normally present in the atmosphere in concentrations of less than 0.001%. Concentra-

tions of 0.1% can be lethal. Carbon monoxide can be emitted from charcoal-burning grills, as well as from automobile exhaust. It is also found in fires, methylene chloride, volcanic gas, and cigarette smoke. Because of the last, carbon monoxide levels in the bloodstream (normally present in concentrations of 1–3% from the degradation of hemoglobin) can be elevated in cigarette smokers to levels of 6% to 7%.

12. D. Headaches are a frequent symptom following carbon monoxide poisoning and can occur with concentrations of less than 10%. Although well-known, the classic cherry-red color on the lips is rarely seen, as it usually requires carboxyhemoglobin levels of 30% to 40% to be evident. In any patient suspected of having experienced carbon monoxide poisoning, 100% oxygen should be immediately administered. Such therapy can shorten the half-life of carbon monoxide in the bloodstream from 320 minutes to 80 to 90 minutes. Steroids have not been proved effective for the treatment of carbon monoxide poisoning and may reduce the oxygen toxicity seizure threshold if hyperbaric oxygen treatments are used. About 75 percent of affected individuals are recovered within 1 year of the carbon monoxide poisoning insult.

13. C. For most patients, symptoms following decompression occur within 6 hours. Symptoms occur within 12 hours in 97 percent of patients. Nearly 80 percent of patients with decompression sickness have neurologic symptoms, the most common being paresthesias. The patient should be placed in a slight Trendelenburg position on the left side to prevent a left ventricular coalescence of gas bubbles and resulting systemic embolization. Air embolism is a more serious form of decompression injury, probably resulting from lung injury and producing symptoms within 5 minutes of decompression because of occlusion of large vessels. Recompression is the only real definitive treatment.

XIV. Transplantation

193. Transplant Immunology and the Use of Immunosuppressive Agents in Solid Organ Transplantation

1. True or False. Cyclosporine (CSA) acts by inhibiting interleukin-2 (IL-2) synthesis through inhibition of mRNA transcription.

2. True or False. CSA should be given as intravenous bolus therapy.

3. True or False. CSA levels are best obtained as a peak dose after oral administration to best guard against nephrotoxicity.

4. Select the best answer.

A. CSA is primarily excreted in the urine.
B. Oral CSA has a mean bioavailability of 80 percent.
C. Adequate CSA absorption depends on the presence of bile salts.
D. CSA dosing usually has to be increased with time after transplantation.

5. Select the best answer.

A. Drugs that induce the P-450IIIA enzyme (phenytoin, rifampin) can cause increased CSA levels.
B. Drugs that are metabolized by the same enzymes as CSA, such as erythromycin, show competitive enhancement and lead to decreased CSA levels.
C. P-450IIIA enzymes have been isolated from the intestine and may influence oral CSA absorption.
D. CSA metabolism cannot be influenced advantageously.

6. Select the best answer.

A. The major side effect of CSA administration is hepatotoxicity.
B. To avoid nephrotoxicity, CSA dosing must be carefully adjusted in patients with renal failure.
C. CSA nephrotoxicity only develops acutely.
D. Calcium channel blocking agents may be the drugs of choice in the management of hypertension in the transplant patient.

7. Select the best answer.

A. Corticosteroids inhibit IL-2 synthesis.
B. Corticosteroids inhibit chemotaxis of inflammatory cells.

C. Optimal dosing of corticosteroids has been established in the 30 years of their use in treatment of transplant rejection.
D. Steroids can reverse only 30 to 40 percent of rejection episodes in kidney and heart transplant patients.

8. Select the best answer.

A. OKT3 is effective for the treatment of acute cellular rejection episodes.
B. OKT3 is effective in blunting chronic humoral rejection.
C. OKT3 is not effective in treatment of rejection episodes refractory to conventional treatment.
D. OKT3 is administered in a slow intravenous drip to minimize capillary leak syndrome.

194. Critical Care Problems in Kidney Transplant Recipients

1. Select the best answer.

A. Prevention of acute tubular necrosis (ATN) posttransplant begins immediately in the intensive care unit.
B. Patients with low output of urine postoperatively should be vigorously volume resuscitated regardless of renal response.
C. Dialysis is not indicated in the renal transplant recipient, as it will impair graft function.
D. Living related kidney recipients are prone to fewer postoperative complications because of a lesser requirement for immunosuppression.

2. Select the best answer.

A. ATN averages 15 percent in cadaveric kidney recipients.
B. Prognostic factors for ATN are ischemic and immunogenic.
C. ATN has no influence on graft rejection.
D. ATN and acute rejection are managed similarly.

195. Specific Critical Care Problems in Heart, Heart-Lung, and Lung Transplant Recipients

1. True or False. Heart-lung transplants are commonly performed for patients with pulmonary vascular disease.

2. True or False. The transplanted lung remains hypoperfused after transplantation into the recipient with pulmonary hypertension.

3. Select the best answer.

A. Acute failure of a transplanted heart is seen more commonly than acute failure of a transplanted lung.
B. Lung graft failure can be manifested by hypoxemia, pulmonary edema, and even perihilar infiltrates on chest x-ray.

C. Prophylaxis for pulmonary history of deep venous thrombosis is not required.
D. An inferior vena caval filter should not be used in lung transplant recipients because of the possibility of filter migration and disruption of the transplant pulmonary artery vascular anastomosis.

4. Select the best answer.

A. Airway complications are common after heart-lung transplantation.
B. Early airway complications after transplantation are generally attributed to delayed healing caused by steroids.
C. Intraoperative bronchoscopy is not indicated because of the risk of disrupting the newly created anastomosis.
D. Dehiscence of the airway anastomosis occurs 1 week after transplantation.

196. Care of the Pancreas Transplant Recipient

1. True or False. The initial postoperative care of the pancreas transplant recipient should involve maintenance of blood glucose levels below 250 mg per deciliter.

2. True or False. Steroids are useful in the treatment of rejection in the pancreas transplant recipient.

3. Select the best answer.

A. Pancreatic rejection episodes are heralded by hyperamylasemia.
B. The first laboratory derangement seen in rejection of a pancreatic/kidney allograft is a rise in serum sodium.
C. Most rejection episodes in simultaneous kidney/pancreas transplant recipients are heralded by a rise in serum creatinine.
D. Urinary amylase is not useful in the monitoring of pancreatic allograft function.

4. Select the best answer.

A. The pancreas is subject to complications during transplantation that are similar to other solid organs.
B. University of Wisconsin (UW) solution for preservation has contributed to a lower incidence of graft-related complications in pancreas transplantation.
C. Pancreatic allograft thrombosis occurs in up to 9 percent of cases.
D. Since bleeding is a more common occurrence than thrombosis, the use of antiplatelet and anticoagulant drugs is contraindicated in pancreatic transplantation.

197. Management of the Organ Donor

1. True or False. There are 50,000 *potential* brain-dead organ donors per year in the United States, but the AIDS epidemic and the 55-miles-per-hour speed limit have had a significant impact on the number of available donors.

2. True or False. The rate of organ donation is rising such that the overall consent rate for organ donation is currently on the rise.

3. True or False. Transmission of malignancy is rare and has occurred in fewer than 100 transplantation cases out of 150,000 transplants.

4. Select the best answer.

A. Rates of consent from families for organ donation are higher when the discussion of a patient's death is performed separately from the request for organ donation.
B. The order of priority for next of kin is (1) spouse, (2) adult brother or sister, (3) adult son or daughter, (4) either parent, and (5) legal guardian.
C. The order of priority for next of kin is (1) spouse, (2) legal guardian, (3) adult brother or sister, (4) adult son or daughter, and (5) either parent.
D. The order of priority for next of kin is (1) legal guardian, (2) spouse, (3) either parent, (4) adult brother or sister, and (5) adult son or daughter.

5. Select the correct answer. Regarding the pathophysiology of brain death:

A. Resting vagal tone is preserved after brain death.
B. Hypotension after brain death is due to loss of vasomotor tone and peripheral venous pooling.
C. Cardiac dysfunction is uncommon after brain death.
D. The Cushing reflex is seen in brain herniation and consists of hypertension and tachyarrhythmia.

6. Select the correct answer. Regarding the management of the potential organ donor:

A. Hypertension is the most common hemodynamic abnormality seen in brain-dead organ donors.
B. The usual cause of hypotension in brain-dead organ donors is loss of endogenous catecholamine response to stress.
C. Beta-blockade using short-acting agents is useful in treating the tachyarrhythmias associated with brain death.
D. Electrolyte abnormalities are uncommon in the organ donor.

198. Diagnosis and Treatment of Rejection, Infection, and Malignancy in Transplant Recipients

1. True or False. Ten percent of renal transplant recipients experience at least one episode of acute rejection in the first 6 months posttransplantation.

2. True or False. Since the advent of immunosuppressant therapy with cyclosporine, the clinical signs of acute rejection have become more subtle.

3. Regarding immunosuppressive agents, which of the following statements is false?

A. Corticosteroids bind to a steroid receptor and migrate as a complex to the nucleus, where the action is to upregulate specific mRNA production.

B. Interleukin-2 production is blocked by corticosteroids.
C. OKT3 binds to the CD3 molecule, which leads to downregulation of T cell activity.
D. Azathioprine interferes with nucleic acid synthesis.

4. Which of the following is true about chronic rejection?

A. Chronic rejection is a slow process that is inevitable, well characterized, and well understood.
B. Chronic rejection is characterized by acute graft dysfunction followed by slow return of function, though rarely to baseline levels.
C. The histologic characteristics of chronic rejection are primarily vascular.
D. Chronic rejection is the consequence of tissue-destructive mechanisms that are distinct from acute rejection.

5. Select the correct answer. Regarding cytomegalovirus (CMV) infection:

A. CMV is easy to identify directly in urine and blood.
B. Immunocytochemical identification of CMV is sensitive and specific, but unfortunately it requires several days to see results.
C. Biopsy can be a useful diagnostic tool in the diagnosis of CMV infection.
D. Treatment of CMV infection is the same regardless of the clinical state of the patient.

Answers

Chapter 193

1. True. CSA acts by interrupting the signal transduction of cytokine synthesis in antigen-primed T-lymphocytes. CSA brings about immunosuppression through binding to calcineurin, which is responsible for proper assembly of transcription factor NF-AT. This precludes proper binding of NF-AT to the IL-2 gene in the cell nucleus, and this inhibits mRNA transcription for IL-2 and other cytokines.

2. False. CSA has nephrotoxicity as a major side effect. This nephrotoxicity is especially pronounced after intravenous bolus therapy. For this reason, CSA should be administered by intravenous infusion over 6 hours or as a constant infusion.

3. False. CSA level monitoring is most commonly performed as a steady-state predose level. The time to peak CSA level after oral administration is variable, and the peak level is therefore unreliable and is not usually measured. In addition to allowing for the maintenance of CSA levels within therapeutic ranges, CSA levels and monitoring help ascertain patient compliance and allow for differentiation between allograft dysfunction, allograft rejection, and drug toxicity.

4. C. Oral CSA has a mean bioavailability of 30 percent, but adequate absorption depends on the presence of bile salts. Less than 1 percent of unchanged CSA is excreted in the urine. Factors that impair CSA absorption include cholestasis, short bowel, diarrhea, ileus, gastroparesis, and biliary diversion. These are generally seen early in the postoperative period, so the dosage of CSA must often be reduced with time as the availability of CSA increases.

5. **C.** Drugs that induce P-450IIIA enzymes such as phenytoin and rifampin can cause significantly decreased CSA levels, leading to allograft rejection. Drugs that are similarly metabolized, such as erythromycin, can cause elevated CSA levels. P-450IIIA enzymes have been found in the human intestinal mucosa, and either induction or inhibition of these enzymes can impair or enhance CSA absorption. Inhibitors of CSA metabolism, such as ketoconazole and diltiazem have been shown to decrease CSA dose requirements by 80% and 50%, respectively. Furthermore, there is a suggestion of renal protection with diltiazem.

6. **D.** Although the proper adjustment of CSA dosing is critical to avoid the complication of nephrotoxicity, dosage adjustment is not required in the patient with preexisting renal failure, since 1 percent of CSA is excreted in the urine. CSA nephrotoxicity may develop at any time in the posttransplant period. The acute form is mediated by altered intrarenal hemodynamics. Long-term CSA administration has been associated with histologic evidence of interstitial fibrosis and tubulointerstitial injury. Preliminary evidence suggests that calcium channel blockers may help to ameliorate CSA nephrotoxicity.

7. **B.** Corticosteroids suppress both the alloantigen-specific and nonspecific immune responses through intracytoplasmic binding to a receptor. The steroid-receptor complex then binds to nuclear DNA and modifies mRNA transcription of enzymes and cytokines. Interleukin-1 is the most important cytokine that is inhibited by corticosteroids. Additionally, corticosteroids inhibit chemotaxis of inflammatory cells and production of proinflammatory molecules. In spite of 30 years of steroid use in the treatment of graft rejection, optimal dosages associated with maximum efficiency and minimum toxicity are not well established. Intravenous methylprednisolone reverses 75 to 85 percent of rejection episodes in kidney and heart transplant recipients.

8. **A.** OKT3 is effective in treating acute cellular rejection. It is more effective than steroids as first-line antirejection therapy in kidney and liver transplant patients. OKT3 also has been used effectively to reverse rejection episodes that are refractory to conventional therapy. OKT3 is typically administered as an intravenous bolus of less than 1 minute. Low-dose therapy has been associated with less severe side effects but must be coupled with CD3+ cell monitoring to ensure adequate levels of immunosuppression.

Chapter 194

1. **D.** Prevention of ATN posttransplant begins intraoperatively with liberal hydration including crystalloid and colloid products to avoid hypotension from intravascular volume depletion at the time of unclamping. The patient's cardiac status must always be borne in mind when fluid replacement is managed in the renal transplant patient. If there is no cardiac dysfunction, high-output diuresis is managed with cc/cc replacement. With cardiac dysfunction, replacement should be less than cc/cc. Patients with low-urine output should not be overhydrated, as this can result in volume overload, congestive heart failure, and pulmonary edema. Hyperkalemia and volume overload are indications for dialysis in the kidney transplant recipient.

2. **B.** ATN is the most common cause of impaired kidney function immediately posttransplant. ATN is rare in living related recipients, and incidence in cadav-

eric transplant recipients is 35 percent. Prognostic factors for the development of ATN are ischemic (cold and warm ischemic time, hypertension, hypotension, and vasopressor use) and immunologic (high percentage of antibodies, retransplantation, and poor matching). ATN has an early impact on graft function and also has a detrimental effect on graft survival and postoperative morbidity. Patients with posttransplant ATN have a higher incidence of acute rejection.

Chapter 195

1. **True.** Heart-lung transplants are performed almost exclusively for patients with pulmonary vascular disease with either primary or secondary pulmonary hypertension. A heart-lung transplant may occasionally be performed for septic lung disease with cardiomyopathy, such as in the patient with cystic fibrosis and cardiomyopathy.

2. **False.** Single lung transplantation was initially performed for patients with pulmonary fibrosis. It is now also undertaken for patients with chronic obstructive pulmonary disease and has recently been done in conjunction with repair of congenital heart defects. In patients who undergo single lung transplantation for pulmonary hypertension, reperfusion edema can be seen. This results from elevated blood flow through the transplanted lung. Up to 80 percent of the total blood flow can be seen going to the transplanted lung on perfusion scan in these patients.

3. **B.** Acute failure of a transplanted lung is more commonly seen than acute failure of a transplanted heart. Many of the reasons are related to preoperative considerations, such as suboptimal graft condition, unrecognized donor lung injury, and reperfusion edema in the transplanted lung. Lung graft failure can be manifested by infiltrates on chest x-ray, hypoxemia, and edema with reperfusion. Prophylaxis for pulmonary embolism is routinely employed in the lung transplant recipient, as pulmonary embolism is a devastating complication. The insertion of inferior vena caval filters is advocated in patients with a history of deep venous thrombosis.

4. **B.** Airway complications are more common after single lung or bilateral lung transplantation because the vascular supply to the anastomosis is more tenuous than in the heart-lung recipient. Early complications are related to steroids and delayed healing. It is important to perform intraoperative bronchoscopy to establish a baseline appearance of the bronchial anastomosis. Dehiscence will usually occur 3 to 6 weeks after transplantation. Early signs of dehiscence include pallor of the site, gray or black mucosa at the suture line, suture material apparent within the airway, and herniation of externally wrapped tissue into the lumen of the airway.

Chapter 196

1. **False.** Laboratory monitoring of the pancreas transplant recipient involves glucose determinations every 2 hours. In the early postoperative period, an infusion of regular insulin is employed to maintain plasma glucose levels below 150 mg per deciliter because it has been demonstrated that chronic hyperglycemia is detrimental to beta cells.

2. **False.** All rejection episodes are assumed to be steroid resistant. These data come from the University of Minnesota, where the majority of acute rejection episodes did not respond to initial use of steroids alone or were followed by early second rejection episodes if anti-T cell therapy was not utilized.

3. **C.** The acute rejection of a pancreatic or simultaneous kidney/pancreas transplant is heralded by a decrease in urine amylase and an increase in urine pH as the exocrine function of the pancreatic graft (amylase/bicarbonate) diminishes. However, in the simultaneous kidney/pancreas transplant recipient, the first indication of rejection is often a rise in serum creatinine.

4. **C.** The pancreas is an organ that is prone to a unique series of complications because of its exocrine function and relatively low blood flow. Thrombosis is a particularly devastating complication that can occur secondary to preservation edema from pancreatitis. To minimize graft thrombosis, low-dose heparin and antiplatelet drugs are used in the immediate postoperative period. The risk of bleeding in these patients is not trivial, but it is significantly smaller than the risk of thrombosis of the graft (0.95% versus 6–9%, respectively).

Chapter 197

1. **False.** The number of potential brain-dead organ donors is roughly 8000 as estimated from statistics available for 1992. Of these potential donors, 4521 actually became organ donors. The single most commonly cited reason for lack of organ retrieval is inability to obtain consent. Family refusal or inability to locate and contact family members remains the leading cause for nonuse of potential organ donors.

2. **False.** The overall consent rate for organ donation is dropping even today. This is an especially acute consideration for the intensive care unit physician, who may be a significant liaison between a grieving family and the primary care team. A recent public opinion survey suggested that 69 percent would be interested in donating their own organs and that 93 percent would honor the wishes of a family member if these wishes were clearly stated. The problem is that only 52 percent of these individuals had communicated their wishes to family members. A critical statistic shows that 37 percent of these same people did not comprehend that a brain-dead person should be considered as dead and 42 percent did not know that organ donation costs the family of the deceased nothing.

3. **True.** Transplantation of malignancy via donor organs is very rare, having occurred in fewer than 100 cases in over 150,000 transplants. Donor selection is particularly important in this regard, such that potential donors with most types of cancer are contraindicated as sources of organs. The exceptions are low-grade skin malignancy, carcinoma in situ of the uterine cervix, and low-grade nonglioblastoma primary brain malignancy. It is especially important to ensure that a donor with an assumed primary central nervous system malignancy does not have a metastatic brain lesion. It is also contraindicated to use as donor a patient with a primary brain malignancy who has undergone radiotherapy, chemotherapy, shunting, or craniotomy because of the increased risk for systemic dissemination of tumor cells.

4. **A.** Rates of consent for organ donation are significantly higher if the discussion of brain death occurs and the family is then allowed time to assimilate the

loss of a loved one. The proper order for consent is specified in the Uniform Anatomical Gift Act of 1968 for a donor over age 18: (1) spouse, (2) adult son or daughter, (3) either parent, (4) adult brother or sister, and (5) legal guardian.

5. **B.** The pathophysiology of brain death has been derived from observation and through animal models. Hemodynamic instability seen with brain herniation is the result of autonomic dysfunction secondary to the loss of central neurohumeral regulatory control of vital functions. Increased intracranial pressure leads to worsening brain ischemia and severe systemic hypertension resulting from an excess of catecholamines. A period of transient bradycardia associated with the hypertensive response can be seen early in the process of brain herniation and is termed the Cushing reflex. Cardiac dysfunction is common during and after brain death, and an impairment in coronary blood flow can be seen, which results in cardiac microinfarcts. Within 15 minutes after brain herniation and brain death, catecholamines decrease to below baseline levels.

6. **C.** The management of the potential organ donor is an important part of intensive care unit care. Hypotension and tachyarrhythmias are common in the brain-dead patient. The usual cause of hypotension in these patients is a relative hypovolemia due to vasomotor collapse and common treatments used for increased intracranial pressure, which require minimizing hydration and the use of osmotic diuretics. The state of hydration is critical in these patients. Additionally, drugs used to treat dysrhythmias should be short acting, such as esmolol and nitroprusside. Another commonly used agent is dopamine, which should be used in low doses. Electrolyte abnormalities are common, and hypophosphatemia, hypokalemia, hypocalcemia, and hypomagnesemia should be monitored for and treated. High-dose inotropic support is to be avoided owing to vasoconstrictive effects and the potential for end-organ damage.

Chapter 198

1. **False.** More than half of renal transplant recipients experience at least one acute rejection episode in the first 6 months posttransplantation. In those patients who experience an episode of acute rejection, it is known that 1-year graft survival is decreased.

2. **True.** The diagnosis of acute rejection is based on clinical, biochemical, and histologic features in biopsy specimens. Since the introduction of cyclosporine in the 1980s, the clinical signs of acute rejection, such as graft tenderness and graft swelling have become less obvious. The biochemical markers of rise in serum creatinine and blood urea nitrogen with a fall in urine output are helpful indices of acute rejection, but the differential diagnosis should always include other causes of graft dysfunction, such as hypovolemia, acute tubular necrosis (delayed graft function), ureteral obstruction or urinary leak, and cyclosporine nephrotoxicity.

3. **A.** The commonest immunosuppressive agents act at various sites within the immune system to prevent and treat acute rejection. Adrenal corticosteroids such as oral prednisone and intravenous methylprednisolone bind to a steroid receptor, which migrates intracellularly to the nucleus, where the complex acts to downregulate specific mRNA production. Interleukin-2 production is se-

verely impaired by corticosteroids. Azathioprine is an antimetabolite that interferes with rapidly dividing cells such as lymphocytes through interfering with nucleic acid synthesis. OKT3 is a murine monoclonal antibody that binds to the CD3 molecule and interferes with the actions of T cells in the immune cascade. OKT3 is effective in ongoing rejection because it can inhibit the activity of established effector T cells.

4. C. The cellular mechanisms responsible for chronic rejection are less well understood than those responsible for acute rejection. Chronic rejection usually occurs months to years after transplantation. It is a process characterized by progressive functional deterioration thought to stem from repeated episodes of acute rejection or from small subclinical foci of acute rejection within a graft. Both immunologic and nonimmunologic mechanisms are thought to be involved. Histologically, vascular changes occur with fibrointimal thickening and interstitial fibrosis.

5. C. Early diagnosis of CMV infection is critical because early treatment may limit or decrease the severity of infection. CMV is coated with a beta-2 microglobulin in the blood and urine, so it is not simple to identify its presence directly. Immunocytochemical detection can be accomplished in less than 24 hours with a sensitivity and specificity in active CMV infection of 90 percent or greater. CMV infection also may be identified by histologic analysis of biopsy specimens from the lung, esophagus, liver, or stomach. Identification of intranuclear vital inclusions and giant cells is characteristic of CMV infection. The treatment of CMV infection ranges from observation of the asymptomatic patient on minimal immunosuppression, to the administration of ganciclovir with or without reduction in immunosuppression, and finally to the addition of CMV hyperimmune globulin to ganciclovir therapy in the most severe cases.

XV. Metabolism and Nutrition

199. The Multiple Organ Syndrome

1. Select the correct answer. Nitric oxide synthase inhibition in animal models of septic shock

A. Can reverse hypotension.
B. Can cause liver injury.
C. Can increase mortality.
D. May have adverse effects on the host immune response.
E. Can produce all of the above.

2. Which of the following statements is true?

A. Increased lactate production always indicates that anaerobic metabolism is excessive.
B. Inadequate oxygen utilization is a major factor contributing to the development of the multiple organ dysfunction syndrome in certain high-risk populations.
C. Sepsis is known to decouple oxidative phosphorylation.
D. Direct and indirect measurements of oxygen consumption produce identical values.
E. The enzymes composing the Krebs carboxylic acid cycle are destroyed during sepsis.

3. Which of the following cytokines is **not** considered as important as the others in sepsis and the multiple organ dysfunction syndrome?

A. Tumor necrosis factor alpha (TNF-α).
B. Interleukin-1 (IL-1).
C. Interleukin-6 (IL-6).
D. Interleukin-7 (IL-7).
E. Interleukin-8 (IL-8).

200. Total Parenteral Nutrition

1. True or False. The major clinical consideration regarding total parenteral nutrition (TPN) revolves around energy malnutrition.

2. True or False. Serum albumin is a poor prognostic outcome variable.

3. True or False. The most variable portion of the total energy expenditure is the resting energy expenditure.

4. True or False. Overfeeding of carbohydrates should be a goal of nutrition in the septic or early postoperative patient, primarily for its protein sparing effects.

5. Select the best answer. Regarding fat in the diet of the critically ill patient:

   A. Fatty acid mobilization from peripheral fat stores is suppressed by glucose infusion.
   B. Fatty acid oxidation is increased.
   C. Use of exogenous fat in sick patients does not obviate the negative effects of excess carbohydrate infusion.
   D. Most intensive care unit practitioners supply 30 to 50 percent of the daily caloric requirement as fat.
   E. The total dose is usually limited to approximately 2.5 gm of fat per day.

6. Select the answer that is **false**. Regarding fat infusions:

   A. The most common type of lipid used as a caloric source in TPN is medium-chain triglycerides.
   B. Long-chain triglycerides are not cleared by lipoprotein lipase as efficiently as would be optimal.
   C. Medium-chain triglycerides are more rapidly and efficiently oxidized by carnitine-independent pathways and have less uptake in the reticuloendothelial system.
   D. Medium-chain triglyceride infusions have been shown to increase oxygen demand and change minute ventilation if infused too rapidly.

7. Select the best answer. Regarding glutamine:

   A. Glutamine is required in decreased amounts during severe stress.
   B. Glutamine is normally synthesized in the kidney and stored in skeletal muscle.
   C. Glutamine may have an important clinical role in maintaining the integrity of intestinal mucosa during stress.
   D. Glutamine is routinely available in standard parenteral solutions.

202. Disease-Specific Nutrition

1. True or False. Parenteral formulations designed for use in hypermetabolic patients include high-dose arginine and glutamine.

2. True or False. Regarding dietary manipulation in renal failure, clinical trials comparing essential amino acids alone to a mixture of nonessential and essential amino acids have shown a need of greater than 40 gm of essential amino acids per day.

203. Modulating the Inflammatory Response and Its Associated Immune Dysfunction

1. True or False. Nosocomial infections are typical in the systemic inflammatory response syndrome and multiple organ dysfunction syndrome (SIRS-MODS), which usually begin 7 days postinjury and involve skin organisms.

2. True or False. The mechanisms hypothesized in the development of nosocomial infections with gut flora involve failure of gut barrier functions.

3. True or False. There is no benefit to early enteral feeding regarding timing or route that can improve patient outcome.

ANSWERS

Chapter 199

1. **E.** Nitric oxide is a potent vasodilator that appears to be intimately involved with the pathophysiology of septic shock. In animal models of sepsis, administration of inhibitors of nitric oxide synthase can reverse the systemic hypotension observed in those models. Because of this finding, there was initially a great degree of interest in this inhibition as a potential modality for the treatment of human septic shock. However, subsequent studies have indicated that reversal of hypotension in sepsis is not necessarily beneficial, as liver injury and increased mortality can be observed. Furthermore, nitric oxide appears to be important for the phagocytic functions of macrophages. Thus, inhibition of nitric oxide production could adversely affect the host response to infection.

2. **B.** Altered oxygen metabolism appears to be a key component of sepsis and the multiple organ dysfunction syndrome. It is apparent that inadequate oxygen utilization is a major factor contributing to the development of the multiple organ dysfunction syndrome. While it appears that oxygen consumption is often impaired during sepsis, it is not clear what mechanisms are involved with the process. It does not appear that oxidative phosphorylation is uncoupled, nor is there evidence that the Krebs cycle is dysfunctional. While lactate levels are often elevated when anaerobic conditions exist, lactate increases in sepsis may or may not indicate an anaerobic state, as lactate can be increased in the process of aerobic glycolysis as well. Indirect measurements of oxygen consumption through use of thermodilution cardiac output measurements and the reverse Fick equation often do not equal those observed using exhaled gas analysis. While this difference may be due to the consumption of oxygen by alveolar and other pulmonary cells that may not be reflected by the indirect technique, the actual reasons for such differences are not clearly known.

3. **D.** Several cytokines appear to be involved in the pathophysiologies observed in sepsis and the multiple organ dysfunction syndrome. Those that are currently the focus of intense investigation as likely key mediators are TNF-α, IL-1, IL-6, and IL-8. TNF-α, IL-1, and IL-6 share many biologic activities, activating many of the other inflammatory and coagulation cascades.

Inhibition of the activities of these agents in animal models of sepsis often ameliorates the response. Furthermore, IL-1 and TNF-α appear to be able to stimulate the release of other cytokines. IL-8 is also elevated in septic states and appears to induce the expression of adhesion molecules, among other effects.

Chapter 200

1. **False.** Much of the data in the field of nutritional metabolic reports relate to preexisting protein energy of malnutrition and examine how correcting existing protein energy malnutrition, or reducing potential development, can impact an outcome. It has been suggested that the clinical importance of energy malnutrition is overemphasized. Emphasis should be directed toward the loss of body protein and how this affects physiologic functions in organs such as skeletal muscles, in respiratory function, in wound healing, and in the immune system.

2. **False.** Serum proteins may be distorted because of fluid shifts due to resuscitation. Levels of serum albumin, transferrin, and prealbumin, which normally give a balanced composite view of the patient's serum protein status, may be affected by postresuscitation considerations. During critical illness, the body mass of albumin is redistributed, with a tendency to move from the intravascular space to the extravascular space. Despite the many reasons why serum albumin level may be distorted, it appears to continue to be able to predict poor outcome in the intensive care unit setting.

3. **True.** The most variable portion of the total energy expenditure is the resting energy expenditure. This changes dramatically in the intensive care unit patient. Elevations of resting energy expenditure with acute illness occur in most critical illnesses and may exceed those seen with surgical procedures. In surgical procedures, the resting energy expenditure may increase up to 10 percent in the immediate postoperative period. Head trauma patients have documented resting energy expenditure measurements of 125 percent of predicted values. In spite of these considerations, intensive care unit physicians must demonstrate diligence in feeding to avoid overfeeding the critically ill patient because of untoward effects such as fluid overload, increased carbon dioxide production, increased oxygen consumption, and hepatic steatosis.

4. **False.** Glucose is the primary source of carbohydrates and necessary fuel for brain and bone marrow cells. Although there is a protein sparing effect of glucose in the unstressed starving patient, this diminishes in importance in the critically ill patient. During severe critical illness, there is not a deficit in available glucose, as glucose production is enhanced and glucose oxidation is relatively unimpaired. The maximum rate of glucose oxidation is probably in the range of 7 gm/kg/day. The cost of converting excess glucose supply to storage forms of glycogen and fat is 10 percent of the energy value of glycogen. Once glycogen supplies are repleted, this cost is closer to 30 percent when lipid storage is involved.

5. **D.** The other major caloric source of fuel in critically ill patients is fat. Fatty acid mobilization from peripheral fat stores is increased in the intensive care unit patient population. This is not suppressed by glucose infusion. Fatty acid

oxidation is also increased. As in carbohydrate metabolism, there is a recycling that occurs in fat metabolism, with fatty acids being recycled and transported back to adipose tissue for storage. Fat is a calorically dense, effectively utilized fuel source. Use of exogenous fat in critically ill patients can obviate the negative effects of excess carbohydrate infusion. Most intensive care unit physicians supply 30 to 50 percent of the daily caloric requirement as fat and limit the total dose to 2.5 gm of fat per kilogram per day.

6. **A.** The most common type of lipid used as a caloric source in TPN is long-chain triglycerides in a lipid emulsion derived from soybean or safflower oil. Some reported disadvantages of long-chain triglycerides are their immunosuppressive effects on nutritional function and macrophagocytosis and a general impairment of the function of the reticuloendothelial system. Long-chain triglycerides are not cleared by lipoprotein lipase efficiently. Long-chain triglyceride metabolism is dependent on a carnitine-controlled oxidated pathway, which is impaired in sepsis. An alternative to long-chain triglycerides are medium-chain triglycerides, which are derived from palm and coconut oils, are more rapidly and efficiently oxidized by a carnitine-independent pathway, and have less uptake in the reticuloendothelial system.

7. **C.** Glutamine is a conditionally essential amino acid required during stress situations, when it is increasingly utilized by the body. It is normally synthesized and stored in skeletal muscle and is a major fuel for the intestine and certain bone marrow cells. Glutamine may have an important clinical role in maintaining the integrity of the intestinal mucosa, although the role of glutamine in preventing the intestinal mucosa atrophy that develops during TPN is still being investigated. Glutamine is not standard in commercially available parenteral solutions.

Chapter 202

1. **True.** Specialty amino acid solutions marketed for use in patients for severe metabolic stress include essential, semiessential, and nonessential amino acids with higher concentrations of branched-chain amino acids. Other modifications currently under investigation include high-dose arginine and glutamine. Arginine is provided in currently available standard amino acid products in amounts lower than doses demonstrating immunomodulating properties. Glutamine has limited solubility and stability in solution and so is not available in standard amino acid solutions. It is available as a supplement for an essential amino acid solution marketed for use in renal failure.

2. **False.** Nitrogen metabolism in renal failure is an area of great interest where both quantity and quality of protein must be considered. Patients requiring hemodialysis or peritoneal dialysis have an increased catabolism and loss of protein into the dialysate; therefore, protein restriction is not appropriate. Clinical trials comparing essential amino acids alone to a mixture of nonessential and essential amino acids have had conflicting results. Excessive amounts (> 40 gm of essential amino acids) may cause hyperammonemia. Nonessential acids, such as arginine, ornithine, and citrulline, are necessary for ammonia detoxification, via the urea cycle, without which there may be increased serum ammonia levels.

Chapter 203

1. **False.** Nosocomial infections are typical of SIRS-MODS and usually begin 7 to 10 days postinjury. The major sites are the sinuses, the lower respiratory tract, invasive lines, prosthetic devices, and the urinary tract. The organisms involved tend to be those harbored in the gut. Within a few days of injury, the enteral flora will have colonized the skin, upper gut, and respiratory tract in up to 80 percent of patients.

2. **True.** There are two mechanisms hypothesized through which this colonization of sites with gut flora could occur, both originating from a failure of gut barrier functions. In the first, organisms move up the gut from the colon, to the small bowel, to the stomach, and to the respiratory tract by a direct migration. In the second, organisms translocate through the wall of the gut into regional lymph nodes and then into the systemic circulation.

3. **False.** There appears to be a window within the treatment of critically ill patients where enteral feeding can improve patient outcome. The window of opportunity appears to be sometime between the injury event and the establishment of the systemic inflammatory response. The reduction in infection rate appears to be for both line sepsis and for infections other than line sepsis.

XVI. Pharmacokinetics and Pharmacodynamics

205. Applied Pharmacokinetics: Specific Application for the ICU

True or False. Regarding applied pharmacokinetics in the intensive care unit (ICU):

1. The bioavailability of prodrugs is usually less than 100 percent even though they have been administered intravenously.

2. With constant infusions of a drug, serum concentrations are assumed to have reached steady-state concentrations after three elimination half-lives of the drug.

3. Albumin concentrations will have an insignificant effect on free serum drug concentrations if the free fraction is less than 0.5.

4. Drugs that undergo significant tubular secretion have renal clearance values that are greater than the glomerular filtration rate (GFR).

206. Physiologic Clearance and Pharmacokinetic Parameters to Individualize and Monitor Dosage Regimens of ICU Patients

1. Which of the following drugs does **not** approximate a one-compartment model for its elimination?

A. Gentamicin.
B. Amikacin.
C. Phenytoin.
D. Penicillin.
E. Tobramycin.

True or False. Regarding pharmacokinetics in the ICU:

2. The volume of distribution for aminoglycosides is normally about 60 percent of body weight.

3. The second phase of a two-compartment linear model is attributed to the drug's diffusing into the tissue compartment while being eliminated from the body.
4. Measurement of serum concentrations for drugs with low therapeutic indices is recommended for the critically ill patient.
5. Acidic drugs bind to albumin.
6. Acidic drugs bind to alpha-1-acid-glycoprotein.

Match each of the conditions in the first column with its impact on drug requirements in the second column.

7. Volume resuscitation
8. Hyperdynamic sepsis
9. Aggressive forced diuresis
10. Multiple organ failure
11. Major abdominal surgery
12. Application of plaster casts

A. Increases drug requirements
B. Decreases drug requirements
C. Could increase or decrease drug requirements
D. No effect

207. Antiarrhythmic Agents

1. Select the correct answer. Adenosine
   A. Is not approved as an antiarrhythmic agent by the Food and Drug Administration (FDA).
   B. Is an endogenous pyrimidine nucleoside compound.
   C. Exerts most of its antiarrhythmic effects at the level of the vagal nerve.
   D. Must be given intravenously for its antiarrhythmic effect.
   E. Increases conduction through the atrioventricular (AV) node and enhances automaticity of cardiac pacemakers.

208. Neuromuscular Blocking Agents

1. Which of the following statements regarding muscle relaxants is not true?
   A. The main route of excretion for vecuronium is hepatobiliary clearance.
   B. Nearly 100 percent of pancuronium is metabolized by the liver.
   C. The neuromuscular blocking agents are distributed in the extracellular fluid.
   D. Negligible cerebrospinal fluid penetration occurs with muscle relaxants.
   E. The majority of atracurium undergoes spontaneous decomposition.

2. Select the correct answer. Laudanosine is
   A. A metabolite of succinylcholine.
   B. A contaminant of vecuronium preparations.
   C. Not very lipophilic.
   D. An effective anticonvulsant.
   E. A product of atracurium degradation.

3. Which of the following statements regarding prolonged paralysis (acute generalized neuromyopathy) is not true?

A. The duration of neuromuscular blockade is usually for periods of greater than 5 days.
B. Concomitant corticosteroid use is a common feature.
C. Both atracurium and vecuronium appear to produce the syndrome with equal predilection.
D. Patients in renal failure appear to be at risk for prolonged paralysis.
E. Pancuronium use is involved in many cases.

209. Sedative Agents

1. Which of the following is **not** a property of benzodiazepines?

A. Hypnotic.
B. Anxiolytic.
C. Muscle relaxant.
D. Diuretic.
E. Anticonvulsant.

2. Select the correct answer. Propofol

A. Is a benzodiazepine.
B. Should not be used in the ICU for sedation.
C. Has a long terminal elimination phase.
D. Has not been shown to affect seizure activity.
E. Has no effect on serum triglyceride levels.

3. Which of the following statements regarding haloperidol is **not** true?

A. The mechanism of action is unknown.
B. There is no established therapeutic range for haloperidol when it is used to treat delirium in the ICU.
C. The dosage of haloperidol should be adjusted in renal failure.
D. Intravenous administration of haloperidol is not currently approved by the Food and Drug Administration (FDA).
E. Haloperidol distribution into human body tissues and fluids has not been fully elucidated.

210. Antihypertensive Agents

1. True or False. Propranolol, metoprolol, esmolol, and atenolol all inhibit both $beta_1$- and $beta_2$-adrenergic receptors.

2. True or False. Calcium channel antagonists exert their antihypertensive effects by inhibiting the influx of calcium across the membranes of arterial smooth muscles.

3. True or False. Nitroglycerin is metabolized primarily by the liver.

4. True or False. Patients receiving diuretics are at increased risk of renal dysfunction as a result of angiotensin-converting enzyme (ACE) inhibitor therapy.

211. Theophylline

1. True or False. Theophylline is a smooth muscle relaxant that has been used for many years and whose mechanism of action is well understood.
2. True or False. Pulmonary function has been shown to improve as a direct function of theophylline concentration in otherwise healthy asthmatic patients.
3. True or False. The greatest proportion of theophylline clearance is through metabolism by the liver's cytochrome P-450 system.
4. True or False. Smoking increases the serum theophylline concentration.
5. True or False. Cimetidine increases the serum theophylline concentration.

212. Antimicrobial Agents

1. Which of the following statements regarding vancomycin is not true?

   A. It has a distribution volume of 0.7 liter per kilogram.
   B. It can produce flushing and hypotension if infused rapidly.
   C. It needs to achieve peak serum levels of between 5 and 10 mg per liter for efficacy.
   D. It is mostly eliminated by the kidneys.
   E. It is not absorbed from the gastrointestinal tract.

2. Select the correct answer. Imipenem

   A. Is structurally related to the aminoglycosides.
   B. May need to be given more frequently than normal to hyperdynamic patients.
   C. Has a clearly established therapeutic range.
   D. Is well absorbed following oral administration.
   E. Is primarily metabolized by the liver.

213. Anticonvulsant Drugs

1. The oral bioavailability of phenytoin is

   A. 0 percent.
   B. 10 to 20 percent.
   C. 40 to 50 percent.
   D. 60 to 70 percent.
   E. 90 to 100 percent.

Answers

Chapter 205

1. **True.**

2. **False.**

3. **False.**

4. **True.**

   The bioavailability of intravenously administered drugs is usually assumed to be 100 percent. Exceptions to this concept are drugs that are administered as prodrugs, which need further processing before they are clinically active. An example of a prodrug is chloramphenicol succinate, which is inactive until it is cleaved by the liver to yield active chloramphenicol. Intravenously administered drugs given as a continuous infusion are assumed to have achieved a steady state with respect to the serum concentration values after five elimination half-lives of the drug have elapsed. The same time period is required for the achievement of a steady state when the drugs are given as intermittent infusions. Because the delay in achieving therapeutic concentrations may be disadvantageous with some drugs, a bolus infusion is often administered at the initiation of therapy. Examples of such loading doses are seen in the common methods of administering lidocaine or phenytoin. Most drugs bind to plasma proteins, with about 95 percent of the binding being to either albumin or alpha-acid glycoprotein. The binding is usually reversible, with a constant equilibrium existing between the proportion of free and bound drug existing. Only the free drug is active pharmacologically. Usually, the protein binding capacity is more than enough to remain unsaturated, although exceptions exist, such as with valproic acid and salicylates. If protein binding saturation occurs, the total serum drug concentration can be in the normal range, but the free fraction (i.e., the active component) is increased, thus potentially contributing to toxicity. If the free fraction is greater than 0.5, then less than one-half of the drug is bound, and changes in albumin concentrations will have little effect on free serum concentrations. The factors that influence the renal clearance of a drug are glomerular filtration, active tubular secretion, and passive reabsorption. Drugs that are only filtered by the glomerulus and neither secreted nor reabsorbed have a clearance that is equivalent to the GFR. On the other hand, drugs that have significant tubular secretion will have renal clearance values higher than the GFR, while those drugs that are reabsorbed will have clearance values less than the GFR.

Chapter 206

1. **C.** Most drugs used in the intensive care unit (ICU) follow linear pharmacokinetic principles. This means that a change in serum concentration will be directly proportional to a change in the patient's dosage regimen. Most antibiotics and analgesics used in the ICU follow these linear principles. Phenytoin is nonlinear in epileptic patients. This indicates that there is some enzymatic metabolism of the agent that follows saturation kinetic principles (i.e., Michaelis-Menten concepts). However, in patients who are hyperdynamic, it is possible that a nonlinear drug such as phenytoin could behave in a linear manner.

2. **False.**

3. **False.**

4. **True.**

5. **True.**

6. False.

Total body water is normally about 60 to 70 percent of body weight. Of this, roughly two-thirds is intracellular, and one-third is extracellular. Because of their quarternary amine and highly charged nature, aminoglycosides remain in the extracellular fluid volume. Thus, the volume of distribution for aminoglycosides is normally only about 20 percent of body weight. Linear models commonly used to approximate the behavior of drug concentrations within the body are the one-compartment and two-compartment models. The one-compartment is the simplest to apply and use. It assumes minimal to no tissue uptake and a linear relationship between drug concentration and dosage. A two-compartment model shows a biphasic relationship between drug concentration and time. The first phase occurs as a result of the combination of drug diffusing into the tissue compartment while it is simultaneously being eliminated from the body. The second phase results from only drug elimination from the body. Because of the highly variable physiology that is commonly seen among critically ill patients, it is nearly impossible to apply the assumptions inherent in dosing nomograms for these patients. Therefore, measurement of serum concentrations for drugs with low therapeutic indices is recommended for the critically ill patient. Acidic drugs bind to albumin, which is often decreased in critical illness, whereas basic drugs bind to alpha-1-acid glycoprotein, an acute phase reactant that is often increased in acute critical illness.

7. A.

8. C.

9. B.

10. B.

11. A.

12. D.

A patient's physiologic state can markedly affect the pharmacokinetic parameters that will determine the serum concentration of any administered drugs. The disturbance could be so severe as to produce nontherapeutic drug concentrations, either subtherapeutic if the resulting concentration is too low to produce a pharmacologic effect or potentially toxic if the drug concentration is too high. Volume resuscitation tends to expand the apparent volume of distribution for drugs commonly employed in ICU patients, thus requiring a larger drug dose if effective concentrations are to be ensured. Similarly, patients undergoing major abdominal surgery usually have expanded volume requirements to maintain an adequate circulation during surgery, and thus increased dosage requirements will occur. On the other hand, aggressive forced diuresis will tend to contract a drug's apparent volume of distribution, thus reducing drug requirements. Patients with established multiple organ failure will usually accumulate drug because of diminished clearance, and thus less drug may be necessary. Furthermore, if the liver's synthetic capabilities are impaired, the reduction in albumin and other proteins could reduce the total pool requirements for the drug. Patients with hyperdynamic septic state could have increased or decreased drug requirements, depending on the drug. Flow-limited agents will usually have an expanded volume of distribution and a rapid elimination rate, thereby increasing the dosage requirements. On the other hand, capacity-limited drugs could have either increased or decreased clearance, depending on the effects of the hyperdynamic state on the enzyme system(s) involved. Application of plaster casts may affect the patient's measured body weight, as could other devices (e.g., halo vests, traction systems), and thus affect any dosage system based on that measured "body" weight. However, this does not affect the patient's real dosage requirements when the proper determination of pharmacokinetic parameters is made.

Chapter 207

1. **D.** Adenosine is a synthetic form of a naturally occurring purine nucleoside. In 1989, it was approved by the FDA for the emergency management of supraventricular tachycardia involving the AV node. Adenosine exerts its effects through binding to extracellular purine receptors, affecting ionic movement through cell membranes. It produces an inhibitory effect on the sinus and AV nodes, slowing conduction through the AV node and depressing the automaticity of cardiac pacemakers. Exogenously administered adenosine must be given intravenously to achieve its antiarrhythmic effect.

Chapter 208

1. **B.** The nondepolarizing muscle relaxants contain quarternary ammonium groups, making them unable to cross lipid cell membranes. Thus, their distribution is primarily in the extracellular fluid. Also, because of their quarternary structure, negligible cerebrospinal fluid penetration occurs. The main route of excretion for vecuronium is hepatobiliary clearance, whereas the majority of atracurium undergoes spontaneous decomposition. However, up to 60 percent of pancuronium is excreted unchanged by the kidney, with the remaining 30 to 40 percent being converted by hepatic oxidative enzymes. The 3-OH deacylated metabolite of pancuronium is excreted by the kidney and possesses roughly half the activity of pancuronium as a muscle relaxant. Thus, renal failure can prolong the duration of action of pancuronium. Only about 11 percent of pancuronium and its metabolites is excreted via the biliary tract.

2. **E.** Most atracurium undergoes spontaneous decomposition under physiologic conditions through a reaction known as Hofman elimination. This process cleaves atracurium to produce laudanosine and monoquarternary methacrylate. Laudanosine is a central nervous system stimulant and has a potential to provoke seizure activity, although there is no clinical evidence of drug-related convulsive behavior reported. It is highly lipophilic and could therefore accumulate to a significant degree in central nervous system tissue.

3. **C.** In recent years, there have been many reports of prolonged paralysis or an acute generalized neuromyopathy. It appears to occur more commonly in patients who have been paralyzed for prolonged periods, usually 5 days or more. The coexistence of renal failure or corticosteroid use also seems to increase the likelihood of prolonged paralysis. Pancuronium or vecuronium has been implicated in the majority of cases, but there is no clear evidence that atracurium can produce the syndrome.

Chapter 209

1. **D.** Benzodiazepines are commonly used for sedation in the intensive care unit (ICU). They have hypnotic, anxiolytic, anticonvulsant, muscle relaxant, and antegrade amnesic properties. As there appear to be no benzodiazepine receptors outside of the central nervous system, their predominant effects are therefore produced in the central nervous system, primarily acting in the limbic, thalamic, and hypothalamic areas.

2. **C.** Propofol is an intravenous agent (2,6-diisopropylphenol) that has sedative and hypnotic properties. It is not a benzodiazepine and does not belong to any other standard class of sedative. It has been approved for ICU sedation. Its effects on seizure potential are unclear, in that it has been shown to produce anticonvulsant activity in animals and in humans, and yet there are numerous reports of seizure-like activity following propofol administration. It can elevate serum triglyceride concentrations due to the lipid load of the emulsion carrying the sedative. A three-compartment pharmacokinetic model has been used to describe propofol's elimination, in which the exponential third phase is very long due to the slow elimination of drug remaining in poorly perfused tissues. However, for practical purposes, this does not seem to produce much clinical effect because the second phase is that of a rapid metabolic clearance that eliminates the bulk of the drug, usually leaving the remaining amount to be eliminated by the third phase at a level of drug that is too low to produce a clinical effect.

3. **C.** Haloperidol is a butyrophenone-derived antipsychotic molecule whose exact mechanism of action is unknown. Although intravenous administration is not an FDA-approved route, there is a significant degree of experience and evidence to support the safety of haloperidol lactate administration by the intravenous route. Haloperidol deconoate should not be administered intravenously, however. The therapeutic range for haloperidol in the ICU management of delirium is not established, but serum concentrations of 3 to 20 mg per milliliter appear to be effective in providing antipsychotic activity. The distribution of haloperidol into human tissues and fluids has not been fully determined. Because most of the metabolism of haloperidol is hepatically mediated, no adjustment in haloperidol dosage is necessary in renal failure, but adjustment is important in cases of hepatic dysfunction.

Chapter 210

1. **False.** The beta-adrenergic receptor inhibitors metoprolol, esmolol, and atenolol preferentially inhibit beta$_1$-receptors and are thus considered cardioselective in their activity. However, propranolol inhibits both beta$_1$- and beta$_2$-receptors.

2. **True.** Calcium channel blockers are agents that have antiarrhythmic as well as antihypertensive properties. They exert their antihypertensive effect through inhibition of calcium influx into arterial smooth muscle cells.

3. **True.** Nitroglycerin is metabolized in the liver with a plasma elimination half-life of 1 to 4 minutes to less active dinitro and mononitro forms. Therefore, nitroglycerin dosage should be carefully adjusted in patients with liver dysfunction.

4. **True.** ACE inhibitors can often increase renal blood flow, but the combination of ACE inhibition with diuretic administration can actually raise the blood urea nitrogen and creatinine.

Chapter 211

1. **False.** Although theophylline has been used for many years as a smooth muscle relaxant with a bronchodilatory action, the exact mechanism of that action is not yet clear. Several mechanisms have been proposed, including the inhibition of cyclic adenosine monophosphate phosphodiesterase, inhibition of cellular calcium translocation, inhibition of leukotriene production, reduction in the uptake or metabolism of catecholamines, and blockade of adenosine receptors.

2. **True.** Generally, the therapeutic range for theophylline is 10 to 20 mg per liter. It has been shown in a study of hospitalized but otherwise healthy asthma patients that the peak expiratory flow rate increased in proportion to the logarithm of the serum theophylline concentration.

3. **True.** Roughly 90 percent of circulating theophylline is metabolized by the liver through the cytochrome P-450 system.

4. **False.** Because smoking cigarettes in excess of 20 per day induces the cytochrome P-450 system, theophylline clearance is higher in smokers than nonsmokers. Thus, smokers require about 1.5 to 2 times the daily dose of theophylline that nonsmokers require.

5. **True.** Cimetidine inhibits hepatic microsomal enzyme function and thereby decreases theophylline clearance by 25 to 100 percent, thus tending to increase serum theophylline concentrations.

Chapter 212

1. **C.** Vancomycin is a glycopeptide antibiotic that is effective in the management of infections due to several gram-positive organisms and some anaerobes. It has a relatively large volume of distribution, averaging about 0.7 liter per kilogram, or the amount represented by total body water. It has a peculiar property of producing the "red man syndrome" (rash, vasoflushing, nausea, facial edema, and hypotension) if infused too rapidly. Generally, infusions of 1 gm or more should be infused over a period of 1 hour or more to avoid this syndrome. Peak serum levels for efficacy are generally considered to be between 30 and 40 mg per liter. Vancomycin is mainly eliminated by the kidneys, and thus dosage adjustment is often made in renal failure. Oral administration of vancomycin is effective for the management of pseudomembranous colitis and staphylococcal enterocolitis. However, the drug is not absorbed from the gastrointestinal tract, making it ineffective through the oral route for other systemic infections.

2. **B.** Imipenem is the *N*-formimidoyl derivative of thienamycin, a carbapenem antibiotic that is a structural analogue of beta-lactam antibiotics. There is no established therapeutic range for imipenem, although it is generally thought that the serum concentrations should remain above the minimal inhibitory

concentration (MIC) for the entire dosing interval. Imipenem is not well absorbed following oral administration and is therefore given by either the intravenous or intramuscular route. It is predominantly eliminated by the kidneys. No studies have yet investigated the pharmacokinetics of imipenem in hyperdynamic patients. Because such patients may manifest flow-dependent glomerular filtration, more frequent dosing of imipenem may be necessary to maintain concentrations above the typical bacterial MICs.

Chapter 213

1. **E.** Phenytoin is an anticonvulsant that is also effective for the treatment of digitalis-induced arrhythmias. The therapeutic range for serum phenytoin concentrations is 10 to 20 mg per liter. Oral forms are generally 90 to 100 percent bioavailable, although absorption is slow due to its poor dissolution in acidic fluids. Peak concentrations of phenytoin therefore occur some 3 to 12 hours after an oral dose.

XVII. Dermatologic, Rheumatologic, and Immunologic Problems in the Intensive Care Unit

217. Anaphylaxis

1. Characteristics of anaphylaxis include which of the following?

A. It is a life-threatening form of delayed hypersensitivity.
B. Mast cell mediator release requires IgE binding to cell surface Fab receptor.
C. Preformed mediators are released on cell activation.
D. Mediator release is suppressed by cyclic guanosine monophosphate (GMP) and enhanced by cyclic adenosine monophosphate (AMP).

2. A 12-year-old girl presented to the emergency room with a history of yellow jacket sting approximately 15 minutes earlier. She was anxious, flushed, and rhinorrheic and had a rapid pulse. She reported chest tightness and shortness of breath immediately after the sting, but her breathing seemed to improve on the way to the hospital. A true statement about her condition is

A. The danger of a severe reaction has passed since her breathing has improved.
B. The most common cause of death in anaphylaxis is hemodynamic collapse.
C. This patient should receive epinephrine.
D. Rapid onset of symptoms is a favorable prognostic sign.

3. Penicillin allergy is

A. The most common cause of anaphylaxis in the United States.
B. Associated with cross-reactivity to cephalosporins in 20 to 30 percent of patients.
C. Rarely associated with cross-reactivity to carbapenems.
D. Unlikely with a negative skin test to cephalosporins.

218. Dermatologic Problems in the Intensive Care Unit

True or False. Regarding the toxic shock syndrome:

1. Antibiotic therapy is unnecessary.

2. Vomiting and diarrhea are common.

3. A bacterial exotoxin is the presumed cause.

4. Skin erythema is usually localized.

5. Diffuse muscle tenderness is present.

6. Profound hypotension is characteristic.

7. Select the correct answer. Brown recluse spider bites

A. Can be diagnosed by lymphocyte transformation tests within a few days of envenomation.
B. Respond to topical and systemic steroids with accelerated wound healing.
C. Respond to immediate surgical debridement with less signs and symptoms of systemic toxicity.
D. May produce disseminated intravascular coagulopathy.

219. Collagen Vascular Diseases in the Intensive Care Unit

1. Scleroderma renal crisis is characterized by

A. Microangiopathic hemolytic anemia.
B. Urinary red blood cell casts.
C. Low plasma renin level.
D. Nonoliguric renal failure.

2. A common manifestation of the antiphospholipid syndrome is

A. Increased bleeding tendency.
B. Presence of an active vasculitis.
C. Thrombocytosis.
D. Spontaneous abortions.

Answers

Chapter 217

1. C. Anaphylaxis is a form of immediate hypersensitivity. Initial antigen contact stimulates generation of IgE antibodies with Fab segments that recognize the antigen. These preformed antibodies bind via Fc receptors to mast cells and basophils. The antibodies may remain unbound for weeks. Subsequent antigen exposure can cause release of mediators from mast cells and basophils by binding to the Fab portion of two IgE molecules. This bridging activates secretion preformed primary mediators such as histamine, heparin, neutrophil chemotactic factor, and proteolytic enzymes. The release of mediators is modulated by cyclic AMP and enhanced by cyclic GMP.

2. **C.** The anaphylactic reaction is severe in this patient. Epinephrine is the drug of choice, and she should receive 0.3 to 0.5 ml of a 1:1000 solution (0.3–0.5 mg) subcutaneously. It should be repeated every 5 to 10 minutes if symptoms do not improve. Rapid onset of symptoms correlates with severity of reaction. The major cause of death in anaphylaxis is respiratory failure due to laryngeal edema and bronchospasm. Noncardiogenic edema may also occur.

3. **A.** Penicillin is the most common cause of anaphylaxis in the United States. Approximately 10 percent of the population has a positive skin test to penicillin. Cross-reactivity to cephalosporins occurs in 5.4 to 16.5 percent of the penicillin-allergic population. Unfortunately, skin testing for cephalosporin hypersensitivity is unreliable. Monobactams such as aztreonam do not cross-react with penicillins, but carbapenems such as imipenem show a high degree of in vivo cross-reactivity.

Chapter 218

1. **False.**

2. **True.**

3. **True.**

4. **False.**

5. **True.**

6. **True.**

   Toxic shock syndrome (TSS) is characterized by the acute onset of high fever, diffuse skin erythema, profound hypotension, and vomiting or diarrhea. An exotoxin produced by *Staphylococcus aureus*, TSS toxin 1, is the cause of the acute symptomatology. Muscle tenderness and neurologic symptoms of headache and disorientation are common. Supportive treatment and removal and/or drainage of infected foci are important. Antibiotic therapy directed against *S. aureus* may not affect the course of the acute syndrome, but appropriate antibiotics reduce the risk of bacteremia and recurrent symptoms.

7. **D.** Severe systemic problems including hemolysis and disseminated intravascular coagulopathy may occur after a brown recluse spider bite. The bite may initially go unnoticed, but it may subsequently evolve into a necrotic, ischemic full-thickness lesion over 24 to 48 hours. Enzymes in the spider venom are responsible. The lymphocyte transformation test is specific but will not become positive until 1 month after the bite. Neither corticosteroid treatment nor surgical debridement have improved local healing or systemic toxicity. Oral dapsone has been reported effective, but potential drug toxicity must be closely monitored.

Chapter 219

1. **A.** Scleroderma renal crisis is characterized by accelerated hypertension and renal insufficiency. Oliguria is typical. Increased renin release is triggered presumably by decreased renal cortical blood flow. Vascular constriction and intimal necrosis and fibrosis lead to microangiopathic hemolytic anemia. Modest proteinuria is common, but urinary red blood cell casts typical of glomerulonephritis are not seen. The hypertension and renal insufficiency often respond to angiotensin-converting enzyme inhibitors, sometimes with the addition of calcium channel blockers.

2. **D.** Antiphospholipid antibodies are present in some patients with systemic lupus erythematosus as well as some with other connective tissue disease syndromes and some with no identifiable underlying disease. Antiphospholipids have prothrombotic effects believed caused by promotion of platelet aggregation and thrombus formation and/or effects on plasminogen-activating factor or activation of protein C. The pathologic lesion is thrombosis and embolization, not vasculitis. Thrombocytopenia is common. Spontaneous abortion occurs more frequently in women with antiphospholipid antibodies due to vascular insufficiency and thrombosis in placental vessels.

XVIII. Psychiatric Issues in Intensive Care

221. Diagnosis and Treatment of Agitation and Delirium in the ICU Patient

1. Delirium is

A. Identical to dementia.
B. Irreversible.
C. An organic mental disorder.
D. Distinguished from dementia because dementia also has an altered level of consciousness.

True or False. Regarding delirium:

2. The electroencephalogram (EEG) of a delirious patient is usually abnormal.

3. Atropine is not a likely cause of delirium in an ICU patient.

4. The severity of EEG slowing parallels the intensity of delirium.

5. Benzodiazepines are the treatment of choice for all phases of the alcohol withdrawal syndrome.

6. The delirium associated with narcotic withdrawal can be so severe as to be lethal.

7. Haloperidol is not recommended for the treatment of delirium because it lacks Food and Drug Administration (FDA) approval for such an indication.

8. Extrapyramidal symptoms are common following intravenous haloperidol use.

9. Which of the following drugs is least likely to produce delirium in an ICU patient?

A. Meperidine.
B. Naloxone.
C. Lidocaine.
D. Cimetidine.
E. Penicillin.

222. Recognition and Treatment of Anxiety in the ICU Patient

1. Select the correct answer. Anxiety in the intensive care unit (ICU)

A. Is the most common reason for psychiatric consultation early after admission to the coronary care unit.
B. Is experienced by 10 percent of postoperative coronary artery bypass graft patients.
C. Has no effect on the patient's hemodynamic status.
D. Does not contribute at all to the mortality of patients following myocardial infarction.
E. Is not associated with plasma catecholamine levels.

2. True or False. Anxiety is defined as the sense of dread and foreboding that may occur in response to an external threatening event.

3. True or False. An organic etiology for the anxiety is suggested by its occurrence in the absence of a psychologically charged situation or in conjunction with discrete physical events.

4. True or False. Complex partial seizures do not cause anxiety symptoms.

5. True or False. Panic disorders have been found in 40 to 60 percent of patients with chest pain and normal coronary angiograms.

6. True or False. In patients with overlapping anxiety and depressive syndromes, a single antidepressant medication can often be used for treatment.

7. True or False. ICU patients are commonly overmedicated, thereby suppressing many of the symptoms of anxiety.

8. True or False. Ventilator weaning can often provoke anxiety in the ICU patient.

9. Which of the following benzodiazepines is least likely to produce a significant interdose rebound?

A. Oxazepam.
B. Midazolam.
C. Clonazepam.
D. Lorazepam.

223. Recognition and Treatment of Depression in the ICU

1. Which of the following conditions is **not** a common cause of depression in the intensive care unit (ICU) patient?

A. A reaction to an acute medical illness.
B. A manifestation of a primary affective disorder.

C. A mood disorder associated with organic pathology.
D. A result of the overlap of somatic symptoms of depression and the symptoms of medical illness.
E. A side effect of catecholamine infusions.

2. Which of the following conditions has been shown to be associated with depression?

A. Increased cardiac beat-to-beat variability.
B. Relative insulin resistance.
C. Immune system changes.
D. Decreased ventilatory response to carbon dioxide.
E. All of the above.

3. Which of the following statements regarding establishing the diagnosis of depression is false?

A. The evaluating physician should specifically screen for each of the eight symptoms of depression.
B. Either an increase or a decrease in appetite can constitute one of the symptoms of depression.
C. The potentially depressed patient should be assessed for the presence of suicidal thoughts.
D. The evaluating physician should ask if the patient has a specific plan for a suicide attempt.
E. The evaluating physician should assess the feasibility of the patient's suicide plan and offer suggestions for its improvement.

4. Which of the following conditions can be accompanied by depression?

(1) Hypothyroidism.
(2) Cushing's disease.
(3) Post-stroke states.
(4) Human immunodeficiency virus (HIV) infections.
(5) Parathyroid disturbances.

A. 1, 2, and 3.
B. 1 and 3 only.
C. 2 and 4 only.
D. 4.
E. All.

True or False. Regarding tricyclic antidepressant (TCA) medications:

5. Tricyclic antidepressant medications have type I or quinidine-like antiarrhythmic properties.

6. Polycyclic antidepressant medications are not recommended in the acute post-myocardial infarction phase.

7. There is a lower risk of second-degree or third-degree heart block when TCAs are used in patients with bundle branch blocks.

8. TCAs can decrease premature ventricular contractions.

9. Orthostatic hypotension from TCAs is infrequently observed in medically healthy patients.

224. Suicide

1. The least likelihood for suicidal potential is present in which of the following groups of individuals?

A. Those who have never married.
B. Patients with panic attacks.
C. Married individuals with children.
D. Unemployed individuals.
E. Patients who suffer from substance abuse.

True or False. Regarding suicide:

2. The most important risk factor for suicide is the presence of psychiatric illness.

3. Increasing age is correlated with decreased suicidal risk.

4. Renal dialysis patients have been found to have a suicide rate more than 400 times that of the general population.

5. Asking a patient about the possibility of suicide can have the adverse effect of planting the idea in the patient's mind.

6. Most suicidal intoxicated patients will still be suicidal when the effects of the intoxicants have worn off.

7. Which of the following principles is least important in handling the suicidal patient?

A. Treatment of the underlying problem.
B. Allowing the passage of time.
C. Maintenance of patient safety through the use of physical or chemical restraints.
D. Respect for the patient's wishes to refuse treatment.
E. Allowing the intoxicated patient to become sober before completing the evaluation.

225. Problematic Behaviors of Patients, Family, and Staff in the ICU

1. Which of the following items does not contribute to feelings of helplessness and anxiety on the part of intensive care unit (ICU) patients?

A. Limited communication from the ICU staff regarding the patient's condition.
B. Use of physical or chemical restraints.
C. Being placed in a dependent situation.
D. Open communication regarding the patient's situation and treatment involving both the patient and the family.
E. The absence of denial mechanisms on the part of the patient or family.

2. Which of the following personality types is likely to pit ICU staff members against each other?

A. The oral-dependent (or borderline) personality.
B. The histrionic character.
C. The obsessive character.
D. The noncompliant patient.
E. None of the above.

226. Recognition and Management of Staff Stress in the ICU

True or False. Regarding "burnout":

1. There appears to have been more research on burnout among intensive care unit (ICU) nurses than ICU physicians.

2. Individuals' personalities usually have little or no influence on whether burnout develops compared to the impact of their environment.

3. Studies have shown that ICU nurses have higher burnout rates than non-ICU nurses.

4. A lack of opportunity to share experiences and feelings with other staff members is a leading source of stress for ICU personnel.

5. Uncertainty regarding the operation and function of specialized equipment does not contribute to stress in the ICU.

6. Which of the following features of the "house officer syndrome" is **not** ubiquitous in all house officers at one time or another?

A. Chronic anger.
B. Pervasive cynicism.
C. Suicidal ideation.
D. Episodic cognitive impairment.
E. Family discord.

227. Neuropsychiatric Aspects of Cancer and AIDS in the ICU

True or False. Regarding the neuropsychiatric aspects of cancer:

1. Patients who have previously received chemotherapy that provokes vomiting may become conditioned to avoid treatment.

2. Complex partial seizures are easier to diagnose than are generalized seizures.

3. Generalized seizures are common among cancer patients.

4. Generalized seizures are more common than are complex partial seizures.

5. Akathisia can occur as a side effect of neuroleptic medications.

True or False. Regarding neuropsychiatric syndromes that occur in human immunodeficiency virus (HIV)–infected patients:

6. The most common psychiatric diagnoses in HIV-infected patients are adjustment disorders, major depression, and organic mental disorders.

7. Magnetic resonance imaging is superior to computed tomography in the evaluation of patients with HIV encephalopathy because of its superior capacity to distinguish white matter disease.

8. Seizures in HIV-infected patients can be attributed to a mass lesion in nearly all cases.

9. Akathisia can be produced by agents such as phenothiazines, butyrophenones, and metoclopramide.

10. Suicide rates for AIDS patients are equivalent to that of the general population.

11. Which of the following statements regarding the primary infection syndrome in HIV infection is true?

A. Seroconversion usually occurs some weeks before the appearance of a primary infection syndrome.
B. Primary infection syndrome is insidious in onset.
C. The illness usually takes several months to resolve.
D. The symptoms are similar to those of mononucleosis.
E. Headaches are rare and are mild whenever they occur.

Answers

Chapter 221

1. C. Delirium occurs often in intensive care unit (ICU) patients. It is a reversible organic mental disorder characterized by the acute onset of confusion and an altered level of consciousness. This altered level of consciousness is what distinguishes delirium from dementia, in which confusion exists with a normal level of consciousness.

2. True.

3. False.

4. True.

5. True.

6. False.

7. False.

8. False.

The EEG of a delirious patient is typically abnormal, suggesting a state of cerebral insufficiency and failure of the normal cerebral metabolic processes. The EEG characteristically shows a diffuse, generalized slowing whose severity usually parallels the intensity of the delirium. It is this typical EEG abnormality that is most responsible for characterizing delirium as an organic defect. An abnormality in cholinergic function appears to be involved with the pathophysiology of delirium. Many drugs have been implicated as potential causes of delirium, one of which is atropine. Benzodiazepines, usually chlordiazepoxide in a dosage of 25 to 100 mg four times a day, are the treatment of choice for all phases of the alcohol withdrawal syndrome. Opioid withdrawal is typically treated with replacement and tapering using a long-acting agent such as methadone. Despite the significant degree of uncomfortable agitation that opioid withdrawal can produce, it is not lethal. The treatment of nonspecific delirium is best approached with a neuroleptic such as haloperidol. Although the intravenous use of haloperidol lacks FDA approval, haloperidol has been shown to be effective for treatment of delirium with a high degree of safety in the ICU patient. Interestingly, extrapyramidal symptoms, which commonly occur following oral and intramuscular haloperidol use, appear to be uncommon when the drug is administered intravenously.

9. **B.** Several drugs have been shown capable of producing a delirium syndrome. Most of these appear to evoke the condition through anticholinergic effects. Narcotics such as meperidine and morphine are common and often unrecognized causes of delirium among ICU patients. Naloxone can often be an effective antidote for treatment of delirium under these circumstances. Other classes of drugs that can produce delirium are antiarrhythmics (e.g., lidocaine, procainamide, and quinidine), antibiotics (e.g., penicillin and rifampin), antihistamines (e.g., diphenhydramine, promethazine, cimetidine, and ranitidine), and beta-blockers (e.g., propranolol).

Chapter 222

1. **A.** In ICU patients, anxiety is the most common reason for psychiatric consultation within the first 2 days following admission to a coronary care unit. The reasons for this are multiple. Anxiety is a very common phenomenon among ICU patients, with 60 percent of coronary artery bypass patients and 65 to 85 percent of acute myocardial infarction patients estimated to experience anxiety. Anxiety can have very profound effects on the ICU patient, resulting in increased cardiac output as a result of sympathetic nervous system activity. Elevated levels of catecholamines, free fatty acids, and cortisol often accompany the anxiety associated with acute myocardial infarction. There is evidence that psychiatric consultation and treatment of anxiety are associated with decreased urinary levels of catecholamines and free fatty acids, along with decreased incidence of ventricular arrhythmias and potentially a reduction in mortality.

2. **False.** Fear is defined as the sense of dread and foreboding that may occur in response to an external threatening event. Anxiety differs from fear in that the same sense of foreboding instead derives from an unknown internal stimulus and either is inappropriate or excessive to the reality of the external stimulus or is concerned with a future one.

3. **True.** An organic etiology for the anxiety is suggested by its occurrence in the absence of a psychologically charged situation or in conjunction with discrete physical events.

4. **False.** Complex partial seizures secondary to limbic system irritability can cause anxiety symptoms.

5. **True.** Panic disorders can occasionally be so severe as to be confused with acute myocardial infarction. The condition has been found in 40 to 60 percent of patients with chest pain and normal coronary angiograms.

6. **True.** Depression can often manifest many anxiety-like symptoms. Treatment with a benzodiazepine does not address the depressive etiology and could adversely affect such patients. A single antidepressant medication can often be used for treatment of overlapping anxiety and depressive symptoms.

7. **False.** Despite the common occurrence of anxiety among ICU patients, it appears that undertreatment is the rule in common ICU practice. Only 66 percent of patients admitted for evaluation and treatment of acute myocardial infarction had benzodiazepines prescribed for them during their stay in the coronary care unit; in many, this was only on an as needed basis, and the medication was actually never given.

8. **True.** The presence of mechanical ventilation can often provide psychological support to the patient, and weaning can therefore provoke significant anxiety, often severe enough to interfere with the weaning process itself.

9. **C.** Interdose rebound is less likely with drugs that have a relatively long half-life compared to their dosing frequency. Drugs with an especially short half-life, such as midazolam (Versed, 1–2 hours), are therefore quite likely to produce interdose rebound. Oxazepam (Serax) has a half-life of 5 to 15 hours, and lorazepam (Ativan) has a half-life of 10 to 20 hours, making them also relatively short-acting agents. Of this list, clonazepam (Klonopin) has the longest half-life, ranging from 15 to as long as 50 hours, making it least likely to produce an interdose rebound phenomenon.

Chapter 223

1. **E.** Depression can be seen in the ICU patient and can frequently complicate critical care intensely. There is evidence that depressed patients have poorer survival statistics than do patients who are not depressed. Depression can occur in the ICU patient as a reaction to an acute medical illness. Examples would include driven individuals who are suddenly confronted with their own mortality, as following an acute myocardial infarction, or a young vigorous individual stunned by a permanent traumatic spinal cord paralysis. Depression can also present as a manifestation of a primary affective disorder, as such patients can also develop critical illnesses. Depression can also emerge as a manifestation of organic pathology, as may occur with some brain tumors, and can produce somatic symptoms that may mimic medical illnesses.

2. **E.** Depression is associated with many physiologic changes that can have important consequences in the critically ill patient. Significant cardiac effects can be seen in depressed patients, and recent data suggest that untreated depression is associated with increased cardiac mortality. A possible mechanism for the increased cardiac deaths is suggested by the finding that depressed patients often have increased cardiac beat-to-beat variability. Many endocrine alterations have been identified in depressed patients. These include increased

plasma cortisol, increased plasma and central nervous system metabolites of norepinephrine, and a relative resistance to insulin. Changes in the immune system, specifically decreased T and B cell mitogen responses, have been observed, as has a decreased ventilatory response to carbon dioxide levels.

3. **E.** The diagnosis of depression is based on several clinical findings. To qualify as clinically depressed, a patient must have had a sustained period of a depressed mood for at least 2 weeks in association with at least four (out of a total of eight) neurovegetative symptoms. The eight possible symptoms should each be specifically asked about and evaluated. They are remembered by the mnemonic SIG: E CAPS for (1) *S*leep alteration, (2) decreased *I*nterest, (3) *G*uilt, (4) decreased *E*nergy, (5) decreased *C*oncentration, (6) altered *A*ppetite, (7) *P*sychomotor retardation or agitation, and (8) *S*uicidal ideation. The presence of suicidal ideation, especially if the physician can determine that an actual suicide plan exists, mandates psychiatric consultation.

4. **E.** Various medications and medical conditions can cause depression and other organic affective disorders. Endocrine disorders (e.g., hypothyroidism, Cushing's disease, and parathyroid diseases) are often accompanied by depression. Following cerebrovascular accidents, up to 60 percent of patients with left hemispheric lesions and 15 percent of those with right hemispheric disorders can develop depression. Depression may be the first manifestation of infection from HIV.

5. **True.**

6. **True.**

7. **False.**

8. **True.**

9. **False.**

TCA medications have many potent cardiovascular effects. They exhibit type I (quinidine-like) antiarrhythmic properties and can decrease the rate of premature ventricular contractions. In patients with bundle branch blocks, there is a greater risk of second-degree or third-degree blocks developing when TCAs are used. Because of the many adverse cardiovascular effects that TCAs can produce, they are not recommended for use during the acute phase following a myocardial infarction. The most serious and frequently encountered cardiovascular side effect of TCAs in medically healthy patients is that of orthostatic hypotension, occurring in up to 20 percent of patients receiving TCAs.

Chapter 224

1. **C.** The potential for suicide attempts should be carefully evaluated when certain behaviors suggest that an individual may be experiencing suicidal thoughts. Statistically, different individuals have variable likelihoods of attempting suicide. Individuals with depressive symptoms are at greatest risk, with other groups at risk being those who are substance abusers, those with psychotic illnesses, and those with character disorders and panic disorders. Individuals who have never married, those who have been widowed, the un-

employed, and those without children are also at greater risk to attempt suicide than are married individuals with children.

2. **True.**

3. **False.**

4. **True.**

5. **False.**

6. **False.**

   Suicide and suicide risk can vary significantly from patient to patient. The most important risk factor for suicide is the presence of a psychiatric illness. Patients who suffer from depression, psychoses, substance abuse, character disorders, and panic disorders are all at risk to attempt suicide. Intoxicated patients who exhibited suicidal behavior during a period of intoxication will often no longer be suicidal once they are sober. The elderly and patients with chronic medical conditions are also in high-risk groups for suicide. One study indicated that patients on chronic renal dialysis had an over 400-fold greater suicide rate than did the general population. Contrary to popular belief, questioning a patient as to whether he or she has ever had suicidal thoughts does not produce or promote such ideas. Therefore, because of the significant risk to life that suicide represents, such questions should not be avoided.

7. **D.** The maintenance of patient safety is the key element that must guide the approach to the suicidal patient. Usually, treatment of the underlying problem and allowing for the passage of time will significantly reduce the suicidal potential. Patients who are intoxicated cannot be fairly evaluated for their suicidal risk and should be allowed to sober up before the evaluation is completed. If a patient is judged to be at significant risk for harming himself, physical or chemical restraints are appropriate if their use reduces the risk. The fact that a patient may not desire any treatment or attention for his problems should not influence the decision on how to protect the safety of a self-destructive individual.

Chapter 225

1. **D.** Being placed in an intensive care setting places a patient in a dependent situation by its very nature. The adjunctive use of chemical and physical restraints may occasionally be necessary to protect the patient from harming himself but may accentuate the sense of helplessness and anxiety. Inadequately dealing with the patient's or family's concerns and anxieties by not fully informing them of the patient's status and likely course can contribute to feelings of helplessness. However, denial may provide some protection against anxiety, and there is evidence that "deniers" have more favorable outcomes than "nondeniers." Thus, there may be no benefit in emphasizing bad news, although, in general, the more informed and involved the patient and family are, the less anxiety and helplessness are produced.

2. **A.** Different personality types bring different coping styles to the experience of intensive care. Patients with oral-dependent or borderline personalities are impulsive, afraid of being alone, and expect total care. Also, these patients are

able to present different sides of themselves to different staff members in order to maintain each relationship at the appropriate emotional distance. This can cause the staff to have opposing views regarding the patient's status and care needs. The divisiveness they cause can actually be one of the strongest clues to the presence of a borderline personality type. Histrionic patients tend to manifest their insecurity by dramatizing everything and encouraging staff members to reveal more of themselves. Obsessive patients tend to become paralyzed by anxiety through their excessive analysis of every detail. Noncompliant behaviors on the part of patients tend to evoke collusion, sadism, or denial among staff members.

Chapter 226

1. **True.**

2. **False.**

3. **False.**

4. **True.**

5. **False.**

   Burnout among ICU staff members can be a serious problem affecting hospital resources, morale, and patient care. Burnout appears to develop as the culmination of a sustained and intense response to negative stress. Both physicians and nurses can experience burnout, although the impact can be different because of the different natures of the jobs involved. Because nurses can be exposed to the stressful environment of an ICU on a continuous basis whereas physicians in training tend to rotate through an ICU for a more limited exposure, there has been a greater amount of study and interest regarding burnout affecting nurses than physicians. However, because of a sentinel case where physician sleep deprivation was incriminated as the cause for an unacceptable patient outcome, more attention has been directed recently at physician burnout. Individual personalities may be more predisposed toward burnout than others; for example, it has been found that among a group of family practice residents, those who were more extroverted, perceptive, and intuitive were less likely to experience burnout. Among the many conditions that can produce stress among health care workers are a lack of opportunity to share experiences and emotions with other staff members, the death of a patient, insufficient dedication of time for a patient's emotional support, inadequate training to help with a patient's emotional needs, and unfamiliarity with the use of specialized equipment. While all of these conditions can commonly exist in ICU settings, studies comparing ICU to non-ICU workers have been unable to identify significant differences in the stress levels between the two environments, although the types of conditions producing the stresses may differ. For example, ICU nurses may be more often stressed by changing shifts or schedules, whereas non-ICU nurses are more likely to be stressed when confronting an emergency situation.

6. **C.** The stressful environment and intense pressures that exist during residency training can produce significant effects on the participants. In 1981, Small described the house officer syndrome, which consisted of seven features: episodic cognitive impairment, chronic anger, pervasive cynicism, fam-

ily discord, depression, suicidal ideation, and substance abuse. It is likely that the first four are present in all house officers at one time or another. However, depression, suicidal ideation, and substance abuse are serious conditions that should be identified and effectively managed to avoid serious harm to the resident or to patients.

Chapter 227

1. **True.**

2. **False.**

3. **True.**

4. **False.**

5. **True.**

Cancer and its treatment can often produce neuropsychiatric symptoms. Patients with cancer more commonly have generalized seizures because of the physiologic effects of tumor, infection, or drug treatments. Complex partial seizures, manifested by psychic phenomena, autonomic changes, or unusual sensory experiences, are more common than are generalized seizures, although they are more difficult to diagnose. The treatment that cancer patients receive can produce a variety of neuropsychiatric behaviors. Patients who have previously received chemotherapy that produces nausea and vomiting as a side effect can later become nauseated at the prospect of a recurrent treatment, becoming conditioned on occasion to avoid therapy altogether. Akathisia, a sense of restlessness, can be produced by neuroleptic medications such as phenothiazines, butyrophenones, and metoclopramide used for the treatment of nausea, anxiety, or agitation in cancer patients.

6. **True.**

7. **True.**

8. **False.**

9. **True.**

10. **False.**

The nature of HIV infection and its treatment often promotes the development of a myriad of neuropsychiatric symptoms. The most common neuropsychiatric disorders in HIV-infected patients are adjustment disorders, major depression, and organic mental disorders. HIV encephalopathy is a syndrome involving affective, behavioral, cognitive, and motor abnormalities. Magnetic resonance imaging can distinguish white matter disease better than computed tomography and thus may be preferable in the evaluation of patients with HIV encephalopathy. HIV-infected patients develop seizures as a result of a mass lesion in roughly one-third of cases, HIV encephalopathy in another third, with unknown causes being responsible for the remainder. Akathisia, a feeling of restlessness, can be produced by agents such as phenothiazines, butyrophenones, and metoclopramide. Suicide rates for AIDS patients have been shown in one study to be up to 66 times higher than that of the general population.

11. D. Primary infection syndrome in HIV infection is an acute mononucleosis-like illness. It occurs within a few weeks of exposure to HIV. Seroconversion usually occurs several weeks after the resolution of the acute syndrome. The illness is usually self-limited after its acute onset, usually resolving within 3 weeks. Headaches may be severe enough to be consistent with the diagnosis of meningitis.